S0-ASO-094

PHARMACEUTICAL
DOSAGE FORMS

PHARMACEUTICAL DOSAGE FORMS

Parenteral Medications

In Two Volumes
VOLUME 1

EDITED BY

Kenneth E. Avis

University of Tennessee Center for the Health Sciences
Memphis, Tennessee

Leon Lachman

Lachman Consultant Services, Inc.
Garden City, New York

Herbert A. Lieberman

H. H. Lieberman Associates, Inc.
Consultant Services
Livingston, New Jersey

MARCEL DEKKER, INC.   **New York and Basel**

Library of Congress Cataloging in Publication Data

Main entry under title:

Pharmaceutical dosage forms, parenteral medications.

  Includes bibliographies and index.
  1. Solutions (Pharmacy) 2. Parenteral therapy.
3. Pharmacy. I. Avis, Kenneth E., [date]
II. Lachman, Leon, [date]. III. Lieberman,
Herbert A., [date]. [DNLM: 1. Infusions, Parenteral.
2. Technology, Pharmaceutical. WB 354 P536]
RS201.S6P49 1984   615'.191   84-7056
ISBN 0-8247-7084-6 (v. 1)

MARCEL DEKKER, INC.
270 Madison Avenue, New York, New York 10016

Current printing (last digit):
10 9 8 7 6 5 4

PRINTED IN THE UNITED STATES OF AMERICA

Preface

Since parenteral medications are administered directly into body fluids or tissues, the development, manufacture, and control of these dosage forms require unique considerations above and beyond other pharmaceutical dosage forms. These unique and distinctive characteristics of parenteral medications and the technology associated with their manufacture and control of quality are covered in this two-volume series. This technology has changed dramatically in recent years, and continues to change, making it difficult even for the pharmaceutical specialist immersed in the field to keep abreast of new developments. Consequently, there appears a strong need for comprehensive, authoritative coverage of this field in a book or series of books which would act as a teaching tool for the graduate and undergraduate student as well as serving as a reference source for practicing professionals. It is with this concept in mind that the editors planned a rational selection of topics for a two-volume series to adequately cover the subject matter.

The first volume contains a general discussion of parenteral medications, their historical development, and the factors associated with their administration. This is followed by the chapters concerned with biopharmaceutics, preformulation, formulation, and processing of the product. In addition, this volume contains chapters devoted to a discussion on the parameters that affect the design and operation of a parenteral manufacturing facility and crucial personnel considerations.

The second volume, to be published at a later date, covers material science (glass, rubber, and plastic), including packaging, labeling, record-keeping, and regulations. In addition, an extensive treatment of medical devices, their manufacture and assurance of quality, is presented. Further, the second volume will contain a thorough consideration of the distinctive characteristics of the processing and handling of parenteral medications in hospital practice.

Such a thorough treatment of parenteral medications has not been previously undertaken, nor has there been a textbook concerned with parenteral dosage forms in which such an impressive group of knowledgeable people has been assembled to write about their particular areas of expertise. The preparation of the manuscript for this two-volume treatise required many years of effort, and at times, because of the commitments of the writers to other responsibilities, proceeded at an agonizingly slow pace. The editors believe that in conjunction with the experts in their particular fields, the resulting volumes provide a resource of information concerning the formulation, manufacture, and control of parenteral products that has long been lacking.

The editors wish to extend their special appreciation to each of the authors in this book, for they have given extensively of their time and energies in preparing their chapters. The acceptability and usefulness of this text is largely attributed to the herculean efforts of each of them. Their forebearance with our constant demands for modifications and revisions is deeply appreciated. Our hopes are that their labor and our judgment regarding the choice of material have resulted in a book that will be useful to all students and practitioners in the field of parenteral medications.

Kenneth E. Avis
Leon Lachman
Herbert A. Lieberman

Contents

Preface   iii
Contributors   viii
Contents of Pharmaceutical Dosage Forms: Parenteral Medications, Volume 2   x
Contents of Pharmaceutical Dosage Forms: Tablets, Volumes 1-3   xi

Chapter 1.   The Dosage Form and Its Historical Development   1

             Kenneth E. Avis and Beth G. Morris

             I.   The Dosage Form   1
             II. History of Parenteral Medications   4
                  Appendix A: Glossary of Terms   9
                  Appendix B: Highlights in the History of Parenteral
                  Medications   10
                  References   11

Chapter 2.   Parenteral Drug Administration: Routes, Precautions,
             Problems, and Complications   13

             Richard J. Duma and Michael J. Akers

             I.   General Indications for Parenteral Administration
                  of Drugs   13
             II. Pharmaceutical Factors Affecting Parenteral
                  Administration   14
             III. Specific Routes of Administration   16
             IV. Distribution of Parenterally Administered Agents   33
             V.   Precautions, Problems, Hazards, and Complications
                  Associated with Parenteral Drug Administration   35
             VI. Methods and Devices for Aiding in Drug Delivery   42
                  References   44

Chapter 3.   Biopharmaceutics of Injectable Medication   47

             Sol Motola

             I.   Physicochemical and Physiological Factors Affecting
                  Drug Absorption by Injection: An Overview   48

II.   Application of Pharmacokinetics to Biopharmaceutic
      Investigations: Pharmacokinetic Models   65
III. Summary   85
      References   86

Chapter 4.   Preformulation Research of Parenteral Medications   89

Sol Motola and Shreeram Agharkar

I.   Drug Substance Physicochemical Properties   90
II.   Accelerated Stability Evaluation   112
III. General Modes of Drug Degradation   121
IV.   Preformulation Screening of Parenteral Packaging
      Components   125
V.   Summary   128
      References   135

Chapter 5.   Formulation of Small Volume Parenterals   139

Patrick P. DeLuca and James C. Boylan

I.   Formulation Principles   140
II.   Container Effects on Formulation   185
III. Stability Evaluation   192
IV.   Process Effects   198
      References   199

Chapter 6.   The Processing of Small Volume Parenterals and Related
             Sterile Products   203

Joel Benton Portnoff, Richard J. Harwood, and Edward
William Sunbery

I.   Preliminary Stages in the Processing of Small Volume
      Parenterals   205
II.   Manufacture of the Product   229
III. Packaging and Sealing   254
IV.   Inspection of the Final Product   261
V.   Labeling   261
VI.   Conclusion   262
      Appendix: List of Suppliers   262
      References   262

Chapter 7.   Manufacturing of Large Volume Parenterals   265

Nicholas J. Kartinos and Michael J. Groves

I.   Fluid Dynamics and Heat Flow   266
II.   Water: The Essential Raw Material   277
III. Raw Materials   281
IV.   Batch Mixing   284
V.   Filtration   287
VI.   Cleaning Process Equipment and Lines   303
VII. Containers and Closures   307
VIII. Filling   311
IX.   Sealing   311

X.   New Directions   312
     References   313

Chapter 8.   Records and Reports   315

             David C. Fry

     I.   Purpose of Records and Reports   315
     II.   Record Content   317
     III. Record Maintenance and Retrieval   321
     IV.   Record Systems   324
     V.   Reports   349
           References   353

Chapter 9.   Environmental Factors in the Design of a Parenteral
             Production Facility   355

             A. Michael Keller

     I.   Site Selection   355
     II.   Facility Area Use Planning   358
     III. Design Concepts   369
           References   424

Chapter 10. Personnel: The Key Factor in Clean Room Operations   427

             Cecelia J. Luna

     I.   Contamination   427
     II.   Personnel Characteristics   429
     III. Selection of Clean Room Personnel   433
     IV.   Personnel Factors Required to Control Contamination   435
     V.   Personnel Practices and Procedures   439
     VI.   Training Program for Clean Room Employees   442
     VII. Management Role in Clean Room Operations   451
           References   454

Index   457

Contributors

Shreeram Agharkar, B. Sc., M. S., Ph. D.   Section Leader, Sterile Products
Formulation Research and Development, Schering Corporation, Bloomfield, New
Jersey

Michael J. Akers, Ph. D.   Research Scientist, Parenteral Products Development,
Eli Lilly and Company, Indianapolis, Indiana

Kenneth E. Avis, D. Sc.*   Goodman Professor and Chief, Division of Parenteral
Medications, Department of Medicinal Chemistry, University of Tennessee Center
for the Health Sciences, Memphis, Tennessee

James C. Boylan, Ph. D.[†]   Director, Pharmaceutical Development, G. D. Searle
& Company, Skokie, Illinois

Patrick P. DeLuca, B. S., M. S., Ph. D.   Professor and Associate Dean, College
of Pharmacy, University of Kentucky, Lexington, Kentucky

Richard J. Duma, M. D., Ph. D.   Chairman, Division of Infectious Diseases,
Professor of Medicine, Pathology and Microbiology, Medical College of Virginia,
Virginia Commonwealth University, Richmond, Virginia

David C. Fry, B. S.[‡]   Manager, Compliance Audits, Compliance Assurance,
Bristol Laboratories, Division of Bristol-Myers Company, Syracuse, New York

---

Present affiliations:

*Goodman Professor and Chairman, Department of Pharmaceutics, University of
Tennessee Center for the Health Sciences, Memphis, Tennessee

[†]Director, Scientific Services, Hospital Products Division, Abbott Laboratories,
North Chicago, Illinois

[‡]Director of Regulatory Affairs—Marketed Products, Bristol Laboratories, Division
of Bristol-Myers Company, Syracuse, New York

Michael J. Groves, Ph.D.*   Associate Director, Pharmaceutical Development, Travenol Laboratories, Inc., Morton Grove, Illinois

Richard J. Harwood, Ph.D.[†]   Research Fellow, Pharmaceutical Research, Merck, Sharp and Dohme Research Laboratories, West Point, Pennsylvania

Nicholas J. Kartinos, B.S., M.A., Ph.D.   Director, Research and Development, Special Activities, Corporate Research and Development, Travenol Laboratories, Inc., Morton Grove, Illinois

A. Michael Keller, P.E.   Director of Engineering, Syntex Agribusiness, Des Moines, Iowa

Leon Lachman, Ph.D.   President, Lachman Consultant Services, Inc., Garden City, New York

Herbert A. Lieberman, Ph.D.   President, H. H. Lieberman Associates, Inc., Consultant Services, Livingston, New Jersey

Cecelia J. Luna   Training Supervisor, GMP Training Department, E. R. Squibb & Sons, Inc., New Brunswick, New Jersey

Beth G. Morris, B.S., R.Ph.[‡]   Health Care Associate Trainee, Division of Parenteral Medications, Department of Medicinal Chemistry, University of Tennessee Center for the Health Sciences, Memphis, Tennessee

Sol Motola, B.S., Ph.D.[‡]   Associate Director, Pharmaceutical Research and Development, Schering Corporation, Bloomfield, New Jersey

Joel Benton Portnoff, B.S., M.S.   Senior Research Fellow, Pharmaceutical Development, Merck, Sharp and Dohme Research Laboratories, West Point, Pennsylvania

Edward William Sunbery, B.S.   Research Pharmacist, Pharmaceutical Development, Merck, Sharp and Dohme Research Laboratories, West Point, Pennsylvania

Present affiliations:

*Professor and Head, Department of Pharmaceutics, College of Pharmacy, University of Illinois at Chicago, Chicago, Illinois

[†]Department Manager, Pharmaceutical Development, New Product Development, William H. Rohrer, Inc., Fort Washington, Pennsylvania

[‡]Staff Pharmacist, Department of Pharmacy, Memorial Hospital, Hollywood, Florida

[‡]Director, Pharmaceutical Research and Development, Merck Frosst Canada, Inc., Pointe Claire-Dorval, Quebec, Canada

Contents of Pharmaceutical Dosage Forms: Parenteral Medications, Volume 2

1. Industrial Sterilization: A Review of Current Principles and Practices, Frank J. Marino and Floyd Benjamin

2. Formulation for Large Volume Parenterals, Levit J. Demorest

3. Glass Containers for Parenterals, Frank R. Bacon

4. Plastic Containers for Parenterals, Donald D. Solomon, Raymond W. Jurgens, Jr., and K. Lim Wong

5. Elastomeric Closures for Parenterals, Edward J. Smith and Robert J. Nash

6. Particulate Matter, Patrick P. DeLuca and Julius Z. Knapp

7. Environmental Control in Parenteral Drug Manufacturing, Franco DeVecchi

8. Quality Assurance, Samir A. Hanna

9. Federal Regulation of Parenterals, Jonas L. Bassen and Bernard T. Loftus

10. Medical Devices: Design, Manufacture, and Quality Control, David H. Wayt

11. Quality Assurance for Parenteral Devices, Carl W. Bruch

12. Regulatory and GMP Considerations for Medical Devices, Larry R. Pilot

13. Parenteral Products in Hospital Practice, John W. Levchuk

Contents of Pharmaceutical Dosage Forms: Tablets, Volumes 1–3

edited by Herbert A. Lieberman and Leon Lachman

VOLUME 1

1. Preformulation Testing, Deodatt A. Wadke and Harold Jacobson

2. Tablet Formulation and Design, Gilbert S. Banker, Garnet E. Peck, and George J. Baley

3. Compressed Tablets, Bhogi B. Sheth, Fred J. Bandelin, and Ralph F. Shangraw

4. Compression-Coated and Layer Tablets, William C. Gunsel

5. Effervescent Tablets, Raymond Mohrle

6. Special Tablets: Sublingual and Buccal Tablets, James W. Conine and Michael J. Pikal

7. Chewable Tablets, Jahan B. Daruwala

8. Medicated Lozenges, David Peters

VOLUME 2

1. Mixing, Russell J. Lantz, Jr., and Joseph B. Schwartz

2. Drying, Michael A. Zoglio and Jens T. Carstensen

3. Size Reduction, Russell J. Lantz, Jr.

4. Compression, Eugene L. Parrott

5. Granulation and Tablet Characteristics, Dale E. Fonner, Neil R. Anderson, and Gilbert S. Banker

6. Bioavailability in Tablet Technology, James W. McGinity, Salomon A. Stavchansky, and Alfred Martin

7. Pharmaceutical Tablet Compression Tooling, George F. Loeffler

VOLUME 3

1. Principles of Improved Tablet Production System Design, Neil R. Anderson, Gilbert S. Banker, and Garnet E. Peck

2. Pan Coating of Tablets and Granules, Stuart C. Porter, Charles H. Bruno, and Gerald J. Jackson

3. Particle-Coating Methods, Dale E. Wurster

4. Sustained Drug Release from Tablets and Particles through Coating, Joseph M. Conrad and Joseph R. Robinson

5. The Pharmaceutical Pilot Plant, Charles I. Jarowski

6. Tablet Production, Charles T. Lay and Frank W. Burans

7. Stability/Kinetics, Samir A. Hanna

8. Quality Assurance, Samir A. Hanna

1

The Dosage Form and Its Historical Development

KENNETH E. AVIS and BETH G. MORRIS

University of Tennessee Center for the Health Sciences
Memphis, Tennessee

I. THE DOSAGE FORM

When Christopher Wren sharpened the hollow quill of a feather, attached it to an animal bladder, and used this crude device to inject an equally crude extract of opium into the vein of a dog in 1656, neither he nor his contemporaries could have envisioned the developments that have brought to humankind the clean, pure products and the sophisticated devices used today to inject medications parenterally. Striking as these improvements are, we cannot rest complacently on such achievements since each advance in technology may reveal deficiencies not previously recognized. These become a challenge to be overcome, and thus progress is made toward producing an ever more nearly perfect product, a goal that is both challenging and elusive.

Unquestionably, the parenteral dosage forms available today meet standards of quality far higher than was dreamed possible even a few years ago. They are assuming an increasingly important role in patient health care, particularly in the institutional setting. Because of the risks involved when they are injected through the skin and mucous membranes, most parenterals are administered by professional members of the health care team. In some instances, where patients must receive frequent injections, the patient or members of the family, are taught to maintain asepsis and to develop the technique for administering the injection, but such exceptions must be limited.

A parenteral dosage form may be selected in preference to an oral dosage form for a number of reasons. The characteristics of the drug may determine this choice. For example, should the drug be degraded by digestive processes in the gastrointestinal tract, the drug should not be administered orally. Frequently, the condition of the patient requires parenteral administration. For example, the oral route must not be used if the patient is unconscious or otherwise unable to swallow. If action from the drug must be obtained rapidly, an injection can produce an effect in a few seconds. Control of drug level in the body usually favors administration by the parenteral route. The health care professionals who normally administer parenteral dosage forms can be expected to be more accurate and reliable in the amount, site, and schedule of administration than an untrained layperson can be. The control of dosage of a drug relative to the response of

host tissue usually can be more precisely achieved following parenteral administration than following oral administration, parenteral administration permitting
greater predictability and reproducibility of drug absorption. Also, new drugs in
preliminary phases of clinical trial sometimes are prepared in parenteral form
since it is possible to control dosage more precisely, the absorption is more predictable and repeatable, and side effects can be observed and controlled more
closely. Consequently, a better controlled and defined study of therapeutic effects
and potential side effects can be performed. However, it should be noted that as
early as possible in the development of a drug, the appropriate dosage form should
be determined so that data can be collected for that dosage form.

A. Distinctive Characteristics

Like all dosage forms, parenteral preparations must offer a drug in a form that
is convenient, safe, and effective for the patient. But because the route of administration is by injection, parenterals must meet standards of purity and freedom
from contamination that are far higher than those for any other dosage form. In
fact, they must be as nearly perfect as possible within the achievements of present
technology. Therefore, each manufacturer of parenterals has the responsibility
to guard intensely the quality of every parenteral product and each of its packaging
units. The manufacturer of the devices by which parenterals are administered has
a similar responsibility, one that begins with the selection and procurement of the
raw materials, extends through each step of the manufacturing process, and includes the testing and release of the finished product. Similarly, a major responsibility is placed on all those members of the health professions who manipulate
or utilize these products, including their administration to the patient.
      Legally and organizationally, emphasis has been placed on controlling the
quality of these preparations during the manufacturing process. It is regrettable
that the handling and administration of these products has been given less attention.
Even the purest, cleanest product can be rendered highly contaminated and unsafe
for use should improper handling occur during administration to the patient. Therefore, it behooves every person involved in the manufacture and ultimate use of
parenterals to be highly informed about the appropriate and necessary conditions
for handling these distinctive dosage forms.
      Since parenterals must be of especially high purity, achieving that goal re-
quires beginning with appropriate standards for the raw materials. Carefully
drawn specifications must be delineated for the degree of quality required for all
raw materials utilized. This applies not only to product ingredients but to container materials and those utilized in devices for administering the parenteral.
Usually, specifications required for a given component must be carefully developed
and rigidly adhered to at a much higher level than for the same ingredient used in
other types of dosage forms or in other commercial applications. Trace contaminants present in the raw material or subsequently released from it have been
known to exert acute or chronic toxicity in the patient when the product is used.
In such instances, refinement and purification are required to eliminate the contaminant. Further, the manufacturing process must be carefully controlled so that
contamination is not introduced. Examples of such contamination include the extraction of iron from stainless steel transfer pipes or reaction vessels, and the
pickup of particulate matter from the environment or the inclusion of tiny metal
shavings from operating equipment. Biological contamination may include microorganisms picked up from the environment or people during processing, or the development of pyrogens from the growth of viable microorganisms from ineffective

cleaning of equipment at some stage in the process. Such examples illustrate the exceptional attention and care that must be given throughout the process to maintain the freedom from contamination that is so essential and distinctive for parenterals.

B. Dosage Form Perspectives

When patients receive an injection, they are intensely concerned about the procedure and the dosage form of the drug. Their concern may be due to the real or imagined pain from the injection, but probably, at least in part, it is due to a conscious or subconscious awareness that this is a "special" dosage form. They know that such dosage forms are normally given only by health care professionals, and they are conscious of the extra care used in preparation for the injection. On the other hand, patients may be acutely ill when parenterals are administered. In such instances patients may be in no condition to exercise concern.

Health care professionals, particularly physicians, dentists, nurses, and pharmacists, should know the benefits from giving drugs by injection as well as the risks if an inferior or a contaminated parenteral is administered. They should know that such a dosage form must be free from toxic chemical contaminants, particulate matter, living microorganisms, and pyrogens. Although the human body is normally remarkably resilient to adverse conditions, many disease states greatly reduce the ability of the body to overcome additional adversity. Therefore, nothing should be done to impair the potential recovery of the patient. Health care professionals normally utilize parenterals and devices prepared by the pharmaceutical and related industries. As such, they have the responsibility to maintain the high standard of quality "built" into the product by the manufacturer. They must exercise discretion in selecting products of impeccable quality and reliability and then must utilize equally high standards in their use and administration. Unfortunately, health care professionals sometimes appear not to understand what constitutes, in the hospital setting, standards complementary to those of the manufacturers of parenterals.

Manufacturers of parenteral products and administration devices have made outstanding technological advancements, particularly in the last 30 years. Raw materials are being made more pure, process equipment operates more cleanly and reliably, analytical methods are more accurate and definitive, environmental conditions are more controllable, and composite historical data are available more readily and quickly. Part of this improvement is the result of an impetus from the U.S. Food and Drug Administration, but much has come as a result of the commitment of the personnel of the industry to produce high-quality products by constantly seeking to improve their own methods and to utilize proven technological improvements from other fields.

The U.S. Food and Drug Administration (FDA) has been charged by Congress with the responsibility to protect the public and to see that drugs, dosage forms, and devices are safe and effective. For many years adulterated drugs and dosage forms were subject to seizure and the manufacturer to criminal prosecution, but more recently Congress has given the FDA authority to inspect manufacturing operations and facilities to determine whether or not the practices being utilized meet current standards (known as current good manufacturing practices or CGMPs) deemed necessary to assure the quality required for the product. This awesome responsibility has been undertaken quite seriously by the FDA and has aided in the improvement of the quality of drugs, dosage forms, and devices produced by small as well as large manufacturers. There is debate, today, however, as to whether some of the CGMPs reflect current good practices or idealized concepts.

Another arm of the federal government which exercises significant interest in the use of parenterals and devices is the Centers for Disease Control (CDC). The CDC has developed an extensive program for monitoring nosocomial infections throughout the nation. Therefore, the CDC is likely to be the first group to become aware of an infectious condition affecting patients in hospitals nationwide, from whatever source. The CDC was thus first to detect recent infectious conditions that arose in certain large volume parenterals (LVPs). Although the CDC has no regulatory power, it provides a very useful and needed alarm system for early identification of developing infectious problems in hospitals across the nation. The CDC also performs selected research functions and develops guidelines for hospital functions to control infections.

Closely associated, but independent of the federal government is the United States Pharmacopeia (USP). The Congress, in the Pure Food and Drug Act, recognized the USP and National Formulary (now a part of the USP) as the compendia responsible for establishing standards for drugs and dosage forms. Therefore, many standards for parenterals are included in the USP and must be met by those products purporting to be of USP quality and, by inference, for many others. Standards in the USP are generally minimal in nature; that is, they provide the minimum specifications, which often are exceeded in practice. Nevertheless, USP standards play a very important role in maintaining the quality of parenteral products.

Many persons and groups have a vital interest in parenteral products and in devices for their administration. The discussion above has highlighted the perspective of some of those with the greatest interest. It should not be construed that this brief account covers all groups or all interests.

Understanding parenteral dosage forms will be heightened by a review of their development. The following historical account will give the reader such a review.

II. HISTORY OF PARENTERAL MEDICATIONS

The development of parenteral medications as useful dosage forms has occurred almost entirely during the past half century. Their role in the treatment and control of disease today has escalated to one of exceptional importance. However, this development would not have been possible without the investigations performed by our predecessors, whose work we often would label as very crude, even primitive. A review of some of those beginnings will help us appreciate the current status of this critical dosage form [1-10].

Our very early ancestors believed disease to be caused by the entrance of evil spirits into the body. With time, we began to gain some understanding of disease, its causes, and treatment. The ancient Egyptians developed the technology to prepare medicinal substances in several different forms, among which was their so-called "injection," in actuality an enema. This accomplishment was recorded in the Papyrus Ebers around 1550 B.C. However, it was not until the discovery of the circulation of blood by William Harvey in 1616 that the possibility of phlebotomy or venesection could be contemplated.

The first attempts at parenteral therapy in ancient times apparently were blood transfusions tried by the Egyptians, but these efforts failed. In 1492, Pope Innocent was said to have received a transfusion from three young boys, but some believe that it was performed enterally rather than parenterally. The first parenteral blood transfusion to be performed without any doubt of its validity was in 1654 by Francesco Folli. Others, such as Richard Lower in 1663, Jean Baptiste Davis in 1667, and Blundell in 1818, tested their skills in performing transfusions, but their results were deadly. Later, discovery of the blood groups, sterilization, and the sodium citrate method of anticoagulation were instrumental in paving the road for progress in this area of parenteral therapy.

Introducing drugs into the body through the skin possibly was conceived by observing the bites of venomous snakes and insects and their effects on the body. Probably similar observations explain the use of poisoned arrows, a crude precursor of parenteral therapy, used to kill enemies and prey in Africa, South America, and other parts of the world. In 1656, Christopher Wren first injected medicinal substances into animals with a goose quill and pig's bladder. But it was J. D. Major and Johannes Elsholtz who first successfully injected humans in 1662, using solutions of opium, purging agents, jalap resins, arsenic, snail water, and others. Only the previous year Elsholtz had concluded that intravascular injections were of value for the treatment of diseases. However, after 1662 the practice of intravenous injection slowed to a standstill until the late eighteenth century.

The next major advancement came in the early 1850s, when Alexander Wood was credited as being the first to give subcutaneous injections using a true hypodermic syringe, originated in 1836 by G. V. LaFargue. Charles Hunter contributed to the development of this route of parenteral administration by noting the effectiveness of the subcutaneous route for systemic absorption and coining the word "hypodermic." Unfortunately, pain and irritation were commonly associated with the subcutaneous administration of drugs; it was for this reason that in the late nineteenth century, Alfred Luton introduced the intramuscular route for the injection of acidic, irritant, or slowly absorbed drugs. It was Felix Balzer who coined the word "intramuscular."

With the development of these two routes of administration, investigators began turning their attention to the devices used for injection. A syringe developed by Robert Koch in 1888 was the first that could be sterilized, and this was a great improvement over the instruments used by earlier workers. The first all-glass syringe was built by Karl Schneider in 1896. Further improvements are credited to Ralph Walsh and Joseph Payne, who built the early prototypes of the current cartridge syringe. Wyeth Laboratories obtained from the Bartos Company in 1943 the design for the first practical disposable syringe, the Tubex.® Pressure-type syringes, utilizing compressed air, were developed in 1930 and used during the Spanish Civil War. The most recent versions have been the Hypospray and Hypodermic Jet Injection Apparatus, which operate on the jet injection principle without the aid of a needle. These are used most extensively for the rapid vaccination of large numbers of people.

Brief mention should be made of the historical developments of vaccines. Centuries ago, inoculation was performed in the Far East by infecting a small wound with the pus from a smallpox sore. In 1716, Cotton Mather was told by his slaves of their practice of immunization against smallpox. This was 80 years before the discovery of the first smallpox vaccine by Edward Jenner. In 1954 the modern era of virus vaccines began with the Salk vaccine, a killed polio virus. Shortly thereafter, the first living attenuated virus vaccine was developed by Sabin. Since then, many preparations have been developed and marketed.

With the subcutaneous and intramuscular routes of injection having been firmly established during the nineteenth century, it is only fitting that the intravenous route should have a similar evolution. In 1831, W. B. O'Shaughnessy contemplated the water, saline, and alkali deficits in the blood of cholera victims. Hoping to follow up on O'Shaughnessy's work, Thomas Latts used normal saline in treating diarrhea in cholera patients and, in essence, was the first to employ intravenous infusion as a successful mode of rational therapy. Ironically, the first recognition of the role of isotonicity did not occur until 1880, and it was noted by a pharmacist named L. Wolff. Nevertheless, therapy with intravenous solutions at this time was still relatively crude. In 1924, in a paper to the American Surgeons Association, Rudolph Matas discussed the inadequacies of some of the methods used for fluid therapy (oral, proctoclysis, hypodermoclysis, etc.), and made mention of an intravenous method, giving 4000 to 5000 ml of 5% dextrose in water every 24 hr. Concurrently, he discussed the problems of air emboli and thromboses with his new method [11]. This work was the beginning of modern intravenous fluid therapy.

The practice of intravenous feeding soon followed intravenous fluid therapy. In 1843, Claude Bernard used sugar solutions, milk, and egg whites to feed animals intravenously, and by the end of the nineteenth century, it was a widely accepted practice. Do not be mistaken in believing that all efforts in intravenous nutrition were instant successes. Kausch suffered defeat in 1911 when he attempted the first postoperative intravenous injections of glucose. However, with Murlin and Riche leading the way in 1915 with their animal studies on the intravenous administration of fat, Yamakawa was able to introduce in 1920 the use of emusified fat in humans. Work was continued in the 1950s to perfect the intravenous use of fat emulsions for their caloric content. Although the Food and Drug Administration removed intravenous fat emulsions from the market in 1964, due primarily to capillary occlusion in the lungs, this method of nutrition has survived, and today, the use of the emulsion Intralipid® is widespread [12].

Somewhat parallel to the development of intravenous fat emulsions was hyperalimentation by intravenous infusion. The groundwork for the parenteral use of protein hydrolysates in humans began in 1937 when W. C. Rose identified the amino acids necessary for the growth and development of rats. S. J. Dudrick also pioneered this area in 1965 with juvenile beagle dogs. Complications arose with this method, foremost being the concern that peripheral veins were unable to tolerate such concentrated solutions. Dudrick and others solved this dilemma by developing a safe method for long-term catheterization of the subclavian vein, which, because of its large diameter and blood volume, permitted infusion of highly concentrated solutions without damage to vein walls [13]. Shortly thereafter, in June 1967, the first clinical use of hyperalimentation solutions occurred in an infant suffering from gastrointestinal abnormalities. Subsequently, hyperalimentation has proven to be a lifesaving mode of therapy.

An important process in the preparation of parenteral medications is filtration. Although researchers have found evidence of filtration methods in ancient Chinese writings, in Egyptian tomb illustrations, Carthaginian records, and preChristian Hebrew scrolls, the modern era of filtering parenteral solutions probably began in 1855 when Fick produced "ultrafilter" membranes on ceramic thimbles by dipping them in a solution of nitrocellulose in ether. In 1891, Nordtmeyer of Germany introduced the filtering medium kieselguhr. A few years later R. Zsigmondy and W. Bachmann developed methods for commercial production of nitrocellulose membranes and in 1918 coined the term "membrane filter." In a further development, a method of determining the pore size of membrane filters was developed by H. Beckhold early in the twentieth century by measuring the filter's "bubble point." Application of the membrane filtering technique to the purification of liquids apparently was done first by the United States Biological Laboratories at Fort Detrick, Maryland. However, problems arose with the use of nitrocellulose filters such that other materials, particularly cellulose nitrate and acetate, were investigated. Today, these esters of cellulose, as well as other polymer materials, including polyethylene, polyvinyl chloride, nylon, and cellulose triacetate are being successfully used to produce membrane filters with varying properties and controllable pore size.

A different utilization of filtration vital in parenteral therapy is hemodialysis. About 120 years ago Thomas Graham of England separated solutions into their component parts with a device called the dialyzer. This concept was applied in 1913 to the first external blood dialyzer, the "artificial kidney." During World War II, the first sustained use of hemodialysis occurred in Holland in a life-and-death situation [14]. It has also been used to filter excess drugs out of the blood of drug-overdosed patients.

Aseptic technique and sterilization are two of the most important process steps in the preparation of parenteral medications. Louis Pasteur and Joseph Lister began the development of sterilization as a means of eliminating living pathogenic microorganisms during the 1860s. Pasteur, known as the father of bacteriology, was responsible for establishing the basis for aseptic technique in handling sterile instruments and solutions. Lister became known as the father of modern antiseptic surgery and published the first paper on surgical antisepsis in 1867. However, physicians generally neglected to recognize the importance of their work and continued to practice using unclean procedures and nonsterile equipment. Ernst von Bergman reevaluated surgical practices and, in 1886, was the first to sterilize instruments using steam. Problems were also encountered in preventing the growth of fungus in hypodermic solutions which had been prepared but not used immediately. Boiling became the accepted method of accomplishing this task by 1870, to be followed by the addition of preservatives, such as 1/6% carbolic acid in 1873 and chloroform water and salicylic acid in 1877. Another method for controlling fungal growth was developed by Stanislaus Limousin and L. Friedlander in 1886, that of filtering the solution through a Chamberland filter into a glass container which could be heat-sealed. This container was the first ampul. Later developments included the first modern type of autoclave designed by Charles Chamberland in 1884, the discovery of formaldehyde in 1859, the discovery of the sterilant ethylene oxide in 1944, and the first use of Bacillus subtilis var. niger spore strips as sterilization indicators in 1944. Radiation, such as ultraviolet light, has been used as a means of sterilization since the early 1940s.

Radiopharmaceuticals are a quite recent and unique type of parenteral. Their development began with the introduction of the concept of radioactivity by Henri Becquerel in 1896 through his work with uranium. Two years later, Marie and Pierre Curie extended Becquerel's work and isolated radium. With these remarkable developments, it was a natural step for Wickham and Degrais to use radium intravenously for the treatment of disease in 1911. The first human diagnostic study came in 1926 when Blumgart, Yens, and Weiss used radioisotopes to determine arm-to-arm circulation time. Today the majority of radioisotopes are produced by nuclear reactors, the first reactor being built in Chicago by Enrico Fermi in 1942. Since the ideal diagnostic radiopharmaceutical must have a short half-life, it must be used near the reactor or a means must be found to produce the radiodiagnostic agent remote from the reactor and close to the point of use. This problem has been resolved by the development of radioisotope generators, the first being produced in 1951. Today, generators are being used to provide the radioactive drugs required in nuclear medicine practice in hospitals worldwide.

The problem of pyrogenic reactions to intravenous injection had been observed as early as 1911 when Wechselman noted an increase in temperature and chills in patients receiving injections of arsphenamine. Meanwhile, E. C. Holt and W. J. Penhold noted that freshly distilled water did not produce an increase in temperature if allowed to stand 48 hr before injection [15]. In 1923, Florence Seibert discovered that the drug fevers referred to by Wechselman were caused by bacteria-produced pyrogens. Her studies were extended to the development of the rabbit test for pyrogens, still the USP test method. While looking for a quicker and simpler pyrogen test for radiopharmaceuticals, J. F. Cooper and his associates, in 1969, developed the limulus test, a test for bacterial endotoxin using Limulus amebocyte lysate [16]. In studies thus far, the limulus test has proven to be more sensitive than the rabbit test.

The critical need for ultraclean facilities for assembling components of vehicles to be used for the exploration of space resulted in a new "clean room" technology, the original clean rooms having appeared in the United States around 1952. HEPA filters, first developed by the United States Biological Laboratories at Fort Detrick, Maryland, during the early 1940s, were used at this time primarily in the air-conditioning units in clean rooms. Then in 1961, W. J. Whitfield developed the concept of laminar airflow, using HEPA-filtered air to sweep a confined space [17]. Thus an ultraclean space was provided as long as the air flowed through the space. This development was subsequently applied to the provision of an environment in which sterile products could be prepared with a markedly upgraded standard for processing. This development was a key in stimulating similar improvements in various technologies associated with the preparation of parenterals and other sterile products, during the 1970s in particular. Today parenterals are made to standards of excellence undreamed of a few decades ago.

Inevitably, written standards and regulations were promulgated together with the developing technology for drugs and drug preparations. In the United States, the first pharmacopeia was published in 1778 for the sole use of the Military Hospital of the United States Army. Later, through the efforts of Lyman Spalding, the first book to be published as a standard for national use was the United States Pharmacopeia (USP) in 1820. A second book of standards was originally published as the National Formulary of Unofficial Preparations in 1888, becoming the National Formulary (NF) when it was designated as an official compendium in 1906. However, it was not until the fifth edition of the National Formulary in 1926 that the first parenterals were accepted, followed by acceptance in the British Pharmacopeia in 1932.

The USP and the NF did not have legal status until identified as official compendia in the Pure Food and Drug Act of 1906. This was the first significant effort by the U.S. government to regulate drugs, although an act to regulate shipment of biological products was passed in 1902. Many amendments of the Act of 1906 were passed over the succeeding years until a complete revision was prepared and passed by Congress in 1938 as the Food, Drug and Cosmetic Act. This Act also established the Food and Drug Administration to enforce the Act. The Durham-Humphrey Amendment of 1952 differentiated between prescription legend and over-the-counter drugs. Then, in 1962, authority was given to the FDA to establish current good manufacturing practices (CGMPs) regulations. Subsequently, these became standards of practice for the pharmaceutical industry, with parenteral preparations receiving singular attention because of the critical quality standards required for their safety. During the most recent years revisions have been in various stages of progress almost continuously because of the continuous changes in technology. Further, there has been considerable debate as to the role of the FDA in writing the CGMPs, centering particularly on whether the FDA should set standards and objectives or, in addition, state how to achieve them. Generally, the industry has felt that the FDA should not tell the industry how to reach the standards and objectives set. The revised CGMPs of 1978 seem to agree essentially with the industry's position and that of the Parenteral Drug Association, a professional organization founded in 1946 and committed to the promotion of technical advancement in the parenteral specialty field.

Thus we have seen that the crude beginning of parenteral therapy of over three centuries ago remained largely a medical curiosity until about 50 years ago. However, during these recent relatively few years, the technology has developed rapidly until the parenterals of today are a highly sophisticated dosage form meeting very high standards of quality, which, with its implications for patient safety, has brought about very stringent regulations to attempt to assure that quality.

APPENDIX A: GLOSSARY OF TERMS

Adulterated: the presence of an impurity which lowers the quality of a preparation and may endanger the well-being of the patient/user.

Ampul: an all-glass hermetically sealed container for a parenteral or other sterile product.

Aseptic: literally, "without sepsis." Used to designate a practical level of sterility; that is, a condition in which every reasonable means has been used to destroy or eliminate viable microorganisms, but with the recognition that an absolute condition has not been achieved.

Clean: a relative term designating freedom from contamination. When used with parenteral medications, "clean" normally designates a highly efficient cleanliness level. An attempt to define cleanliness with respect to processing rooms is found in Federal Standard 209B*, wherein three levels of clean rooms are defined on the basis of particulate matter of specific size suspended in the air space.

Current good manufacturing practices (CGMPs): the regulations promulgated by the U.S. Food and Drug Administration under the authority of the Federal Food, Drug and Cosmetic Act as amended in 1962 and revised in 1971. They attempt to state the practices considered to be current and good for the manufacturing of drug products.

Dosage form: the drug, vehicle, and/or excipients in a form suitable for conveying the drug for administration to the patient.

Large volume parenteral (LVP): a liquid intended for infusion and hermetically sealed in a container of greater than 100 ml volume.

Multiple-dose vial: a container, usually of glass, having a relatively large opening closed by means of a rubber stopper which permits the insertion of a sharp needle and the withdrawing of a part of the contents. The stopper reseals when the needle is withdrawn to maintain the integrity of the package.

---

*Federal Standard No. 209B, General Services Administration, Washington, D.C. 20407, April 24, 1973.

National Coordinating Committee on Large Volume Parenterals (NCCLVP): a committee composed of representatives from national organizations charged with the responsibility to identify and, when possible, propose solutions to problems associated with large volume parenterals (LVPs).

Nosocomial: associated with a hospital; thus nosocomial infections would be those related to hospital practice or the institution.

Parenteral: derived from "para enteron," meaning "other than by means of the intestine." The dosage form for conveying a drug by means of injection through the skin or mucous membranes.

Pyrogen: the fever-producing lipid associated with a polysaccharide or polypeptide of microbial origin.

Small volume parenteral (SVP): a parenteral preparation hermetically sealed in a container of 100 ml or less volume.

Sterile: traditionally defined in absolute terms as the state of freedom from all viable microorganisms. Recognized today as definable in terms of the probability that an item(s) is free from all viable microorganisms.

Sterilization: a process designed to completely eliminate or destroy all living microorganisms.

APPENDIX B: HIGHLIGHTS IN THE HISTORY OF
              PARENTERAL MEDICATIONS

1616   William Harvey discovered the circulation of blood.

1656   Christopher Wren injected medicinal substances into animals with a goose quill and pig's bladder.

1662   J. D. Major and Johannes Elsholtz successfully injected humans with medicinal substances such as opium solutions.

1796   Edward Jenner developed the smallpox vaccine.

1820   The United States Pharmacopeia (USP) was published as a standard for national use.

1836   The hypodermic syringe was originated by G. V. LaFargue.

Early 1850s Alexander Wood gave subcutaneous injections using a true hypodermic syringe.

1860s   Louis Pasteur and Joseph Lister began the development of sterilization as a means of eliminating living microorganisms.

1884   The autoclave was designed by Charles Chamberland.

Late 1800s   Alfred Luton introduced the intramuscular route of administration of drugs.

1906   The Pure Food and Drug Act was enacted by Congress, giving both the USP and the National Formulary legal status.

1918   R. Zsigmondy and W. Bachman coined the term "membrane filter" after developing the methods for commercial production of nitrocellulose membranes.

1923   Florence Seibert discovered that the drug fevers noted by Wechselman in 1911 were caused by bacteria-produced pyrogens.

1924   Work done by Rudolph Matas was the beginning of modern intravenous fluid therapy.

1926   Parenterals were accepted for inclusion in the fifth edition of the National Formulary.

1938   The Food, Drug and Cosmetic Act was passed by Congress and established the Food and Drug Administration (FDA).

1944   The sterilant ethylene oxide was discovered.

1946   The Parenteral Drug Association was founded.

1961   W. J. Whitfield developed the concept of laminar airflow.

1962   Authority was given to the FDA to establish current good manufacturing practices (CGMPs) regulations, with parenteral preparations receiving particular attention.

1965   S. J. Dudrick pioneered parenteral hyperalimentation with his studies on beagle dogs.

REFERENCES

1. Andrews, G. A., in Radiopharmacy (M. Tubis and W. Wolf, eds.), Wiley, New York, 1976, pp. 3-17.
2. Ansel, H. C., Introduction to Pharmaceutical Dosage Forms, Lea & Febiger, Philadelphia, 1972, pp. 4-17.
3. Brown, H. M., Ann. Med. Hist., 7:177-197 (1917-1918).
4. Chase, G. D., in Remington's Pharmaceutical Sciences, 16th ed. (A. Osol, ed.), Mack, Easton, Pa., 1975, p. 439.
5. Gelman, C., Anal. Chem., 37:29A (May, 1965).
6. Griffenhagan, G. B., Bull. Parenter. Drug Assoc., 16(2):12-19 (1962).
7. Howard-Jones, N., Sci. Am., 224(1):96 (1971).
8. Miller, L. C., Bull. Parenter. Drug Assoc., 10(5):1-8 (1956).
9. Rodwin, R. M., Food Drug Cosmet. Law J., 31:211 (1976).
10. Van Itallie, P. H., ed., Pulse Pharm., 19(1):9-12 (1965).

11. Mengoli, L. R., <u>Am. J. Surg.</u>, <u>121</u>:311 (Mar. 1971).
12. Mueller, J. R., <u>Bull. Parenter. Drug Assoc.</u>, <u>21</u>:225 (1967).
13. Dudrick, S. J., <u>Am. J. Hosp. Pharm.</u>, <u>28</u>(2):82 (1971).
14. Friedlander, H. Z., and Rickles, R. N., <u>Anal. Chem.</u>, <u>37</u>:27A (July 1965).
15. Welch, H., Calvery, H. D., McCloskey, W. T., and Price, C. W., <u>J. Am.</u>
     <u>Pharm. Assoc.</u>, Sci. Ed., <u>32</u>:65 (Mar. 1943).
16. Cooper, J. F., Hochstein, H. D., and Seligmann, E. G., Jr., <u>Bull. Parenter.</u>
     <u>Drug Assoc.</u>, 26:153 (1972).
17. Whitfield, W. J., <u>Bull. Parenter. Drug Assoc.</u>, 21:37 (1967).

2

Parenteral Drug Administration: Routes, Precautions, Problems, and Complications

RICHARD J. DUMA

Medical College of Virginia
Virginia Commonwealth University
Richmond, Virginia

MICHAEL J. AKERS

Eli Lilly and Company
Indianapolis, Indiana

Parenteral administration of drugs, in its broadest scope, includes any route of administration in which the given drug does not initially enter the alimentary canal. Parenteral, from "para enteron" (Greek), means "to avoid the intestines." Thus drugs applied topically to the eye, ear, and skin or even inhaled may be considered broadly as parenterals; however, medical and pharmacy practioners of today generally limit the classification of parenterals to include only those drugs administered directly into tissues, tissue spaces, or compartments by injection or infusion.

The development of techniques for parenteral administration, as well as their employment, have expanded significantly in recent years and continue to do so. Some of these techniques have offered distinct advantages in the science of therapeutics and drug administration; however, many have not been without risks to patients and not without limitations.

This chapter is an attempt to review and to update the current usage of parenteral drugs and the methods of their administration and to describe the trends of existing technology in the field.

I. GENERAL INDICATIONS FOR PARENTERAL ADMINISTRATION OF DRUGS

The parenteral routes of drug administration are indicated for one or more of the following reasons:

1. To ensure delivery of adequate concentrations of the drug in question to diseased tissues or target areas of the body, especially when inadequate or marginal transport of that drug into the tissues or target areas is anticipated. Example: Direct intraventricular injection of drugs (e.g., antibiotics such as the aminoglycosides) which cross the "blood-brain-meninges barrier" poorly may be used in certain patients with bacterial or fungal meningitis and/or ventriculitis.
2. To permit the user to exert direct control over certain pharmacologic parameters, such as the time of drug onset, serum peak and trough levels, tissue

concentrations, and rate of elimination of the drug from the body. Example: Intravenous or direct cardiointraventricular routes may be desirable to achieve immediate effects in emergencies such as might occur in the control of life-threatening hypotension, hypertension, or arrhythmias; or intramuscular routes may be desirable to obtain protracted or sustained effects, such as with insulin in the therapy of diabetes mellitus.

3. To allow the therapist, when outpatient management is desirable, to guarantee dosage and drug compliance, especially when the patient cannot be relied upon to self-medicate. Example: The use of long-acting (monthly) intramuscular penicillins may be used to manage children prophylactically for rheumatic heart disease in order to prevent Group A streptococcal pharyngitis.

4. To deliver a biologic effect that cannot be achieved through oral administration, perhaps because of nonabsorbance from the alimentary canal or degradation by gastric acidity. Example: Insulin and certain penicillins, which may be destroyed by gastric acid or digestive secretions, are given parenterally. Similarly, polyene antibiotics (such as the antifungal agent amphotericin B) which are nonabsorbable are given intravenously.

5. To administer a drug when the desired route (e.g., oral) may not be available. Example: In patients who are aspirating or who have had the upper gastrointestinal tract stream diverted or removed (e.g., because of a carcinoma) a parenteral route may be necessary.

6. To provide a local effect when it is desirable to minimize or avoid systemic toxic effects or reactions. Example: Methotrexate may be given intrathecally to patients with leukemia and leukemic involvement of the meninges to avoid the systemic, toxic effects that would occur if an intravenous route was employed.

7. To administer drugs to the unconscious, uncooperative, or uncontrollable patient. Example: Patients with uncontrollable grand mal seizures often will not cooperate in the oral administration of drugs or will be at risk to aspirate if compelled to take medicines by mouth. Similarly, patients unconscious from narcotic abuse, anesthetic usage, or trauma, or uncooperative patients such as those suffering delerium tremens or a psychosis, may be satisfactorily managed by using parenteral routes.

8. To permit rapid correction of fluid and electrolyte imbalances and to supply short- or long-term nutritional needs (hyperalimentation or parenteral feeding). Example: Patients suffering severe dehydration or electrolyte depletion for a variety of reasons (e.g., heat stroke) can be rapidly corrected with intravenous electrolyte solutions; and patients whose intestinal tracts have been resected for one reason or another may be intravenously "fed" a complete diet of all the necessary amino acids, glucose, minerals, and vitamins for prolonged and indefinite periods of time.

9. To achieve a desired local effect. Example: Local anesthetics for tooth extractions or local anti-inflammatory agents for inflamed joints may be injected directly into the site in question to avoid systemic effects or "systemic" dosages.

II. PHARMACEUTICAL FACTORS AFFECTING PARENTERAL ADMINISTRATION

Certain pharmaceutical characteristics dictate the method or route of parenteral administration, and once the dosage form is injected or infused, influence the rate and extent of drug availability. These characteristics will be reviewed briefly in this section, but the reader is also referred to Chapter 3 for a more detailed treatment of the biopharmaceutical factors affecting parenteral drug availability.

A. Solubility of the Drug and Volume of the Injection

A drug must be completely solubilized, preferably in water, before it can be administered by intravenous injection. Both the extent of drug solubility in its intended vehicle and the dose required for the desired therapeutic effect will determine the volume of the injection. Parenteral routes other than the intravenous one have limitations regarding the maximum volume of medication administered (e.g., intradermal, intramuscular, intraocular, intraventricular, and intrathecal, to name a few).

B. Vehicle Characteristics

Drugs in aqueous vehicles may be administered by any parenteral route, whereas drugs in nonaqueous vehicles, which may or may not be water miscible, are administered most frequently by the intramuscular route. The intravenous route may be used for a few drugs in mixed solvent systems (e.g., diazepam, digoxin, and phenytoin), but precautions must be applied in adjusting the rate of drug infusion to avoid drug precipitation at the site of infusion. Large volume parenteral fat emulsions are also available by the intravenous route. Nonaqueous vehicles which are more viscous than water vehicles will affect the rate of injection through a small-gage needle and the rate of absorption from the injection site.

C. pH and Osmolality of Injectable Solutions

Ideally, administered injections should be formulated at a pH and osmolality similar to that of biological fluids. Unfortunately, this is not possible for many parenteral dosage forms, as many parenteral drugs are unstable at neutral pH. Therefore, such drugs are formulated at the pH at which they are most stable. For example, diazoxide (a nondiuretic benzothiadiazine derivative) is formulated at a pH of 11.6, the pH at which it is most stable. Many parenteral drugs are salt forms of weak bases. Thus the pH of a dosage form containing the salt of a weak base may be as low as 2.0 (e.g., tetracycline hydrochloride), or the pH of a dosage form containing the salt of a weak acid may be as high as 12.0 (e.g., Dilantin®) in order to maintain the active ingredient in solution. Although dosage forms with extreme pH values may be administered by any parenteral route, the rate and volume of injection must be controlled to minimize pain and irritation to the patient and damage to the surrounding tissues.

Certain parenteral formulations are hyperosmotic with biological fluids and contain a relatively high dose of active ingredient(s) in order to achieve a desired level of biological activity. For example, water-soluble contrast media, spinal anesthetics, ophthalmic sodium sulfacetamide, diazoxide, and osmotic diuretics are a few hypertonic parenteral formulations containing high drug concentrations to achieve an appropriate biological action(s). Products of parenteral nutrition are formulated or admixed with high concentrations of amino acids, dextrose, and other essential ingredients, resulting in very hypertonic solutions. These solutions, called hyperalimentation solutions, are so hypertonic that they must be administered via a large vein such as the subclavian. The blood in this vein enters directly into the heart, which allows the hypertonic solution to be rapidly diluted by a still larger volume of blood.

Generally, hypertonic parenteral dosage forms are contraindicated for subcutaneous or intramuscular injections. Whereas blood and tears can tolerate a range of osmolality, other biological fluids, such as the vitreous humor, can tolerate only very narrow ranges of osmotic values from an injected medication. Therefore, although stability and solubility problems may prevent dosage forms from being formulated at physiological pH, they should be formulated with solute contents approximately equal to those of biological fluids.

D. Type of Dosage Form

Parenteral dosage forms include solutions, suspensions, and sterile solids for reconstitution. If the dosage form is a suspension, it may be administered only by the intramuscular or subcutaneous route. Particles should not be present in dosage forms administered intravenously or by other parenteral routes in which the medication enters directly into a biological fluid or sensitive tissue (e.g., brain or eye). Reconstituted solids should be completely dissolved in the reconstituting diluent before they are administered intravenously.

E. Formulation Ingredients

As discussed in Chapter 5, parenteral formulations may contain various active and inactive excipients other than the main therapeutic agent, for a variety of reasons. For multidose parenterals, antimicrobial agents are added to the formulation for the preservation of sterility. However, these agents may be contraindicated in medications to be administered into the cerebrospinal fluid or intraocular fluid because of the toxicity they may produce. Several parenteral formulations contain surface-active agents (such as polysorbate 80) to maintain drug solubility in the solution vehicle. Surface-active agents are known to alter membrane permeability, so their presence must be recognized when administering such dosage forms by the subcutaneous or intramuscular routes.

The expanding field of sustained and prolonged release of drug delivery employs various formulations and additives that at times aid in achieving the desired duration of drug action. These additives are primarily high-molecular-weight polymers or oily solvents. Formulations containing these macromolecules are administered by the subcutaneous or intramuscular routes to permit the delayed release of the active ingredient within deeper tissues of the body.

III. SPECIFIC ROUTES OF ADMINISTRATION

Three primary routes of parenteral administration are commonly employed: intramuscular, intravenous, and subcutaneous. These three routes satisfy to a large extent the four principal reasons for administering parenterals: (1) for therapy (definitive or palliative), (2) for prevention, (3) for diagnosis, and (4) for temporarily altering tissue function(s) in order to facilitate other forms of therapy. Besides these three primary routes, additional ones are utilized under special circumstances: for example, subconjunctival, intraocular, intrathecal, intra-articular, and so on. In the sections to follow, the primary and special routes of parenteral administration are reviewed, in alphabetical order. Each review will include four subheadings: description, indications, precautions, and method of drug or fluid delivery.

A. Primary Routes

　　1. Intramuscular

　　Description. Injection directly into the body of a relaxed muscle.

　　Indications. The intramuscular (i.m.) route is one of the most popular and convenient routes available, both for the administrator and for the patient [1], especially for a child [2]. Therefore, whenever it is possible and practicable, the intramuscular route is used. The intramuscular route provides a means for prolonged release of drugs formulated as aqueous or oily solutions or suspensions. The intramuscular route is preferred over the subcutaneous route when a rapid rate of absorption is desired and over the intravenous route when for one reason or another the drug cannot be administered directly into the vascular compartment. Many factors affect the rate of drug absorption from an intramuscular injection [2]; they will be discussed later in this chapter. Drugs commonly injected by intramuscular administration include lidocaine, cephalosporins, aminoglycosides, diazepam, phenytoin, insoluble salts of penicillin G (procaine penicillin G), corticosteroids, narcotics, narcotic antagonists, and contraceptive steroids, to name a few.

　　Precautions. Although intramuscular injections are much easier to administer than other injections, the main precaution is to avoid entering a blood vessel (especially an artery), which might lead to infusion of a toxic agent or a toxic vehicle directly to an organ or tissue. This can be prevented usually by pulling back on the plunger of the syringe; if blood does not appear, the needle is probably not in a vessel. Also, the accidental striking of or injection into a peripheral nerve may result in a peripheral nerve palsy with or without sensory damage. Occasionally, when a large bolus of drug is injected into the muscle, local damage or muscle infarction may result, leading to a sterile abscess or to elevation of serum levels of muscle enzymes. The latter complication may present confusing diagnostic problems, especially in patients under suspicion of having a myocardial infarction or hepatitis.

　　If materials contaminated with microorganisms are injected, a septic abscess may result. Therefore, appropriate precautions must be taken to ensure sterility prior to injection. In patients with poor hygiene or skin care, microorganisms from the skin flora may be punched in by the needle at the time of injection, resulting in staphylococcal or streptococcal abscesses; and rarely in such situations as gas gangrene [3] (especially if epinephrine is injected) or tetanus [4].

　　An important note of caution: the intramuscular route should never be employed in patients with significant heart failure or shock, when uptake into the vascular compartment may be expectantly poor. This caution should be followed especially if immediately high serum or plasma concentrations of the drug are desired or if rapid distribution to a distal organ is mandatory.

　　Method. Various muscle sites are available for delivery (Fig. 1), including the gluteal, deltoid, triceps, pectoral, and vastus lateralis muscles. In adults the site of choice often is the gluteal muscle, because large volumes of drug may be injected and tolerated. However, the vastus lateralis of the thigh may also be used because it not only tolerates large volumes of medication, but it is also away from any major vessels or nerves. For rapid absorption and small volumes (<2 ml), the deltoid muscle is preferred, as some studies suggest that blood flow in the deltoid muscle is 7% greater than that of the vastus lateralis and 17% greater than that of the gluteus maximus [5]. In infants and small children, the vastus lateralis of the thigh is often preferred because it is better developed than other muscle groups.

　　With intramuscular injections a beveled, 19 to 22 gauge (Table 1), 1 to 2 in. long, stainless steel needle is used and no more than 5 ml of fluid is injected,

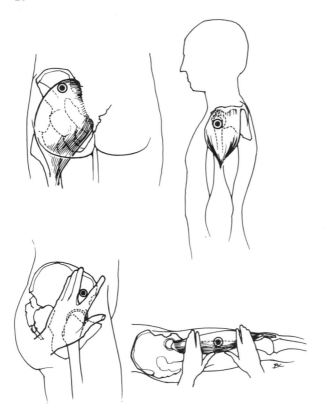

Figure 1 Some common sites employed for intramuscular injections. Upper left:
posterior gluteal, located in the outer upper quadrant about 2 in. below the iliac
crest. Upper right: deltoid, located about 2 in. below the acromion process. Lower left: ventrogluteal, located in the triangle formed by one finger on the anterior
superior iliac spine and the other on the iliac crest. Lower right: vastus lateralis,
located along the middle third and lateral aspect of the thigh. The "bull's-eye" indicates the approximate site of injection.

depending on the site selected. The skin is first cleaned with alcohol or a suitable
disinfectant, and the plunger on the syringe is always retracted prior to injection to
be sure that the needle is not in a vessel. For deep intramuscular injections, as
might be used for irritating medications such as iron preparations, a "z-track" injection method is employed.

2. Intravenous

Description. Injections or infusions directly into a vein.

Indications. Intravenous (i.v.) administration of drugs, fluids, and/or electrolytes is one of the most common parenteral routes employed in hospitals today. It is
especially convenient for rapidly infusing large volumes of fluid. The most common
indication for use of this route are: (1) to guarantee delivery and distribution when
hypotension or shock exists; (2) to restore rapidly electrolyte and fluid balance;
(3) to achieve an immediate pharmacologic effect, especially in emergencies, such

Table 1 Needle Selection

Injection site	Length range (in.)	Gauge range
Intra-abdominal	4 to 6	14 to 18
Intra-articular	1 to 3	19 to 22
Intracardiac	4 to 6	18 to 21
Intradermal	1/4 to 5/8	24 to 26
Intraocular		
Anterior chamber	1 to 3	25
Intravitreal	1 to 3	25
Retrobulbar	1-1/2	25
Subconjunctial	1-1/2	25
Intrapleural	5 to 6	13 to 18
Intrathecal		
Adult	3 to 5	20 to 22
Pediatric	1 to 1-1/2	25
Neonatal	1/2 to 1	27
Intravenous		
Metal needle	1 to 2	15 to 25
Winged needle	3/4 to 1-1/2	16 to 23
Plastic needle	3 to 5	15 to 21
Intracatheter	11-1/2	15 to 21
In-lying catheter	12, 26	14, 15
Hypodermoclysis		
Adult	2	19
Pediatric	1 to 1-1/2	20 to 22
Subcutaneous	1/4 to 5/8	24 to 25

as the treatment of certain arrythmias or of seizures; (4) to treat serious, life-threatening infections or conditions; (5) to provide continuous nutrition (hyperalimentation) when patients are unable to be fed by mouth; and (6) to avoid complications which might result if other administration routes were employed (e.g., hematomas at the site of intramuscular injections in a patient with a bleeding diathesis). In addition, the intravenous route may be used for a variety of other purposes, such as plasmapheresis, blood transfusion, and hemodynamic monitoring, to name a few.

Precautions: A large number and variety of complications may occur using the intravenous route. A few of these are: (1) thrombosis with or without complicating infection at the site of injection or infusion; (2) injection of microorganisms, toxins, particulate matter, or air; (3) the occurrence of physical or chemical incompatibilities between agents prior to or at the time of injection; (4) uncontrolled or excessive administration of drugs or fluids; and (5) extravasation of injections or infusions at the site of administration. When indwelling catheters are utilized, rarely the catheter tip may break off and lodge in a major vessel, in the heart, or in the lung.

Method. The upper extremities are chosen whenever possible for the site of injection or infusion. As many venous sites as possible should be preserved for future use; thus the most peripheral veins (e.g., these over the hand) are selected for initial use. When arm sites are no longer available, the leg veins (femoral and saphenous) or dorsal foot veins may be utilized; and in small children the scalp veins.

Selection of a vein depends on the size of the needle intended for use, type of fluids to be infused, flow rate anticipated, volume to be received, concomitant medications to be given, degree of patient mobility desired, and of course the skill of the person performing the venipuncture or catheterization. The veins in the antecubital fossa are among the most commonly chosen, because they are large and readily punctured. Other veins utilized commonly are basilic, cephalic, radial at the wrist, and the metacarpal and dorsal venous plexuses.

Needles are generally preferred to indwelling intravenous catheters, as the risk of infection is believed to be less [6]. Even after apparent exhaustion of all available venous sites, surgical cut-downs of deep veins with insertion of catheters may be performed. When long-term, repeated usage is expected or when prolonged infusion is anticipated, the subclavian or internal jugular (central veins) in the upper chest may be utilized. For peripheral veins and single or short-term usage, a 1 to 2 in. long, beveled, 18 to 22 gauge (Table 1), stainless steel needle is commonly used. The needle is inserted percutaneously into the vein after cleaning the skin and preparing it aseptically. Usually, a tourniquet is applied proximal to the site of insertion in order to congest the vein, thus dilating it and rendering it easy for entry. For long-term and/or repeated intravenous administration, a sterile plastic catheter may be inserted into the vein percutaneously through or over the needle that was used for the initial puncture. The needle is then removed and the catheter is left in place. The indwelling needle or catheter, whichever is utilized, is anchored to the extremity or body by means of appropriate, sterile occlusive or nonocclusive dressings, often impregnated with an antibiotic ointment. Indwelling catheters may contain a heparin lock to ensure against clotting and loss of patency through venous thrombosis.

3. Subcutaneous

Description. Injection into the loose connective and adipose tissue beneath the skin (dermis).

Indications. This route may be utilized if drugs cannot be administered orally because of lack of absorption from or inactivation by the contents of the gastrointestinal tract, if the patient is unable to ingest medications by mouth or if self-medication of parenterals (e.g., insulin) is desired. Drugs are more rapidly and more predictably absorbed by this route than by the oral one, but absorption is slower and less predictable than by the intramuscular route. Medications commonly administered subcutaneously (s.c.) include insulin, vaccines, narcotics, epinephrine, and vitamin B_{12}. As with the intramuscular route, if heart failure, shock, or vascular collapse exist, this route should not be depended upon.

Hypodermoclysis (Sec. III.B.1) is a special form of subcutaneous administration, namely, the infusion of large amounts of fluid into the subcutaneous tissues when intravenous sites are not available. This form of administration is rarely (if ever) used today but in the recent past was a common mode of replenishment of fluid and electrolytes in infants and elderly patients.

Precautions. Medications that are highly acidic, alkaline, or irritating, causing the production of pain, inflammation, and/or necrosis of tissues, should not be administered by this route. Infection, as with all parenteral injections, may occur, particularly in a patient with poor skin hygiene and particularly in situations where self-administration is practiced.

Methods. Generally, a beveled, 24 to 25 gauge (Table 1), 1/4 to 5/8 in. long, stainless steel needle is utilized. The volume injected generally does not exceed 0.5 to 1.5 ml. Injection sites include the abdomen at the level of the umbilicus, the upper back, the upper arms, and the lateral upper hips [7]. The skin over the site of administration should be cleaned prior to injection with a 70% alcohol sponge. Prior to injection, aspiration should be attempted to be certain that the needle has not inadvertently entered a vessel. If blood does not appear in the syringe when the plunger is retracted, it is safe to inject.

B. Secondary Routes

1. Hypodermoclysis

Description. The use of the subcutaneous route of administration for infusion of large volumes of solution into the subcutaneous tissue is called hypodermoclysis (see Sec. III.A.3).

Indications. Although infrequently practiced today, administration of fluids by hypodermoclysis may be indicated when a slow rate of absorption is desirable or if no suitable veins are available (e.g., with infant and geriatric patients). Fluids such as lactated Ringer's, dextrose 2.5% in 0.45% saline, and normal saline may be injected for maintenance or restoration of fluid and electrolyte balance.

Precautions. Injections must be given slowly to avoid distention of tissues. Hypertonic solutions, electrolyte-free fluids, amino acids, fat emulsions, and those differing significantly from body pH should not be used. Local infections are common and may be a problem. If hypotonic nonelectrolyte solutions are infused, large amounts of fluid can be drawn from the vascular compartment, resulting in decreased plasma volume and shock.

Method. A slightly larger needle is used than that for normal subcutaneous injections (Table 1). The site of injection usually chosen is at the interior or lateral portion of the thigh, although in infants the best site is in the subcutaneous tissue at the base of either scapulae. The rate of infusion depends on how well the fluid is absorbed. An enzyme (hyaluronidase) may be injected concomitantly to hasten absorption.

2. Intra-abdominal (Intraperitoneal)

Description. Injection or infusion directly into the peritoneal cavity via a needle or indwelling catheter or directly into an abdominal organ, such as the liver, kidney, or bladder.

Indications. The intra-abdominal route may be employed to treat local or widespread intra-abdominal disease due to infection or tumor (carcinomatosis); to dialyse and remove various cumulative toxic substances from the body when severe renal failure prohibits removal (peritoneal dialysis); and to determine the patency, as well as the structure, of various vascular or collecting systems (e.g., percutaneous intrahepatic or intrarenal injection of radiopaque contrast material).

Precautions. Infection (peritonitis) and hemorrhage are two of the major complications following intra-abdominal injections or infusions. The source of infection may be extrinsic (e.g., from skin or contaminated drugs or infusates) or intrinsic (e.g., from puncture of the bowel). The risk of infection is enhanced if an indwelling catheter, rather than a single injection using a sterile needle, is utilized. The longer the indwelling catheter remains in place, the greater the risk of infection. Such infections are particularly difficult to treat, especially in the presence of ascites; thus every precaution should be taken to prevent them. In addition, an aseptic peritonitis may be induced if the agent or fluid injected is highly irritable or contains endotoxin [8].

The chance of inducing hemorrhage is related generally to the size of the needle employed, the anatomical site selected for injection, the skill of the technician, and any tendencies of the patient to bleed (i.e., coagulation problems). If hemorrhage is induced, it may be difficult to control and may require surgical intervention and repair.

Peritoneal dialysis has special problems associated with it [9], such as hypotension from rapid removal of large quantities of fluid, heart failure from fluid overload, electrolyte disturbances, and chemically induced peritonitis or pancreatitis. Drugs injected into the intraperitoneal space are usually absorbed into the vascular compartment, but in some circumstances unpredictably so, thus posing an uncontrolled risk of toxicity or therapeutic failure; intraperitoneal insertion of aminoglycosides is not advised for this reason.

Method. After suitable aseptic preparation of the skin, a 16 or 18 gauge (Table 1), stainless steel needle is inserted through the anterior abdominal wall just lateral to the rectus muscles. If ascites is present, there is little risk of bowel puncture; however, if the peritoneal cavity is "dry," puncture of the bowel may occur (indicated by aspiration of fecal contents). Bowel puncture may be avoided by shallow punctures and withdrawing on the plunger while advancing the needle.

In peritoneal dialysis, a large, suitably sized catheter is inserted through a trochar which has been placed through the skin following a small incision in the midline just below the umbilicus (Fig. 2). The catheter is blunt-ended and contains many pores on its lateral aspects to abet fluid exchange without clogging. Suitable dressings must be employed to prevent ingress of microorganisms from the skin into the peritoneum via the potential space created between the catheter and the superficial tissues through which it passes. The catheter must be securely anchored to the abdomen with tape. A variety of dialysis kits are commercially available to simplify this procedure.

Intrahepatic injection is accomplished by percutaneous insertion of a needle in the right upper quadrant anteriorly, just below the last rib. A suitable radiopaque dye is injected into the liver substance itself; and because of the many bile canaliculi and ducts which exist in the tissue, the contrast material will find its way into the collecting system and thus can be photographed to document patency. A similar method may be used in studying the kidney, where contrast material may be injected into the renal parenchyma through a needle or catheter inserted percutaneously through the flank ("antegrade pyelogram").

3. Intra-arterial

Description. Injection or infusion into an artery which leads directly to the target organ.

Indications. The intra-arterial route is employed generally for diagnostic purposes, such as injecting radiopaque substances for roentgenographic studies of the vascular supply of various organs or tissues (e.g., coronary, cerebral, pulmonary, renal, enteric, or peripheral arteries). Almost every artery is approachable by arterial catheterization; virtually none are inaccessible to the skilled surgeon or radiologist.

Usage of the intra-arterial route for treatment purposes is infrequent and limited generally to organ-specific chemotherapy, such as treating certain localized

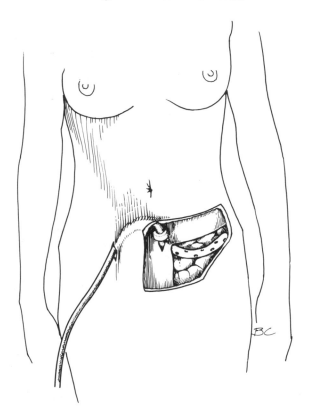

Figure 2   Catheter inserted for peritoneal dialysis. Note the subcutaneous tunneling of the catheter prior to entry into the peritoneal cavity to prevent microorganisms from gaining easy access to the cavity.

cancers (e.g., malignant melanomas of the lower extremities), where regional per- fusion with high concentrations of toxic drugs (which when given intravenously may be associated with serious systemic reactions) can be achieved.

Precautions. This route can be extremely hazardous, because products ad- ministered intra-arterially are not adequately diluted nor are they filtered by the lungs, liver, or kidneys before contact with peripheral tissue(s) or vital organs nourished by the artery. Products contaminated with microorganisms, endotoxin, and/or particulate matter may result in serious complications or reactions, such as infection (either intra-arterial or extra-arterial) or arterial thromboembolism or vasospasm, which may result in ischemia, infarction, or gangrene of the tissues or organs supplied. In addition, if the technique of entry is faulty, damage to the arterial intima and vessel wall may occur; so that either serious hemorrhagic ex- travasation may result or a dissecting aneurysm may be produced. If air is infused accidentally, air embolism with consequent ischemia and/or infarction of the tissue supplied may occur, an event which usually does not occur when small amounts of air are infused into the venous system.

Method. Either a suitably sized, smooth bore, stainless steel needle or a short, flexible, plastic catheter is surgically inserted into the desired artery or a lengthy catheter is guided over a stylet or needle through a percutaneous entry sight (sometimes under fluoroscopy) until the desired artery, organ, or tissue is reached; or the skin over the artery may be punctured directly, and the needle then inserted into the artery. Also, an open operative incision through the skin may be made (a "cut-down"), by which the artery is surgically exposed and under direct visualization is entered; a catheter is then inserted into the artery and sewn in place. Regardless of the method used, strict aseptic technique is practiced and appropriate occlusive or nonocclusive dressings are employed.

4. Intra-articular

Description. Injection or infusion into the synovial sacs of various accessible joints. An excellent description of this route of administration is contained in the book by Steinbrocker and Neustadt [10].

Indications. Antibiotics, lidocaine, and corticosteroid esters may be administered into bodily joints for the treatment of infections, pain, inflammation, or other problems resulting from inflammatory diseases (e.g., rheumatoid arthritis or trauma). Some agents are administered in single injections and some (e.g., antibiotics) via continuous infusion and "bathing" of the joint. Usually, the intra-articular approach is utilized when no more than one or two joints are involved. Often it supplements systemic therapy since, when the synovium is inflamed, it is highly vascularized, permitting a multitude of agents to enter with ease from the intravascular compartment.

Precautions. Iatrogenic infection is always a threat following intra-articular injection. The consequences of such infection may be destruction of the joint. Administration of corticosteroids is particularly troublesome because if serious infection does occur, recognition may be delayed due to suppression of the local inflammatory response; thus destruction of the joint and the cartilage may occur before the therapist is aware of a complicating infection. Severe, recurrent, intra-articular hemorrhage may be produced if a bleeding diathesis, such as hemophilia or severe hypoprothrombinemia, is present. Ordinarily, such blood is resorbed, but with recurrent hemorrhage eventual destruction of weight-bearing joints may occur. If the therapist is inexperienced, tendons may be ruptured if injected inadvertently.

Method. The anatomy and a roentgenograph of the joint to be entered should be studied prior to injection [11]. Entry should be at the point where the synovial cavity is most superficial and free of large vessels and nerves. The site of skin entry is cleaned and prepared as with any surgical procedure; strict aseptic technique is mandatory. Procaine infiltration is often unnecessary, especially if effusions are present. A sterile, 19-22 gauge (Table 1), stainless steel needle attached to a syringe is inserted into the synovial cavity. Fluid is first removed to ensure that the needle is within the joint space. The syringe is changed, and one containing the material to be injected is attached. If more than light pressure on the plunger is necessary, the needle is probably not in the joint space.

Intra-articular injections are easily accomplished in the knee, ankle, wrist, elbow, shoulder, phalangeal, sternoclavicular, and acromioclavicular joints; however, the hip joint is entered with difficulty. Joints deformed by any disease process (e.g., rheumatoid arthritis or trauma) may be more difficult to enter and inject.

5. Intracardiac

Description. Injection directly into chambers of the heart.

Indications. The use of this route is not recommended since better methods of delivery are available. Nevertheless, under unusual circumstances and in certain emergency situations, such as cardiac arrest, in which drugs may have to reach the myocardium immediately, intracardiac injections may be used. Myocardial activity may have to be stimulated or controlled following cardiac standstill or ventricular fibrillation, respectively.

Precautions. The heart muscle, coronary arteries, or the conducting system may be damaged by the trauma of an injecting needle or by the drug injected. Various arrhythmias, some of which may be fatal (e.g., ventricular fibrillation) may be precipitated. Occasionally, hemorrhage into the myocardium or pericardium may result, leading to infarction or pericardial tamponade, respectively. If extracardiac structures such as the lung are inadvertently punctured, a pneumothorax may result and breathing may be impaired. Occasionally, when the xiphoid approach is used, the liver may be lacerated.

Method. The heart is approached from either of two directions: anterolaterally, in the anterior axillary line at the fifth or sixth intercostal space (in which case the needle is aimed upward toward the opposite scapula); or medially, just beneath the xiphoid process of the manubrium (in which case the needle is aimed upward toward the scapula on the same side). Selection of the route may be influenced by the presence of left or right ventricular hypertrophy, the former being better suited for the anterolateral approach and the latter being better suited for the medial approach, or any anatomical derangements of the chest which may exist. Generally, a beveled, 18 to 21 gauge (Table 1), 4 to 6 in. long, stainless steel needle is used. An electrode may be attached to the needle to indicate when the myocardium is reached; however, in emergency situations this luxury may not be available.

6. Intracisternal

Description. Injection directly into the cisternal space surrounding the base of the brain.

Indications. This route is employed mainly for diagnostic purposes. It is used when intracranial pressures are elevated and the risk of herniation of the brain exists if fluid is removed from the lumbar sac. Diseases involving the cisterns generally extend to nearby, contiguous structures; and for reasons explained in Section III.B.13, these diseases are better treated by utilizing the intraventricular route. Rarely, in order to locate and define a particular disease process, especially a spinal tumor or abscess, various contrast materials are injected into the cisterns. Usually, though, materials are injected below in the lumbar sac to study these cavities and any related pathology.

Precautions. Many of the precautions concerning the use of the intraventricular route are applicable to the use of the intracisternal route, particularly as regards aseptic practices and the threat of physicochemical irritation of the substances injected.

One very serious drawback to the use of this route is the danger of producing permanent, serious, neurologic injury or death by pithing the midbrain. The space entered is relatively small, and insertion of a needle into it should be attempted only when other routes may not be used and only by the most experienced personnel. Most neurosurgeons are abandoning the intracisternal route in favor of entering the subarachnoid space just caudal to the cisterna magnum, between the first and second cervical vertebrae. In this instance a lateral approach is used, and if the needle is inserted too far, pithing of the cord may not result in death or serious neurologic injury.

Method. For intracisternal puncture the patient is placed in a head-down position and the entry approach is posterior between the occiput and the first cervical vertebrae. The cisterna magnum is entered. Care is exercised to continue aspirating with a syringe while inserting the needle, so as to halt insertion the moment that fluid is obtained, thus minimizing the danger of a medullary pith. To repeat, only experienced personnel should attempt this procedure, and other alternative avenues of entry should be considered first (see Secs. III.B.11 and III.B.13).

7. Intradermal (Intracutaneous)

Description. Injection into the dermis (to be distinguished from subcutaneous), located just beneath and adjacent to the epidermis.

Indications. A number of diagnostic agents, antigens (e.g., tuberculin) and vaccines (e.g., smallpox) are administered by this route. The volume of fluid injected generally does not exceed 0.1 ml. Absorption by the intradermal route is very slow.

Precautions. Infections may complicate the procedure, but are unusual.

Method. Generally a beveled, 26 gauge (Table 1), 3/8 in. long, stainless steel needle is utilized. The skin at the site of administration should be cleaned prior to injection with 70% alcohol. Certainty of intradermal injection is evident by the appearance of a localized swelling of the skin, giving the appearance of an orange peel. The most common mistakes in intradermal injections are injecting beneath the skin rather than into it or permitting materials to leak out of the needle tip if it is not inserted completely into the skin. Both may result in false negative skin tests.

8. Intralesional

Description. Injection of medication directly into or around a lesion, usually located in or on the skin or soft tissues, to achieve a therapeutic effect.

Indications. Injection of substances into or around lesions have been particularly useful when a potent local effect is desired. It has been used in neutralizing various toxins, such as tetanus, in which situations injections of antitoxin in and around the wound have been employed. A similar therapeutic usefulness has been assumed for rabies, with direct injections of antisera into and around the site of the bite. Dermatologists have commonly used this route to treat psoriasis, lichen simplex, sarcoid, lichen planus hypertrophicus, herpes zoster (and post-zoster neuralgia), and cystic or nodular acne with local steroids [12]. Keloids have also been handled frequently with such local injections, but usually with higher doses of steroids.

Precautions. The most frequent complications have been infections, usually from newly introduced organisms of nosocomial origin. Although at times difficult, depending on the type of lesion being injected, a sterile field should be prepared through which to inject. With infectious diseases, local spread of the process being treated may occur. Finally, in such anaerobic infections as tetanus, further anaerobiasis may be encouraged by occlusion of small vessels by the injected materials, thus defeating the purpose of eliminating the infection.

Method. Generally, a fine 24 to 26 gauge (Table 1), stainless steel needle with a calibrated syringe (e.g., a tuberculin for accurate calibration) is employed. Small volumes (<1 ml) are injected. Occasionally, a jet injector is utilized. However, if antitoxin or antisera are to be infiltrated in and around a wound, larger syringes with larger needles may be employed. The entire procedure should utilize aseptic practices.

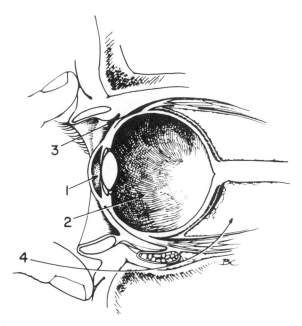

Figure 3   Injection sites for the eye.   1, anterior chamber; 2, vitreous humor;
3, retrobulbar; 4, subconjunctival.

9. Intraocular

Description.   Four types of intraocular injections are utilized (Fig. 3):

1. Anterior chamber: Injection or irrigation directly into the anterior chamber of
    the eye.
2. Intravitreal: Injection directly into the vitreous cavity of the eye.
3. Retrobulbar: Injection around (not into) the posterior segment of the globe.
4. Subconjunctival: Although included under this heading, subconjunctival (and ret-
    robulbar) injections are not intraocular.   Instead, such injections are given be-
    neath the conjunctiva, so that medication diffuses through the limbus and sclera
    into the eye.

Indications.   Such routes are used in the treatment of infections and inflammatory diseases of the eye which are not treated effectively by topical or systemic drug
administration for anesthesia of the globe (retrobulbar) and occasionally for pupillary
dilation with cycloplegics and mydriatics.   Entry of drugs into the eye is frought with
difficulty, as intraocular transport and diffusion are poor.   Intraocular injections
are complemented frequently by intravenous infusions of the therapeutic drugs employed.   Selection of the type of intraocular injection depends on the disease present
and the precise location of that disease within the eye.

Precautions.   Extreme care and precise technique are required to minimize
or prevent damage to the eye, especially to the corneal endothelium.   Complications
that can occur, depending on the route selected, are optic nerve damage, hemor-
rage, retinal detachment, retinal necrosis, cataracts, and injection of the drug
directly into the circulation with consequent systemic effects.   Infection is always
a threat and must be avoided at all costs, as such infections may result in rapid

destruction of the eye and/or blindness. The volume of solution that may be injected into the eye is severely restricted, generally to not more than 0.1 to 0.2 ml. Since an excellent knowledge of the anatomy and function of the eye is required, only an ophthalmologist should attempt these procedures.

Method. The anterior chamber (containing the aqueous humor) is entered at a point located on the edge of the cornea (the limbus) with a 25 gauge or smaller, stainless steel needle, withdrawing a volume of fluid prior to injection equal to that to be instilled. For intraocular injections excluding the anterior chamber, a drop of 1:100,000 epinephrine may be placed on the iris to dilate the pupil. Great care must be taken not to inject or damage the lens, as a cataract may result.

Entry into the vitreous humor is accomplished by injection through the pars plana (junction of retina and ciliary body) with a 25 gauge stainless steel needle. The vitreous appears to be an inert fluid which is not replaced once removed. During injection, great care must be taken not to detach the retina. Again, a volume of fluid equal to that to be injected must be removed before instillation. Generally, not more than 0.1 ml may be injected. Injection of steroids into this chamber can be dangerous, resulting in destruction of the retina (retinal necrosis).

Entering the retrobulbar space involves insertion of the needle at the junction of the lateral and medial third of the orbital rim and then advancing the needle toward the apex of the orbit. Care must be taken not to inject the optic nerve directly. A 1-1/2 in. long, 25 gage stainless steel needle is generally employed. Subconjunctival injections generally do not exceed volumes of 0.5 ml. This route is especially used in treating corneal abscesses. Injection of the sub-Tenon fascia is utilized for the treatment of uveitis (e.g., secondary to localized sarcoidosis) or chronic cyclitis. Again, care must be taken not to inject or nick the globe.

10. Intrapleural

Description. Usually, single injection into the pleural cavity. Occasionally, if indwelling chest tubes are inserted surgically, this route may be used for irrigation purposes or for repeated injections of drugs.

Indications. Occasionally, infections or malignancies involving the pleural cavity, particularly if the disease process is impairing respiratory function, are treated by this route. Enzymes (e.g., streptokinase and streptodornase) may be injected to liquify thick empyemas which may not be removed by aspiration or resorbed naturally. If left untreated, such empyemas may result in fibrosis, adhesions, thickening of the pleura, and restriction of breathing. Also, carcinomatous spread or mesotheliomas involving the pleura are treated by local intrapleural injection of antitumor or sclerosing agents, especially if recurrent effusions are a problem.

Precautions. The complications most frequently resulting from intrapleural injections are pneumothorax (collapse of the lung), intrapleural hemorrhage, and/or superimposed infection. The latter is more common when chest tubes are permitted to remain in place for prolonged periods of time.

Method. For needle punctures, the pleural cavity is most easily entered posterolaterally by having the patient sitting up and leaning forward over the back of a chair or table (Fig. 4). The level of entry selected is based on radiologic findings. If fluid is present in the pleural cavity, an entry site below the fluid level is used to minimize the risk of pneumothorax or puncture of the visceral pleura. Generally, a sharply beveled, 13 to 18 gauge (Table 1), stainless steel needle is selected, and

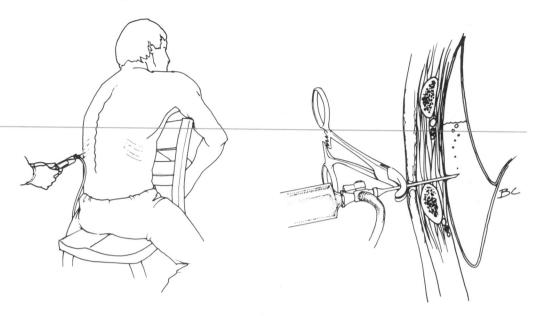

Figure 4   Pleural tap. The needle should be inserted above the rib to avoid puncturing the intercostal vessels. Note the hemostat to stabilize the position of the
needle (see the text for more details).

a two-way stopcock is attached between the syringe and the needle; the stopcock enables one to remove fluid, while permitting injection of medications without producing a pneumothorax. The thicker the fluid, the larger the bore of the needle used.
Care must be taken not to permit air to enter the needle (or syringe) while it is in
place, or a pneumothorax will result. Before entry into the pleural cavity, the skin
is cleaned and draped as for any surgical procedure, and liberal quantities of a local
anesthetic are injected around the lower rib margin in and around the periosteum at
the site selected for entry. Entry is made by inserting the needle until its tip en-
counters a rib, then sliding the needle tip over the rib (to avoid puncture of intercostal arteries located along the inferior margin of the ribs), while at the same time
withdrawing on the plunger of the syringe. As soon as fluid is withdrawn, a clamp
or hemostat is placed on the needle at a point where it will buttress against the skin.
This maneuver permits the therapist to secure the placement of the needle by applying continual, gentle pressure, thus preventing the needle from advancing into the
lung or slipping out of the pleural space. A roentgenogram of the chest should be
taken after withdrawal of the needle to ensure that a pneumothorax has not been
produced.

11. Intrathecal

Description. Injection or infusion directly into the lumbar sac (intrathecal)
located at the caudal end of the spinal cord.

Indications. This route is employed more for diagnostic than for therapeutic
purposes. However, when diseases, particularly infections and tumors, involve
the subarachnoid space along the cord, this route is also utilized for therapy [13].

Treatment frequently consists of injecting or infusing the appropriate chemothera-
peutic agent into the lumbar sac, and depending on the weight of the substance injected, tilting the patient to encourage distribution over the hemispheres. This form
of chemotherapy is often employed to complement some form of systemic intravenous
therapy. However, in the treatment of meningitis, the value of using this route is
controversial and remains to be proven.

Infusion of radiopaque substances via the intrathecal route is valuable in assessing the patency of the subarachnoid space around the cord and base of the brain.
Spinal epidural abscesses and tumors involving or compressing the subarachnoid
space or areas nearby are diagnosed generally with this procedure. Also, anesthetics may be injected into the subarachnoid space around the lower spinal column for
certain surgical procedures limited to areas innervated by nerves below the determined level of anesthesia.

Precautions. The same precautions for intraventricular administration (Sec.
III. B. 13) apply to use of the intrathecal route. In addition, a real threat of tonsilar
or brain stem herniation (and possibly death) exists if this procedure is performed
while intracranial pressure is elevated. Great care must be exercised to avoid this
complication, which usually occurs 1 to 2 hr or sooner after removal of fluid. Pre-
ventative measures, such as performing the tap with the patient's head lower than
the feet, using a small bore (e.g., 22 gauge) needle, not removing an excessive
amount of fluid, keeping the bevel of the needle parallel with the dural fibers so as
to part rather than cut them (thus reducing the chance of continual leak after removal of the needle), avoiding overhydration, and inserting an intravenous access line
prior to the tap in the event herniation should occur. (Infusion of steroids or
mannitol-urea intravenously may rapidly reduce intracranial pressure.) Another
problem with intrathecal injection is the frequency with which the subarachnoid space
is missed and second sacs or extrathecal spaces are created.

Method. A 3.5 in. long, smooth-bore, beveled, 20 to 22 gauge (Table 1), stainless steel spinal needle is used for adults. The patient's skin is prepared as in any
surgical procedure, taking the greatest caution to use aseptic technique. The needle
is inserted posteriorly at the midline into any space below the third lumbar spinal
process. The patient is in the lateral decubitus position with head, back, and thighs
flexed. If intracranial pressure is diffusely elevated, the special precautions outlined above should be taken, but if intracranial masses are suspected, this procedure should not be done.

12. Intrauterine

Description. Infusion or injection via a needle inserted percutaneously into
the pregnant uterus.

Indications. Injection or infusion of certain substances, such as 20% saline,
prostaglandin E, or urea, into the pregnant uterus is used usually after the six-
teenth week of pregnancy to induce labor in medical abortions or to deliver a still-
born fetus. Although most abortions are performed best using surgical techniques,
in the hands of the relatively inexperienced physician, medical abortions via intrau-
terine injections are useful. In addition, contrast material for roentgenographic
studies may be injected to aid in the study of potential congenital anomalies.

Precautions. Infection (amnionitis and myometritis) is the most common complication accompanying this approach. If 20% saline is unexpectedly infused intravenously into a patient, death can result. Fortunately, this is a rare complication.

Occasionally, a disseminated intravascular coagulopathy (DIC) syndrome may result, and some patients may go on to have significant bleeding. Incomplete emptying of the uterus may also occur, resulting in all the problems that may accompany this event. Possibly, in inexperienced hands, an ovarian cyst or the bladder may be injected.

Method. Following a surgical preparatory cleansing, halfway between the umbilicus and the symphysis pubis in the midline, a 18 to 20 gauge, 3.5 in. long, beveled-tip, sterile, stainless steel spinal needle is inserted into the uterus. (The point of entry may be anesthetized locally with 1% xylocaine.) Approximately 150 to 200 ml of 20% saline is then infused into the uterus over a 10 min or longer period. Afterward, the needle is removed and expulsion of fetal material is awaited.

13. Intraventricular

Description. Injection or infusion directly into the lateral ventricles of the brain.

Indications. This route is employed mainly in the treatment of infections (such as bacterial or fungal meningitis and/or ventriculitis) or of malignancies (such as leukemic infiltrates of the meninges or carcinomatoses) involving the membranes and cerebrospinal fluid surrounding the central nervous system. It is used especially in situations where the drugs involved are known to diffuse or pass poorly from the vascular compartment into the ventricles and subarachnoid space and/or where reduction of systemic side effects from a particular agent are desired (e.g., in the treatment of fungal meningitis with amphotericin B or in the therapy of leukemic infiltrates with methotrexate). Often, therapy via this route is complemented by the intravenous administration of the same agent which has been injected into the ventricles.

In the treatment of diseases of these areas, the intraventricular route often is preferred over the intracisternal (Sec. III.B.6) or intrathecal (Sec. III.B.11), since the flow of cerebrospinal fluid is unidirectional and originates principally in the choroid plexus of the lateral ventricles. The fluid then pursues a path through the third and fourth ventricles out the foramina of Luschka and Magendie into the posterior fossa at the level of the pons, down over the spinal cord, and then finally reversing itself to flow up over the cerebral hemispheres (Fig. 5). Intrathecal or intracisternal injections do not result in distribution of the drug into the ventricular space; thus disease within the ventricles (ventriculitis) would not be treated by these routes. In addition, the ventricle provides a large fluid space in which to inject drugs, thereby diluting such drugs in a large volume of cerebrospinal fluid, thus minimizing potential, localized physicochemical irritation to the cells lining the ventricle and subsequent damage from a host reaction (chemical ventriculitis). In addition, if intracranial pressures are excessive, the risk of brain stem herniation may be avoided.

Radiopaque, radiolabeled, or dye substances may be injected into the intraventricular space for studies of either the anatomy or patency of the system or for studies of the flow of cerebrospinal fluid.

Precautions. Since cerebrospinal fluid bathes such critical organs as the brain and spinal cord and since one of its functions is believed to be a protective or cushioning fluid for these organs, any disturbance of this fluid or the membranes containing it may be deleterious and possibly lethal. Any foreign material, chemical or biological, when injected into the system may precipitate an inflammatory response anywhere or everywhere within the system. Strict aseptic techniques should be adhered to when entering the ventricles to prevent iatrogenic infections, and care

should be exercised to be certain that the substances injected or infused are not irritating to the cells lining the ventricular or subarachnoid spaces. If irritating drugs
are injected, ventriculitis or myelitis may result (sometimes progressive), producing obstruction of the system (hydrocephalus) or permanent neurological injury.
The vehicles employed for intraventricular injection should have physical characteristics as close to the cerebrospinal fluid as possible. Often the patient's cerebrospinal fluid may be withdrawn and used as a vehicle. Elliott's B solution is recommended [14]. If the ventricles are small or almost closed due to intracerebral edema, these spaces may be difficult to locate, and undesirable intracerebral injection
of the drug with subsequent neurologic injury may result. In addition, hemorrhages
(subdural, epidural, intraventricular, or intracerebral) may occur, and in children
following repeated injections, porencephaly may result. If the ventricular needle is
inserted too far, passing through the ventricles, damage to the basal ganglia, thala-
mus, or other vital structures may occur. The procedure should be carried out
only by experienced personnel.

Methods. A 3.5 in. long, smooth-bore, 18 gauge, stainless steel, blunt-ended
ventricular needle is used. The patient's skin is prepared as in any surgical procedure, taking the greatest caution to maintain strict aseptic technique. A twist drill
puncture of the cranium is first performed, generally over the coronal suture about
2 cm from the midline and in line with the ipsilateral pupil. The needle, which is a

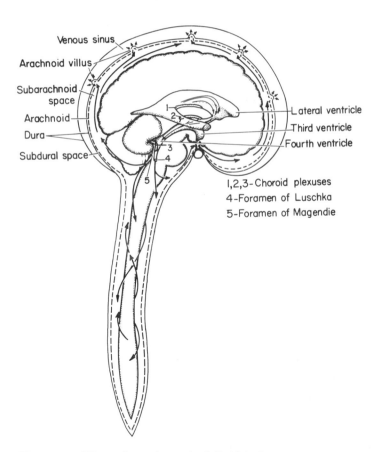

Figure 5   Flow of cerebrospinal fluid in humans.

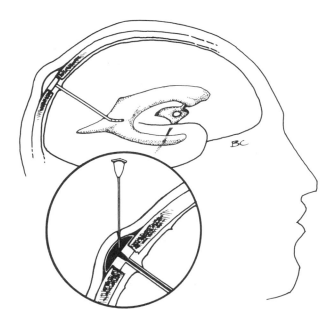

Figure 6   Subcutaneous reservoir with access to the lateral ventricles of the brain. This device is often employed when repeated injections over a long period of time are anticipated. It has the advantage of permitting sampling with relative ease.

special blunt, open-ended needle, is passed through the frontal lobe into the lateral ventricle. When repeated injections or infusions are required, use of an Ommaya [15] or Rickam reservoir or similar silicone, elastomer, subcutaneous reservoir is recommended (Fig. 6). Surgical placement of the reservoir may be accomplished in a variety of ways. Often with these devices no local anesthetic is required for reinjection, and the system may be sampled and injected repeatedly with minimum disturbance to the patient and with reduced risk of infection.

IV. DISTRIBUTION OF PARENTERALLY ADMINISTERED AGENTS

Substances administered intramuscularly, intravenously, or subcutaneously enter the circulatory system via the lymphatic and/or venous transport system. Before being pumped into the arterial circulation by the heart, such substances must first pass through the lungs. The capillary beds of the lungs serve as both a filter and in some instances as a reservoir if the substance injected partitions into the tissues of the lung and is subsequently released back into the circulatory system. In Benet's schematic depiction of drug distribution [16], the lung serves both as a distribution and an elimination organ. The lung also may serve as a site for the metabolism of certain agents.

    After intravenous injection or infusion, drugs that enter the lungs are distributed throughout its entire volume of distribution, provided that the partition of the drug is favorable. A portion of the drug may be cleared by exhalation, especially for those with high vapor pressures. After an intramuscular or subcutaneous injection, absorbed drugs also may be distributed from the lungs; however, injection at these sites is associated with a lag time between the time of injection and their appearance in the blood.

Various factors affect the distribution of drugs which have been injected subcutaneously or intramuscularly into the general circulation. (For a more detailed discussion of distribution, the reader is referred to Chapter 3.)

Solubility of the Drug. Drugs need to be solubilized completely before they can permeate muscle or tissue barriers and enter the circulatory system. Two types of solubility are important: solubility in the dosage form vehicle and solubility in body fluids. For drugs administered as solutions, dosage form solubility is obviated. However, for drugs administered as suspensions, the rate of drug dissolution from the dosage form vehicle, as well as solubility in tissue fluids at the injection site, largely determines the absorption rate of the drug. Dissolution rates of injected drug suspensions depend on the size of the drug particles, pH of the fluids at the injection site, the polymorphic character of the drug crystals, and the diffusion coefficient of the drug. At higher viscosities the diffusion coefficient of the drug is reduced. Once the drug is in solution from the dosage form, its solubility in fluids in the subcutaneous tissues or muscles is dependent on its partition coefficient and its degree of ionization as dictated by the pH of fluids existing at the injection site.

Partition Coefficient of the Drug. The lower the lipid solubility of the drug, the lower will be its partition coefficient, and the slower will be its rate of absorption into the blood stream from the site of injection.

Rate of Blood Flow at the Injection Site. A well-known fact is that the greater the blood flow in the capillary network to and from the site of injection, the higher will be the rate of drug absorption. Injections into the muscles of the lateral thighs or buttocks are associated with slower and lower drug absorption (because of less vascularity and higher fat content) than injections in the deltoid muscles. Factors that increase blood flow, such as exercise, increase drug absorption after intramuscular or subcutaneous injections. On the other hand, factors that retard blood flow, such as vasoconstrictors like epinephrine, if administered concurrently at the site of injection, decrease the rate of drug absorption.

Degradation of the Drug at the Injection Site. Distribution of biologically active drug is retarded if the drug is metabolized or in other ways degraded at the site of injection.

Particle Size of the Drug. The size of suspended drug particles affects their dissolution rate in the dosage form. The larger the particle size, the slower the dissolution rate, as less surface area of the drug is available for interaction with body fluids. Slightly soluble drugs, such as diazepam, phenytoin, and digoxin, are known to precipitate in body fluids following injection because, although sufficiently soluble in their cosolvent dosage form, they are not soluble in aqueous body fluids. The precipitated particles may dissolve eventually, but the rate of dissolution is slow.

Formulation Ingredients. Materials added to drug dosage formulations to aid in resuspendability (such as cellulose derivatives), to aid in solubilization (such as glycerin), and/or to aid in enhancing stability (such as antioxidants) potentially may affect distribution from the site of administration. Such effects may be manifested in diverse ways, such as complexation, which reduces the rate of drug dissolution, and as increased viscosity, which retards the transport of the drug from the injection site to the systemic circulation.

V. PRECAUTIONS, PROBLEMS, HAZARDS, AND COMPLICATIONS ASSOCIATED WITH PARENTERAL DRUG ADMINISTRATION

The precautions necessary to ensure the safe and successful administration of an agent parenterally have been discussed under the specific routes of administration employed (Sec. III). Although in many instances precautions are unique to the route to be utilized, several points deserve emphasis and repetition: namely, good aseptic technique and sterile practices; careful examination of the product beforehand to identify potential or real contamination by microorganisms or toxins; attention to detail in regards to correct dosage, mixing, potential drug interaction, and storage, cautious and intelligent handling of accessory or delivery devices necessary to accomplish the task of injection or infusion or to monitor the patient's situation; selection of correct equipment to accomplish the job; a careful history from the patient with regard to risk factors (e.g., bleeding diathesis, previous reactions, predisposition to infection, etc.); and a careful observation of the patient during and after parenteral administration.

The need for good practices in storage and handling of parenteral drugs or infusions cannot be overemphasized. From the moment a drug or infusate is manufactured, its purity and sterility are constantly threatened by handling or storage errors. Such problems are not unique to manufacturers but extend throughout the life of the product in all areas of delivery, receiving, and distribution; from the truck that delivers the product, to the hospital pharmacy that receives it, to the hospital ward where final delivery to the individual patient takes place. Difficulties encountered may range from gross excesses in storage temperatures, to outdated shelf lives, to subtle hairline cracks (Fig. 7A) invisible to the naked eye but which may be present in product containers [6,17] and lead to microbial contamination (Fig. 7B).

On the other hand, errors or problems in admixture compounding usually occur at the hospital pharmacy or ward level. Over recent years, hospital pharmacies have introduced "central additive programs" as a method of reducing such errors [18]. Here a sterile parenteral product received from the manufacturer is mixed in a central location (usually in the pharmacy) with whatever agents or fluid formulas physicians may prescribe. The central location is away from trafficked areas, and admixing is performed under a laminar flow hood using careful aseptic techniques and practices. Complex formulas are often generated to satisfy the therapeutic needs of an extremely difficult medical or surgical problem (e.g., hyperalimentation). After formulation, the product is shipped to the hospital ward for administration to the patient. Such central additive programs reduce the high risk of compounding and contaminating errors which may occur when large numbers of different people with different skills are compounding or admixing such products on a hospital ward. However, central additive programs must be alert to possible errors in procedure [19], which when they occur, may be multiplied manyfold, often resulting in problems of epidemic proportions. For example, common source epidemics of sepsis from central additive programs have not been unusual [20-22].

In addition, people conducting central additive programs must appreciate that quality control for such programs is virtually impossible to perform in an econom-

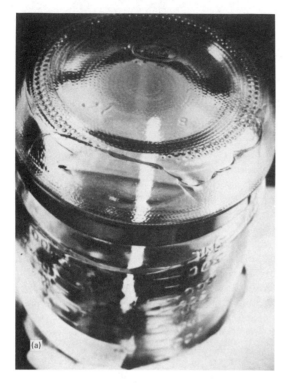

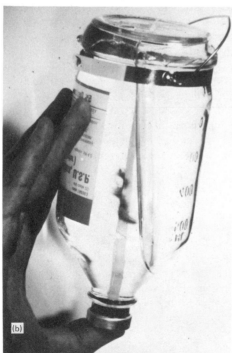

Figure 7   Bottle of intravenous fluid with a hairline crack at its base (a) containing a fungus ball of <u>Aspergillus</u> (b), probably acquired from careless handling or poor storage.

ical and statistically meaningful manner, especially for "low-frequency" problems.
Thus, carefully formulated, sterile products "guaranteed" with a manufacturer's
label may no longer be valid once the product has been adulterated or violated at
the pharmacy or hospital level.

The problems of parenteral administration per se have also been pointed out
or implied earlier in the discussions of the techniques or methods utilized for each
of the routes employed. However, in addition to these problems, further difficulties exist in securing properly trained, highly intelligent, motivated health care
personnel to employ correctly and responsibly the complicated methods often utilized
in the modern hospital or clinic setting. Such personnel, in addition to being expensive and scarce, must be constantly updated on new techniques and problems (continual education). Similarly, some of the devices employed in administration are
not only expensive but also scarce (notably certain plastics), and in some instances
possess inherent or generated problems (e.g., low-level contamination, design
flaws, hairline cracks in materials, etc.) too difficult to identify with 100% assurance with even the best quality control techniques. The actively engaged therapist
must always be alert to real and potential dangers associated with such delivery
systems.

The hazards and complications of parenteral drug administration are numerous and varied but may be considered in terms of their consequence as either general or specific. General hazards or complications are at risk of occurring regardless of the agent or class of drugs being administered, whereas specific hazards
or complications are unique or peculiar to certain agents and methods of administration. An important fact to remember about all parenteral injections is that if a
reaction or adverse side effect of any sort occurs, it is usually impossible to re-
trieve or locally neutralize the offending agent, whereas with oral agents, recovery
or expulsion of the medication is possible.

A. General Hazards or Complications

Many complications associated with parenteral drug administration have already
been noted or described under the individual descriptions of the various parenteral
routes available. The most important of these, common to most forms of therapy,
but particularly to intravenous administration, are summarized in Table 2.

Sepsis may result from microorganisms (notably bacteria or fungi) contaminating the product or delivery system prior to or during use (Fig. 8) or from microorganisms colonizing the patient's skin, which are either dragged into the injection
or infusion site at the time of puncture or, if an intravenous line is present, mi-
grate from the skin into the vein along a fibrin sleeve between the infusion catheter
or needle and the tissues of the body. If bacteremia or fungemia from a distant,
unrelated source should occur, circulating microorganisms may alight upon any
indwelling foreign device (catheter or needle), establishing residence there as a
local infection. This infection may subsequently reseed the bloodstream to produce
a vicious cycle of infection. Resulting sepsis may be localized [e.g., at the site of
injection or infusion (forming an abscess)], it may be systemic (producing septicemia and metastatic infections), or it may be both local and systemic.

The specific microorganisms involved vary considerably but generally are
the same as those indigenous to the locale through which the infusion or injection
passes. For example, since Staphylococcus aureus is commonly found on the skin
of the upper extremities, intravenous infusions passing through the skin in these
regions may be expected to become secondarily infected or colonized by these bacteria. S. epidermidis, Candida spp., streptococci, Acinetobacter calcoaceticus,

Table 2   Summary of General Precautions, Problems, and Complications
of Parenteral Drug Administration

Sepsis: toxemia and toxin injection; may be localized, systemic, and/or metastatic

Thrombosis: limited to intravenous or intra-arterial administration

Phlebitis: principally with intravenous administration

Bleeding: usually related to patient's condition (e.g., bleeding diathesis) but can
          occur from iatrogenic damage of vessels

Particulate matter: most serious in intravenous or intra-arterial administration,
          but can precipitate foreign body reaction at any tissue site

Incompatibilities: physical and chemical; most threatening when they occur in the
          vascular compartments

Physicochemical properties: extremes of pH and osmolality

Hypersensitivity reactions: immediate and delayed

Overdosage: either drugs or fluids

Air emboli: limited to intravenous or intra-arterial usage

Fever and toxicity: may be due to localized or systemic administration; may be
          secondary to allergic or toxic reaction

Infiltration and extravasation: limited generally to intravenous or intra-arterial
          usage

Costs: greater than oral; sometimes very expensive

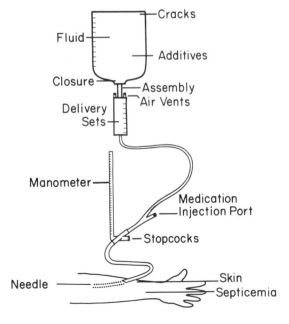

Figure 8   Various sites or entry ports where intravenous administration systems
can become contaminated.

and a variety of Gram-negative bacilli (Pseudomonas, Serratia, Escherichia coli, Enterobacter, Klebsiella, and Proteus) are other pathogenic microorganisms frequently encountered. Since such infections generally occur in a nosocomial setting, the responsible microorganisms often are resistant to most antibiotics and thus are difficult to manage or cure.

Indwelling, in-line, bacteria-retaining filters (pore size 0.22 to 0.45 μm) have been utilized in intravenous infusion systems in an attempt to remove contaminating bacteria or fungi [23]. However, the value and cost-effectiveness of such filters remain to be proven. Ideally, little doubt exists as to the potential usefulness of such filters; however, they are costly, may at times clog up and delay infusion, may leak and themselves become contaminated, and they may represent another device introduced into the system that may in itself become contaminated at the manufacturing or insertional steps. In addition, such filters do not remove toxins elaborated by contaminating bacteria.

Toxemia may result when a biological toxin contaminates the medicinal preparation and is inadvertently infused or injected. The result(s) of injecting or infusing such toxins depends on the nature and quantity of the toxin and the body compartment or tissue into which it is injected. The most common toxin contaminating most materials is endotoxin, a pharmacologically active lipopolysaccharide present in the cell walls of most Gram-negative bacilli. When inoculated intravenously, endotoxins cause fever, leukopenia, circulatory collapse, capillary hemorrhages, necrosis of tumors, and the Schwartzman phenomenon. Tests (e.g., rabbit or limulus lysate) for detecting the presence of endotoxins are available but are not routinely performed in the hospital.

Occasionally, even refrigerated biologicals may be contaminated by microorganisms (psychrophilic bacteria) that produce endotoxin. In such situations, appropriate cultures inoculated at low temperatures have to be performed before isolation of the responsible microorganisms and proof of what occurred are achieved. Since the organisms grow only at low temperatures and not at 37°C (body temperature), blood cultures from the patient will be of no value. The problem is not one of bacteremia resulting from contamination, but rather of toxemia from an infusion or injection of endotoxin.

Injections of substances contaminated by S. aureus may result in serious toxic shock syndromes, such as occurred in the Bundaberg disaster of 1928, in which 12 of 21 children inoculated with a vial of diphtheria toxin-antitoxin died [24]. In this regard, biological substances which might serve as ideal media for the growth of microorganisms should be stored and handled with extra caution. Aspergillus, a highly ubiquitous, aerial fungus with many species, is another organism that may contaminate medications or fluids and that may elaborate a potent toxin. One species, A. flavus, is notorious for elaborating such a toxin; and infusion of it, were it to contaminate biological materials, could result in sudden death.

Thrombosis of a vein (or veins) may occur with any intravenous infusion or injection. Generally, it is limited to the site of administration; however, the thrombus may propagate proximally (and distally) for a considerable length. Two serious complications may result from venous thrombosis: emboli which may travel to the lung, resulting in pulmonary infarction, and secondary infection, which may result in septicemia, multiple pulmonary septic emboli, endocarditis, and/or pneumonia.

Thrombosis of an artery is a more serious complication than that of a vein; and if collateral circulation is inadequate, gangrene of the tissues supplied by the artery may result.

Some important factors responsible for thrombosis are pH; physicochemical irritability of the drugs infused, resulting in venospasm or arteriospasm; drug insolubility or precipitation; particulate matter; infection; osmolality; selection of too small a vessel for injection of a large quantity of drug; prolonged injection; trauma per se; and the presence of a foreign body within the vein or artery (e.g., a plastic catheter). In certain people and in certain disease states (e.g., systemic lupus erythematosis), an inherent propensity to develop thrombosis at the slightest irritation may exist.

Phlebitis may occur following any infusion or injection; however, this condition is more commonly associated with intravenous infusions than with injections, particularly if the device for infusion remains in the same vein for more than a few days. Phlebitis may or may not be associated with infection within the vein and may or may not result in thrombosis. If thrombosis complicates phlebitis, all the consequences of thrombosis may result. The same factors that enhance the risk of thrombosis developing also enhance the risk of phlebitis occurring. In addition, low pH, hyperosmotic infusates, and infusion of particulates appear to increase the risk of phlebitis [25]. Most investigators conclude that thrombophlebitis is primarily a physicochemical phenomenon, and multiple factors appear to predispose to its development [6]. However, some studies have suggested that the incidence of phlebitis may depend more on the personnel administering the parenteral substances and on their technical skills than on the materials injected or the devices used for delivery [26].

Bleeding may occur if a vessel(s) is damaged or ruptured or if the patient has a serious bleeding diathesis (e.g., platelet deficiency). If a bleeding tendency exists, the intravenous route may be safer than the intramuscular, because bleeding may be controlled. Patients with hemophilia or with vitamin K or platelet deficiencies should be given antihemophilic globulin, vitamin K, or platelet transfusions, respectively, prior to parenteral administration to minimize such risks.

Particulate matter may contaminate a wide range of drugs, vehicles, or parenteral fluids [27]. Particles greater than 7 μm in diameter are more threatening than those smaller, because they may occlude the pulmonary capillaries (which are about 7 μm in diameter), resulting in multiple pulmonary infarctions. Also, the infusion of large quantities of particulate matter has been associated with an increased incidence of phlebitis. The composition of such particles has ranged from glass to rubber, fibers, crystals, and even to pieces of insects. Occasionally, in the past, such particles have consisted of asbestos, a known carcinogen [28].

Physicochemical properties of the drug injection, such as pH and osmotic pressure, may cause potentially damaging results on tissues at injection sites, especially if the injectable product possesses a highly acidic or alkaline pH and/or a solution of hypo- or hyperosmolality [29].

Drug incompatibilities may result in loss of biologic activity when such an effect may be critically needed, in unexpected adverse side effects, in a precipitate being formed which when infused might aggregate platelets, in anaphylactoid reactions resulting in shock, and/or in multiple, minute, pulmonary infarctions. A variety of texts or reference sources contain listings of many of the incompatibilities that might occur.

Hypersensitivity reactions may be associated with almost any drug. These reactions, which always follow previous exposure to the agents, are to be distinguished from drug intolerance and idiosyncrasies. Hypersensitivity reactions are divided into immediate and delayed, the former being associated with a "wheal-and-flare" skin lesion (urticaria), anaphylaxis, and/or an Arthus reaction (e.g., serum sickness), while the latter results in a tuberculin-type reaction. A drug reaction may mimic sepsis, and fever commonly develops. Generalized anaphylaxis is the most feared reaction and must be dealt with promptly. This condition follows parenteral administration of a drug much more commonly than it follows oral administration. The initial signs and symptoms are pruritis, hyperemia of the skin, angioedema, nausea, vomiting, vascular collapse, and shock. Fortunately, this type of reaction is infrequent.

Overdosage of drug and fluid overload are ever-present threats from intravenous administration, but they can be prevented if careful attention is paid to management. When a drug is injected by the parenteral route, it should be appreciated that it cannot be easily retrieved or neutralized before serious damage occurs. Fluid overload carries with it the possible consequences of heart failure and pulmonary edema. Often, when patients require prolonged fluid administration, pulmonary capillary wedge or central venous pressures are monitored to ensure against such complications developing.

Air emboli result principally from intravenous infusions, particularly if perfusion pumps are inserted into the system to ensure delivery. Small amounts of air are not harmful; however, as little as 10 ml may be fatal. Such emboli produce their most serious consequences when they enter and occlude the cerebral or coronary arteries. Care should be taken to purge all air bubbles from the syringe or intravenous line prior to starting an infusion and to ensure that the system utilized remains airtight throughout therapy. The following measures may be taken to reduce the risk of this complication or its consequences: (1) discontinue the infusion before the tubing is empty; (2) make sure that all attachments fit tightly; (3) be careful to clamp off the first bottle to empty in a Y-type setup; (4) the extremity receiving the infusion should not be elevated above the heart (thus creating negative venous pressure); and (5) permitting the infusing tubing to drop below the level of the extremity if emptying occurs unobserved. If air embolism occurs, the patient is placed on the left side with the head down and oxygen is made available.

Fever and toxicity may result from sterile abscesses produced from intramuscular injections, from injection of a poorly soluble drug, from pyrogenic material injected or infused, from the presence of contaminating endotoxin (which is pyrogenic), or from a hypersensitivity reaction (a reaction of the host) to the agent injected.

Infiltration or extravasation may occur with the administration of any infusion. Infiltration is the infusion or injection of a substance into a tissue, usually unintentionally when applied to parenteral administration; extravasation is the leakage of a substance or body fluid (e.g., blood) from a compartment (usually vessel) into surrounding tissues or spaces. The severity or the consequences resulting from either will usually depend on the reaction of the host to the particular drug or fluid infiltrating or extravasating, to the volume of infiltrating or extravasating fluid, and to the direct toxic effect of the infiltrated substance(s) on the host tissue(s). Hypertonic dextrose, solutions with pH differences from that of the body, and potassium solutions may cause considerable pain if extravasation occurs. Complications, such as infection, phlebitis, thrombosis, or necrosis of the infiltrated tissue, may ensue after any infiltration.

The cost of parenteral administration is greater than that of drug administration by other routes. The strict purity, sterility, and quality requirements enforced for parenteral solutes and solvents; the special packaging requirements (e.g., Type I glass); the special environmental conditions required for manufacturing parenterals; and the extra manufacturing processes and quality control that are required, such as filtration, sterilization, sterility, and pyrogen testing, all contribute to the added costs of parenteral dosage forms. Additionally, administration devices, such as catheters, tubings, and pumps, and the skilled personnel required to administer parenterals correctly, continuously, and safely add to the cost.

B. Specific Hazards or Complications

Specific hazards or complications are too numerous and varied to be enumerated
or discussed in detail in this chapter. They are unique or peculiar to the agents or
drugs injected or infused, and they may consist of anything from obvious adverse
side effects idiosyncratic to the agent administered (e.g., thrombocytopenia, anemia,
or neutropenia), to immunosuppression (cell mediated or humoral or both), to arrhythmias (which might occur only when the drug is injected parenterally), or to
pain (which usually occurs locally and may be worse with some drugs than with
others). An array of problems unique to parenteral feeding (hyperalimentation)
are reported, varying with the different fluid formulas used and with the basic
caloric source utilized (lipid emulsion versus amino acids and glucose). The practicing physician or pharmacist engaged in administering drugs or fluids by the parenteral route should consult appropriate texts [30,31], package inserts, and the
manufacturer for detailed information concerning specific complications. In addition, the American College of Physicians, the United States Pharmacopeia, and the
Food and Drug Administration encourage the reporting of such complications and
maintain records in this regard.

VI. METHODS AND DEVICES FOR AIDING IN
     DRUG DELIVERY

New methods of parenteral drug delivery and a wide variety of devices aiding in
such delivery are being developed and utilized daily in the care of patients in today's
modern hospital, especially in the intensive care areas [32]. Such items include
pumps (both implanted and external), cannulas and catheters, syringes (both disposable and reusable), intravenous final filters, pressure gauging devices, heparin
locks, stopcocks of all sorts, "piggybacks," Y connectors, flow controllers, guide
wires for catheter placement, and reservoirs, to name a few. Since parenteral
medications and body fluids or cavities frequently come into intimate contact with
most of these items, they and their methods of use must be free of contaminating
microorganisms, contaminants, or harmful substances (which may leach out); free
of pyrogens and particulate matter; designed in such a way as to possess no inherent
risks; and utilized with considerable expertise and respect. Since new methods of
delivery and imaginative devices employed in parenteral drug administration are
being developed at an almost exponential rate and are beyond the scope of a thorough analysis by this text, only a few of them will be discussed, and those only
briefly.

     Pumps. When extremely accurate intravenous drug administration is demanded,
pumps may be inserted into the delivery system to provide constant flow rates.
Such demands are commonly seen in parenteral feeding (hyperalimentation) and in
pediatric cases where minute volumes must be carefully administered. However,
pumps are not without problems: for example, air embolism, leaky lines and clot-
ted catheters, intrinsic contamination, alarm failure, fluid overload, electrical
shorts, and complexity of operation, to name a few.
     For external (as distinguished from implanted) pumps, two major types are
employed: piston-cylinder and peristaltic, with the latter subclassified into rotary
and linear. A wide variety of these pumps are available from a variety of manufacturers.

More recently and still very much in the experimental stages are implanted infusion pumps. These appear to be extremely promising, particularly for providing continuous flow with absolute precision, such as in the administration of insulin. With this technique, the self-administration of drugs such as insulin is no longer required. Complications appear to be few, but perhaps the major ones are infection around the pump and pump failure.

Controllers. These devices control the flow of fluid by counting the drops electrically. They are frequently used in intravenous therapy that requires sophisticated monitoring. They work on gravitational principles, add no pressure to the line (since they are not pumps), and are not difficult to manage. Their drop-rate accuracy is about ±2%. They are without the many problems that pumps possess.

Intravenous Retrograde Administration. The retrograde technique eliminates the time-consuming flushing process required in "piggyback" delivery and the need to reset the rate of flow of an intravenous maintenance solution [33]. To an infant additional fluid required to flush out a drug given by piggyback may be enough to upset the fluid balance. With the retrograde technique, a threeway stopcock is attached to both ends of a piece of coiled tubing inserted into the administration system. When medication is infused into the stopcock proximal to the patient, the solution will flow retrograde (away from the patient) into the coil, forcing the ejection of an equal volume of maintenance solution into an empty syringe attached to the other stopcock. The net result is no alteration in the total volume of fluid administered to the patient.

Cannulas and Catheters. A wide variety of cannulas and catheters are available to suit all forms of parenteral therapy; from simple intravenous needles or catheters to complex Swanz-Ganz catheters threaded into the pulmonary capillary bed and left there as a hemodynamic monitoring device. Needles are the most frequently employed of these items; however, in intensive care services, indwelling catheters are heavily relied upon for intravenous therapy.

Needles are made of stainless steel and come in a variety of bore sizes (see Table 1) and lengths, depending on the use intended. The tips are angular and are from beveled to blunted, depending on the intended use. Most needles are disposable, however, those of a more complex nature are generally reusable. For infants, scalp vein needles, often with wing tips ("butterflies") and short attached catheters, are employed. The wing tips are especially valuable in anchoring the needle, which is generally inserted into a tiny scalp vein. Plastic indwelling catheters eliminate the need for repeated intravenous punctures. They also provide a means for continual infusion into an area difficult to reach (e.g., the brain) and in situations that may require continuous, chronic therapy (see Fig. 6). Catheters used for intravenous therapy are made of polyvinyl chloride, Teflon®, or polyethylene and are generally radiopaque, so that they will be visible on x-ray. The major problem with catheters is infection, and those that remain indwelling and pass through the skin may become infected within several days. The longer the catheter remains in place, the greater the risk of infection. Other problems, such as knotting and "break-offs," have been recorded and can be detected by x-ray.

Heparin Locks. These devices are being used with increasing frequency because they permit the patient to move about in the hospital (even go home), and they can be used to remove blood for tests. They consist of a scalp vein infusion device capped by a resealable latex diaphragm. Small amounts of heparin have to be placed in the lock to maintain patency. Perhaps one of the major problems with heparin locks is the incompatibility of heparin with a variety of medications. Thus, before each injection a small amount of sterile sodium chloride has to be infused to flush out the heparin. In addition, attention must be paid to the quantity of heparin used, as concentrations of $\geqslant 1000$ units/ml may cause elevations in the activated partial thromboplastin time and thus coagulation problems.

Final Filters. These devices are either incorporated into the administration system when it is manufactured or are inserted into the line in the hospital setting. Their major value is in removing particulate matter and possibly preventing sepsis. Some believe that they may reduce thrombophlebitis. The pore size utilized is generally 0.45 μm; however, in order to exclude bacteria thoroughly, 0.22 μm must be employed.

A number of problems may be identified with these devices, and their practical value (especially in cost-effectiveness) is not convincingly established. Lines are reported to leak when filters clog up, air locks may be a problem, a question of drug adherence to the filter in some instances still has to be worked out, and sterilization of still another item in the system must be ensured.

In summary, a wide variety of devices and new methods of drug delivery are being employed. Each has its advantages and disadvantages, which have to be carefully weighed by the therapist. In the area of parenteral drug administration, those directly responsible for drug or fluid delivery must not only be knowledgeable about specific therapeutics and pharmacologic advantages of the agents being administered, but must also be aware of many aspects of engineering, physicochemical properties, sterility, and cost-effectiveness of the devices or methods used.

REFERENCES

1. Greenblatt, D. J., and Koch-Weser, J., N. Engl. J. Med., 295:542–546 (1976).
2. Brandt, P. A., Smith, M. E., Ashburn, S. S., and Graves, J., Am. J. Nurs., 72:1402–1406 (1972).
3. Hook, R. V., and Vandevelde, A. G., Ann. Intern. Med., 83:669–670 (1975).
4. Laforce, F. M., Young, L. S., and Bennett, J. V., N. Engl. J. Med., 280: 569–574 (1969).
5. Evans, E. F., Proctor, J. D., Fratkin, M. J., Velandia, J., and Wasserman, A. J., Clin. Pharmacol. Ther., 17:44–47 (1975).
6. Maki, D. G., Goldman, D. A., and Rhame, F. S., Ann. Intern. Med., 79: 867–887 (1973).
7. Fuerst, E. V., Wolff, L. V., and Weitzel, M. H., Fundamentals of Nursing, 5th ed., J. B. Lippincott, Philadelphia, 1974, pp. 343–344.
8. Karanicolas, S., Oreopoulos, D. G., Izatt, Sh., Shimizu, A., Manning, R. F., Sepp, H., deVeber, G. A., and Darby, T., N. Engl. J. Med., 296:1336–1337 (1977).
9. Oreopoulos, D. G., in Strategy in Renal Failure (E. A. Friedman, ed.), Wiley, New York, 1978, Chap. 19.
10. Steinbrocker, O., and Neustadt, D. H., in Arthritis and Musculoskeletal Disorders, Harper & Row, Hagerstown, Md., 1972, pp. 1–14.
11. Hollander, J. L., in Arthritis and Allied Conditions, 7th ed., Lea & Febiger, Philadelphia, 1966, p. 381.

12. Hurley, H. J., Jr., in Dermatology (Moschella, S. L., Pillsbury, D. M., and Hurley, H. J., Jr., eds), Vol. II, Saunders, Philadelphia, 1975, pp. 1608-1640.

13. Allinson, R. R., and Stach, P. E., Drug. Intell. Clin. Pharm., 12:347-359 (1978).

14. Cradock, J. C., Kleinman, L. M., and Davignon, J. P., Bull. Parenter. Drug. Assoc., 31:237-247 (1977).

15. Ratcheson, R. A., and Ommaya, A. K., N. Engl. J. Med., 279:1025-1031 (1968).

16. Benet, L. Z., in Modern Pharmaceutics (G. S. Banker and C. T. Rhodes, eds.), Marcel Dekker, New York, 1979, pp. 183-210.

17. Daisy, J. A., Abrutyn, E. A., and MacGregor, R. R., Ann. Intern. Med., 91:563-565 (1979).

18. Stolar, M. H., Am. J. Hosp. Pharm., 33:225-230 (1976).

19. Saunders, L. H., Mabadeje, S. A., Avis, K. E., Cruze, C. A., III, and Martinez, D. R., Am. J. Hosp. Pharm., 35:531-536 (1978).

20. Joynson, D. H. M., Howells, C. H. L., and Liddington, R., J. Hyg. Camb., 75:87-91 (1975).

21. Davis, A. T., Nadler, H. L., Brown, M. C., Brolnitsky, O., and Francis, B. J., Morb. Mortal. Wkly. Rep., 25:110-115 (1976).

22. Plouffe, J. F., Brown, D. G., Silva, J., Jr., Eck, T., Stricof, R. L., and Fekety, F. R., Jr., Arch. Intern. Med., 137:1686-1689 (1977).

23. Wilmore, D. W., and Dudrick, S. J., Arch. Surg., 99:462-463 (1969).

24. Kellaway, C. H., Burnet, F. M., and Williams, F. E., J. Pathol. Bacteriol., 33:889-912 (1930).

25. Bivins, B. A., Rapp, R. P., DeLuca, P. P., McKean, H., and Griffen, W. O., Jr., Surgery, 85:388-394 (1979).

26. Costentino, F., Bull. Parenter. Drug Assoc., 31:288 (1977).

27. Davis, N. M., Turco, S., and Sively, E., Am. J. Hosp. Pharm., 27:822-826 (1970).

28. Nicholson, W. J., Maggiore, C. J., and Selikoff, I. J., Science, 177:171-173 (1972).

29. Oshida, S., Degawa, K., Takahashi, Y., and Akaishi, S., Tahoku J. Exp. Med., 127:301-316 (1979).

30. Goodman, L. S., and Gilman, A., in The Pharmacological Basis of Therapeutics, 6th ed. (A. G. Gilman, L. S. Goodman, and A. Gilman, eds.), Macmillan, New York, 1980.

31. Physicians' Desk Reference, 36th ed., Medical Economics Company, Oradell, N.J., 1982.

32. Turco, S., and King, R. E., Sterile Dosage Forms, 2nd ed., Lea & Febiger, Philadelphia, 1979, pp. 333-355.

33. Benzine, G., III, and Loggie, J., Pediatrics, 52:420-425 (1973).

3

Biopharmaceutics of Injectable Medication

SOL MOTOLA*

Schering Corporation
Bloomfield, New Jersey

Biopharmaceutics is the subject in pharmaceutical sciences which examines the influence of physicochemical changes in drug and/or formulation design on the absorption of drugs. Over the last two decades this area of research has emerged as one of the most influential factors in guiding the development of pharmaceutical dosage forms. As a result there has been a rapid increase in the number of scientific publications and textbooks on this subject. Pharmacy schools throughout the world now include biopharmaceutics in both undergraduate and graduate programs. Moreover, practically every new drug product introduced during this period has been designed based on biopharmaceutical data.

To date, most biopharmaceutical investigations have been in support of orally administered dosage forms since they are the predominant ones used in current therapy. Although there have been a significant number of studies reported on the rates of absorption, distribution, metabolism, and excretion of parenterally administered drugs, only a few have been designed to elucidate which properties of the injection formulation or injection site influence these rates. The Danish pharmacologist Schou was one of the first to study extensively the physiological factors that influence the absorption of drugs from subcutaneous connective tissue. In a 1961 review article [1], he described, from a pharmacological viewpoint, how the rate of absorption of subcutaneously administered hormones and drugs could be altered depending on the effect the injection had on the physiological condition of the connective tissues, the capillary membrane, and the capillary blood flow at the subcutaneous site.

During the same year, Wagner [2] reviewed the literature comprising the discipline that had just been coined biopharmaceutics by Gerhard Levy. He reviewed important physicochemical factors influencing drug absorption from various modes of administration. Besides correctly predicting the important role this discipline would serve in the future of pharmacy, he suggested many of the areas for study that have influenced biopharmaceutical investigations of injectable dosage forms.

Ballard applied this information to research on intramuscular injections and, from a pharmaceutical viewpoint, published an influential review article dealing with biopharmaceutical factors influencing intramuscular and subcutaneous

*
Present affiliation: Merck Frosst Canada, Inc., Pointe Claire-Dorval, Quebec, Canada.

injections [3]. Although interest continues in this area of research, as noted by periodic reviews [4-7], relatively little new basic information has been uncovered, leaving room for more in-depth studies.

Not long ago, drugs administered by injection were assumed to provide rapid and complete absorption, particularly when compared to oral administration. During the last 20 years, this assumption has been shown not always to be true. These findings [8-13], coupled with more numerous examples of incomplete absorption from oral dosage forms, have stimulated research on (1) drug absorption and how it is affected by the design of the dosage form (biopharmaceutics), (2) the extent to which drugs are biologically available to the bloodstream relative to the amount administered (bioavailability), and (3) the rates and extents to which drugs are absorbed, distributed, metabolized, and excreted by the body (pharmacokinetics).

The aim of this chapter is to provide the formulator of injectable medication with a basic understanding of the major physicochemical and physiological factors currently considered to play an important role in influencing absorption of drugs administered by injection. Selected topics in pharmacokinetics will be covered primarily to demonstrate their utility in the analysis of biopharmaceutical experiments. The overall goal is for the formulator to be able to apply this knowledge in designing injectable dosage formulations that will provide predictable drug delivery to the patient.

I. PHYSICOCHEMICAL AND PHYSIOLOGICAL FACTORS AFFECTING DRUG ABSORPTION BY INJECTION: AN OVERVIEW

An intravascular (intraveneous) injection places a drug directly into the bloodstream, bypassing conventional physicochemical and physiological influences. Injection of a drug into an extravascular site (all others) leads to the initiation of events that collectively make up the absorption process. Depending on the type of formulation administered, varying degrees of a depot are established. Eventual drug absorption into the bloodstream is influenced by several physicochemical and physiological factors, the two considered most important being passive diffusion and blood flow [14-16]. The relative importance of these factors depends on the capillary bed density at the injection site, the physical form of the drug, and the drug's molecular size. Hence an examination of these and other influential physicochemical and physiological factors is important in providing the pharmaceutical formulator with information that can be used to design formulations yielding acceptable absorption characteristics.

A. Physicochemical Factors Affecting Drug Absorption By Injection

As stated, no absorption step is necessary when a drug is adminstered directly into the bloodstream; therefore, there are no physicochemical factors to affect absorption. Drugs given by extravascular injection require an absorption step before they can enter the bloodstream. Even drugs that are administered by the intraspinal (intrathecal) and intracardiac routes and are in very close proximity to the bloodstream must first undergo local penetration and permeation and then penetrate local capillaries in order to reach the bloodstream. At other extravascular sites, such as intramuscular, subcutaneous, and intradermal, the drug is exposed to a relatively small localized region. From such regions, the drug travels to the blood or lymphatic circulation (only for high-molecular-weight molecules) by means of physical penetration and permeation processes which are associated with passive diffusion and partitioning through the capillary membrane and into the bloodstream.

1. Drug Solubility

A major physicochemical criterion for absorption by passive diffusion and partitioning is drug solubility. Regardless of the dosage form administered, a drug must be in solution in an aqueous system for it to be exposed to processes that will eventually result in its absorption into the bloodstream. Only the fraction of drug in solution is available for absorption. Drugs that remain in solution at the injection site are generally absorbed quickly and easily, all other influencing factors being constant.

A critical difference between the pH of the administered drug solution and the physiological pH at the injection site (and/or solubility of the drug in a cosolvent vehicle and in physiological tissue fluid) can cause an unpredicted decrease in absorption due to precipitation of the drug at the injection site. Phenytoin, a commercial brand of diphenylhydantoin, is a very insoluble free acid and is formulated as the sodium salt in a solution of 40% propylene glycol, 10% alcohol, and Water for Injection. The pH must be adjusted to pH 12 with sodium hydroxide to solubilize the drug. The propylene glycol helps to solubilize the free acid fraction available at this pH. When injected into muscle tissue the large difference in pH causes conversion of the sodium salt to the less soluble free acid which precipitates in tissue fluids at the injection site. Simultaneous dilution of the propylene glycol with tissue fluid contributes to free acid precipitation. Most of the drug is therefore available only slowly, depending predominantly on the dissolution rate of diphenylhydantoin crystals. Thus complete absorption takes 4 to 5 days [10]. Similar reductions in bioavailability due to drug precipitation casued by pH and solubility changes have been reported for Diazepam Injection [11], Chlordiazepoxide Injection [12], and Digoxin Injection [13].

2. Passive Diffusion

Passive diffusion involves the spontaneous movement of solute molecules in solution from an area of higher concentration on one side of a semipermeable membrane to an area of lower concentration on the other side of the membrane. In the biological system, a drug in solution passes from the extracellular to the intracellular tissue fluids by passive diffusion.

The rate of passage of a drug through a biological membrane by passive diffusion is affected by several physicochemical factors, such as concentration gradient, partition coefficient, ionization, macromolecular binding, and osmolality, in addition to differences in physical form of the medication.

Concentration Gradient. The rate at which a drug molecule crosses a semipermeable membrane by passive diffusion is described by Fick's law, expressed by the following equation for the unidirectional case:

$$\frac{dq}{dt} = \frac{DA(C_1 - C_2)}{\ell} \tag{1}$$

where

$\frac{dq}{dt}$ = Flux or amount of transfer of substance per unit of time

D = diffusion constant

A = surface area available for diffusion

C_1 = concentration of diffusing substance in extracellular fluid

C_2 = concentration of diffusate in the intracellular fluid

ℓ = thickness of the membrane

For any particular membrane where A and ℓ are constant, the diffusion rate is controlled by $D(C_1 - C_2)$. The magnitude of the diffusion constant D is influenced by the physicochemical properties of the drug molecule and the characteristics of the membrane.

For any given drug in a contained in vitro system, the rate of passive diffusion is controlled by the concentration gradient $(C_1 - C_2)$ which exists between both sides of the membrane. The rate at which drug molecules move from side 1 to side 2 will decrease as the magnitude of C_2 decreases and approaches C_1. When C_1 equals C_2 the system is at equilibrium. This is described mathematically as follows:

$$\frac{dq}{dt} = \frac{D(C_1 - C_2)}{\ell} \tag{2}$$

When $C_1 = C_2$,

$$\frac{dq}{dt} = 0 \tag{3}$$

However, the concentration gradient $(C_1 - C_2)$ does not become a rate-limiting factor in vivo because of unidirectional movement of the drug through the membrane. In this case, as the drug reaches the other side of the membrane it is removed by the blood, leading to distribution, metabolism, and/or excretion. Therefore, C_1 remains considerably greater than C_2 at all times until the transfer is complete. This is referred to as a "sink" condition and Equation (2) reduces to

$$\frac{dq}{dt} = \frac{DC_1}{\ell} \tag{4}$$

Partition Coefficient The distribution of a solute between an aqueous environment and a lipid membrane is analogous to the distribution of a solute between two immiscible solvents such as water and oil. This type of distribution, called partitioning, plays an important role in passive diffusion. The equation that describes partitioning is:

$$\text{Partition coefficient (PC)} = K = \frac{c_a}{c_b} \tag{5}$$

where, by convention,

c_a = concentration of solute in the oil or lipid phase

c_b = concentration of nonionized solute in the aqueous phase at a defined pH

K = partition coefficient

The influence of the partition coefficient on passive diffusion of a drug through a biological membrane can be illustrated by considering the relative transfer of drugs with high and low partition coefficients. A drug with a high partition coefficient (lipid soluble) will pass readily from the aqueous phase into the membrane, whereas one with a low partition coefficient (water soluble) will remain in the aqueous phase and not pass appreciably into the membrane. As stated earlier, in a biological system, diffusion takes place as a unidirectional process; this is equally true for the process of partitioning. The drug with a higher partition coefficient will exhibit a higher rate of diffusion, dq/dt. Thus lipid-soluble drugs are absorbed and distributed more rapidly than are water-soluble drugs.

Ionization   Whereas partitioning of neutral molecules takes place in relation to their oil-water solubility, this is not true for ionized drugs. Ionization has a profound effect on drug absorption, distribution, and excretion. The degree of ionization of an acid or base is determined by the ionization constant of the compound, pK_a, in addition to the pH, temperature, and ionic strength of the solution. Since in a biological system temperature and ionic strength are essentially constant, their influence can be neglected.

The relationship between pH and pK_a can be readily seen by the following derivation. In water, a weak acid, HA, ionizes (or dissociates) according to the following equation:

$$HA + H_2O \rightleftharpoons H_3O^+ + A^- \tag{6}$$

The equilibrium constant for the reaction is written conventionally as

$$K_{eq} = \frac{[H_3O^+][A^-]}{[HA][H_2O]} \tag{7}$$

Since the molar concentration of water (55.3 mol liter^{-1} at 25°C) is much larger than any of the other values and remains essentially constant during the reaction, one can write

$$K_{eq}[H_2O] = K_{ion} = \frac{[H_3O^+][A^-]}{[HA]} \tag{8}$$

Taking the logarithm of both sides of Equation (8) and transposing log K_{ion} and log $[H_3O^+]$ to opposite sides yields

$$-\log[H_3O^+] = -\log K_{ion} + \log \frac{[A-]}{[HA]} \tag{9}$$

By employing conventional definitions for pH and pK_a, Equation (9) becomes

$$pH = pK_a + \log \frac{[A-]}{[HA]} \tag{10}$$

Equation (10), known as the Henderson-Hasselbach equation, is very useful in predicting the ionization properties of weak acids and bases, particularly with respect to their ability to partition into lipids.

A similar equation describes the ionization of a weak base, but by convention, the reaction is written as the ionization of the protonated weak base, BH^+:

$$BH^+ + OH^- \rightleftharpoons B + H_2O \tag{11}$$

yielding

$$pH = pK'_a + \log \frac{[B]}{[BH^+]} \tag{12}$$

where the symbol pK'_a designates the ionization of the protonated base.

Several obvious but important relationships between pH and pK_a can be seen through inspection of Equation (10), particularly as they affect partitioning:

1. When the concentration of acid [HA] equals the concentration of the anion $[A^-]$ in a solution of a weak acid, the ratio $[A^-]/[HA] = 1$. Since $\log 1 = 0$, $pH = pK_a$.

2. The degree of ionization of weak acids and bases changes rapidly as the difference between pH and pK_a becomes greater until the pH value of the solution is 2 units away from pK_a, at which time further changes in pH have little effect on the degree of ionization of the acid or base. This concept can be easily demonstrated by rearranging Equation (10) to the form

$$pH - pK_a = \log \frac{[A^-]}{[HA]} \tag{13}$$

and examining the difference in the ratio $\log [A^-]/[HA]$ as the difference, $pH - pK_a$, goes through changes from 2 to 0.01 as shown below:

$pH - pK_a = \log \frac{[A^-]}{[HA]} =$	2	1	0	0.1	0.01
Ionized form $[A^-]$ =	100	10	1	1	1
Nonionized form [HA] =	1	1	1	10	100

Therefore, if there were a 3 unit difference between pH and pK_a one would only see less than a 1% further change in ionization.

3. When dealing with ionized and nonionized forms of a drug, the relationship to lipid solubility and partition coefficient becomes apparent. The neutral (nonionized) fraction of the drug is more readily partitioned into the nonpolar lipid membrane. During partitioning of the nonionized molecule the fraction of remaining ionized drug rapidly equilibrates so that nonionized drug is again formed and available for partitioning. This dynamic process takes place until the entire drug partitions through the membrane.

When the pH of a medium causes most of the drug to be in the ionized form (e.g., medium pH = 7 for an acidic drug with pK_a = 5), slow absorption can be expected since the partitionable nonionized form constitutes only a small fraction of the total drug, less than 1% in the case above.

A rank order demonstration of the effect of medium pH and drug pK_a on partitioning is shown by the following hypothetical example. A beaker containing a buffer

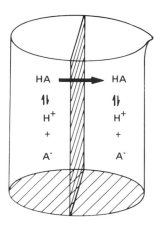

Figure 1 Beaker containing buffer solution in which a semipermeable lipid membrane separates the solution into two compartments. Weak acid HA placed in the left side equilibrates according to Equation (6), allowing only HA to partition through the membrane.

solution is separated equally into two compartments by a semipermeable lipid membrane (see Fig. 1) which allows only the nonionized weak acid (pK_a = 5) to pass through. A quantity of the weak acid drug is dissolved in a negligible volume of buffer solution; the solution is then quickly injected into the left compartment, resulting in a homogeneous solution in that compartment.

After each equilibrium partitioning step takes place (i.e., HA partitions through the membrane, leaving A^- and H^+ behind), the buffer solution on the right side of the membrane (side becoming enriched with HA) is replaced with fresh buffer. The species A^- on the left side reequilibrates with H^+ to form more HA and the process is repeated until eventually all the drug is partitioned as HA.

Referring to the Henderson-Hasselbach equation [Eq. (10)], consider the following two cases, which will demonstrate the effect of pH and pK_a on partitioning.

Case 1: Buffer solution on both sides of the membrane at pH 5. In this case Equation (10) indicate that log $[A^-]/[HA]$ = 1; thus $[A^-]$ = $[HA]$.

Thus 50% of the total weak acid is in the neutral form HA, able to partition through the membrane. The remaining ionized portion, A^-, is unable to partition into lipid.

The hypothetical profile for the system, based on the percent of HA remaining in the left compartment versus the number of equilibrations and buffer solution replacements of the right compartment, is shown in Figure 2. At pH 5 following four equilibrations, only 6% A^- remains in the left compartment (approximately 94% of HA has partitioned).

Case 2: Buffer solution in both compartments at pH 7. Equation (10) now indicates that log $[A^-]/[HA]$ = 100. Substituting these values into Equation (10) yields

$$7 = 5 + \log \frac{100}{1}$$

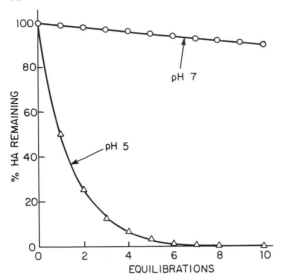

Figure 2 Hypothetical case of comparative partitioning versus number of equilibrations for weak acid HA (pK$_a$ 5), partitioning through a lipid membrane from buffer solutions at pH 5 ($\triangle$) and pH 7 (O).

Therefore, only 0.99 of the total drug, HA + A$^-$, is in the form HA, able to be partitioned.

The hypothetical profile for this system under the conditions stated is shown in Figure 2. In this case at pH 7, after four equilibrations 96% HA remains in the left compartment and only 4% has been able to partition through the membrane. Since 0.99% of the amount of HA present can partition during each equilibration, one can calculate that it would take 95 equilibrations (i.e., 94/0.99) to partition the same amount of HA as was partitioned by four equilibrations at pH 5 in case 1.

These examples are meant to show the relationsip between formulation pH, drug pK$_a'$, and the amounts of partitionable nonionized weak acid or weak base species available for absorption from an injectable solution dosage form.

Binding to Macromolecules Biological fluids contain macromolecules such as proteins which may have affinity for certain drugs. These macromolecules are generally too large to pass through biological membranes by filtration, nor do they have the lipid solubility required for passive diffusion. Therefore, they are confined within their immediate boundaries. When a drug becomes adsorbed or complexed on such macromolecules, its effective "free" concentration of diffusable form becomes lowered. The equation describing this reaction is

$$\text{Drug} + \text{macromolecule} \underset{k_2}{\overset{k_1}{\rightleftharpoons}} \text{drug} - \text{macromolecule complex} \qquad (14)$$

where

$\quad$ k$_1$ = adsorption rate constant

$\quad$ k$_2$ = desorption rate constant

The equilibrium constant is then expressed as

$$K = \frac{[\text{drug - macromolecule}]}{[\text{drug}][\text{macromolecule}]} \tag{15}$$

where K, the association constant, provides a quantitative measure of the affinity of the drug for the particular macromolecule. Significant binding to macromolecules such as serum protein reduces the concentration of free drug in the tissue fluids and hence reduces the rate of passive diffusion by lowering the concentration gradient in accordance with Fick's law [Eq. (1)]. Since binding is an equilibrium process and thus readily reversible, the drug can eventually be desorbed. It is important to note that protein binding reduces the rate of passive diffusion but does not prevent it. Protein binding has a significant effect on passive diffusion when the drug is bound by more than 90% because the desorption rate from the drug–protein complex is usually slower than the diffusion rate of the drug through membranes.

Osmolality   A solution is isoosmotic with tissue fluid when the total number of dissolved particles in the two systems are equal. In general, injectable products are formulated to be isoosmotic to reduce the possibility of irritation that can result if osmotic differences between tissue fluid or red blood cell contents and the injection product are great. The effect of large differences in solution osmolality on passive diffusion can be described by considering the following conditions: (1) hypoosmotic, (2) isoosmotic, and (3) hyperosmotic. When an injection solution is hypoosmotic, it contains fewer solute particles than does the tissue fluid. Based on the law of osmosis, solvent passes from a region of lower concentration of solute to one of higher concentration to reduce the pressure differential caused by the dissolved solute particle imbalance.

Therefore, the extravascular injection of a grossly hypoosmotic solution would cause the movement of fluid away from the repository injection site. In this case, the apparent concentration of drug would increase, resulting in an increase in rate of passive diffusion. Conversely, the extravascular injection of a grossly hyperosmotic solution causes an influx of fluid to the repository injection site, resulting in dilution of drug concentration and an apparent decrease in rate of diffusion. Increasing the osmolality of atropine solutions by the addition of either prolidoxine chloride or sodium chloride led to an apparent reduction in intramuscular absorption, determined by its effect on reduction of heart rate [17]. When an isoosmotic solution is injected, there is no fluid flux either to or away from the injection site, hence no demonstrable effect on passive diffusion.

It is important to differentiate between the terms isotonic and isoosmotic. They are synonymous only when the dissolved solute cannot pass through membranes of red blood cells. However, when such passage does occur, as with aqueous solutions of urea, alcohol, or boric acid, the solution acts as if it were pure water and both solute and solvent pass through the membrane into the red blood cells, causing them to swell and burst (hemolysis). The solution was considered isotonic based on sodium chloride equivalent calculations or as determined by its freezing-point depression; however, it was actually hypotonic or hypoosmotic with respect to red blood cells. The term isotonic should be used only to describe solutions having equal osmotic pressures with respect to a particular membrane. Therefore, it is important to examine the osmotic behavior of new drug substances toward red blood cells before deciding whether an adjustment is to be made. In order to make an isoosmotic aqueous solution of a nonosmotic contributing substance such as urea, an external agent such as sodium chloride, sorbitol, or other osmotic-producing substance must be added at its isotonic level, such as 0.9% sodium chloride.

Volume of Injection From Fick's law, for the sink condition ($C_2 = 0$) it was shown by Equation (4) that $dq/dt = KC_1$. When the volume V_1 of drug solution at the absorption site remains nearly constant, the rate of passive diffusion will be equal to:

$$\frac{dq}{dt} = K\frac{A_1}{V_1} \tag{16}$$

where A_1 is the amount of drug at the site at any time. Thus the diffusion rate is inversely proportional to volume V_1, and absorption rates should increase when volumes decrease [3]. Smaller injected volumes have been reported to enhance drug absorption [18]. Another way of expressing this is to consider the ratio of tissue surface area to volume of injection. An increase in injection volume with a relatively confined area results in a lowering of the tissue surface area-to-volume ratio. Since passive diffusion is directly proportional to surface area, an increase in injection volume should cause a lowering in the rate of passive diffusion. A physiological reason to keep injection volumes small is to help minimize or reduce pain caused by hydrostatic pressure on surrounding tissues.

Differences in Physical Form of Medication Dealing with the premise that the rate of release of a drug from a dosage form is the limiting factor, one can rank the various physical types of injectable dosage forms in order of decreasing rate of drug release following extravascular injection as follows:

Aqueous solution   Fastest release
Aqueous suspension
Oleaginous solution
Oil-in-water emulsion
Water-in-oil emulsion
Oleaginous suspension   Slowest release

Various steps are required before the drug can be released from these dosage forms to surrounding tissue fluids for absorption. The particular steps involved and the speed with which they occur account for the differences in absorption rates. Properly formulated aqueous solutions, which remain in solution in tissue fluid, exhibit the most rapid absorption of drug since no release step is necessary. An examination of physicochemical factors governing drug release from the other dosage formulations listed is important to the formulator.

Aqueous Suspension. This dosage form is the second most commonly administered injectable dosage form, following aqueous solutions. Release of drug from aqueous suspensions can be described as follows:

$$\textbf{DRUG} \xrightarrow{\textit{dissolution}} \textbf{DRUG} \xrightarrow[\textit{partitioning}]{\textit{diffusion}} \textbf{DRUG} \tag{17}$$

solid fine   *dissolved in*   *absorbed*

particles   *tissue fluid*

The rate-determining (slowest) step for the release of drugs from suspension is its dissolution in tissue fluid. The rate of solution of a drug in a fixed volume of liquid is governed by its equilibrium solubility, the surface area of the solid, and the rate of diffusion of solute away from the solid. A general equation expressing this relationship is:

$$\text{Rate of solution} = KS (C_s - C_t) \tag{18}$$

where

C_s = concentration of drug in a saturated solution

C_t = concentration of the solution at time t

S = surface area of the solid drug

K = constant made up of the diffusion constant for the drug in the solution and a rate constant for the transfer of drug to the bulk solution from the solid-liquid interface.

For a particular drug in a vehicle, C_s and K are constants, and therefore the rate of solution is proportional to the surface area of the solid and the concentration of the drug in solution. If the rate of solution is slower than the rate of diffusion, the rate of solution and rate of diffusion will be governed by the surface area of the solid. Thus the particle size of the solid will determine the absorption rate.

Oleaginous Solution. The major factor involved in release from this dosage form is partitioning from the oil phase to tissue fluid. The relatively slow rate of release from oleaginous solutions is attributable to the high oil-water partition coefficient of drugs dissolved in such vehicles and the relatively slow tissue fluid turnover rate.

$$\begin{array}{ccc} & \textit{partitioning} & & \textit{diffusion} & \\ \textbf{DRUG} & \xrightarrow{\hspace{1.5cm}} & \textbf{DRUG} & \xrightarrow{\hspace{1.5cm}} & \textbf{DRUG} \\ \textit{dissolved} & & \textit{dissolved in} & \textit{partitioning} & \textit{absorbed} \\ \textit{in oil} & & \textit{tissue fluid} & & \end{array} \tag{19}$$

Emulsion. A drug will be in the oil or water phase of an emulsion in relation to its solubility and partition coefficient. For acidic and basic drugs, the pH of the aqueous phase and the drug's pK_a value will determine the relative amounts in each phase. The rate of release of drug from oil-in-water and water-in-oil emulsions can be described as follows:

Oil-in-water emulsion. Drugs are generally dissolved in the dispersed oil phase to establish a prolonged release profile. In this case the following scheme can be written:

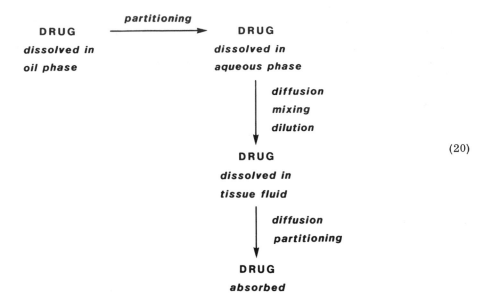

(20)

Drug is partitioned from the internal oil phase to the external aqueous phase, where it can easily pass to tissue fluid. Eventually, the aqueous phase becomes diluted with tissue fluid and the structure of the system breaks down to an oil solution system, previously described.

Water-in-oil emulsion. Assuming that the drug has been dissolved in the aqueous phase, the following scheme can be written:

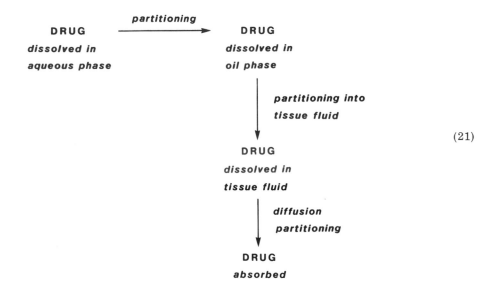

(21)

The partitioning of drug from the aqueous phase to the external oil phase and then to the surrounding tissue fluid will lead to a prolonged release profile for this type of formulation. Because the external phase is oil, little dilution takes place by tissue fluid and the physical nature of the injected liquid should remain intact for a longer time than with the oil-in-water emulsion.

Oleaginous Suspension. This dosage form, normally only administered intramuscularly, provides release of a medicament over periods from weeks to months. For a drug to be absorbed from an oleaginous suspension it must eventually make its way into the aqueous tissue fluid at the injection site. The rate-limiting step in the overall process is drug dissolution (as with aqueous suspensions) either into the oil phase or directly into tissue fluid, depending on its relative solubility. The latter contribution may be small due to the limited surface area of the oil phase brought about by the high surface tension difference between water and oil. Therefore, very little suspended drug is expected to be directly in contact with tissue fluid. The overall scheme for release of drug from an oleaginous suspension can be described as follows:

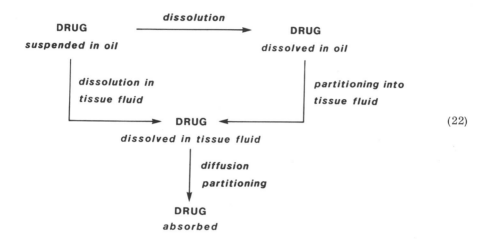

(22)

Contributing to the prolonged release nature of all the formulation types described is the slow movement of fluid through tissues and thus the slow turnover rate of tissue fluid required for the partitioning process.

B. Physiological Factors Affecting Drug Absorption by Injection

    1. Overview of the Circulatory System: Blood and Lymphatic
        Circulation

A simplified overview of the gross anatomy of the circulatory system, with reference to the major differences in blood vessels at the various sites of injection, is important when considering the environment under which physiological processes occur during the absorption of administered drugs. For a drug to exert its expected pharmacological activity, it must make its way into the complex circulatory system either by being administered intravenously or by undergoing absorption from an extravascular site. The drug is then distributed to the body tissues through capillary beds which eventually connect the arteriovenous system; after exerting its pharmacological effect it is eventually excreted and/or metabolized.

As depicted in the schematic diagram of the circulatory system shown in Figure 3, deoxygenated blood (solid lines) from the venous system enters the heart at the right atrium and passes to the right ventricle, from which it is pumped to the lungs. Oxygenated blood returns from the lungs into the left atrium and passes through the left ventricle, from which it is pumped into the aorta. The aorta branches into smaller arteries, which in turn branch into smaller arterioles and

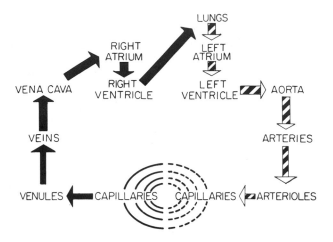

Figure 3 Schematic diagram of the circulatory system.

eventually into microscopic capillaries which exist to varying degrees in all tissues of the body. Once in the capillary bed, the process reverses and blood passes from the capillaries into the venules, which eventually lead to the venous system and ultimately to the vena cava, which empties blood to the right atrium where the loop is completed.

The major purpose of blood circulation is to provide oxygen, nutrients, and added medicaments to the tissues while removing carbon dioxide and other metabolic by-products. It is only through capillaries that this exchange occurs. Arteries and veins act as conduits to and from capillaries. A comparison of volume, rate, and pressure for the various sections of the arteriovenous system is shown in Table 1. This illustrates that capillaries carry only 250 ml or 7% of the blood at any time with a flow rate from 50 to 400 times slower than than of the aorta and vena cava, during which time blood pressure is undergoing a 50-fold decrease.

Table 1 Physical Characteristics of the Arteriovenous System

Anatomical section	Volume (cm^3)	Velocity ($cm\ sec^{-1}$)	Pressure (mmHg)
Aorta	100	40	100
Arteries	325	40–10	100–40
Arterioles	50	10–0.1	40–25
Capillaries	250	0.1	25–12
Venules	300	0.3	12–8
Veins	2200	0.3–5	10–5
Vena cava	300	5–30	2

Source: Adapted from Ref. 19.

The human circulatory system consists of approximately 3.6 billion capillaries with a total cross-sectional area of approximately 4500 cm^2 [20], equating on average to a capillary cross-sectional area of only 1.25 X 10^{-6} cm^2. It is because of this very small cross-sectional area that blood flow is so slow. However, because of this slow blood flow, transfer of nutrients and medicaments is possible. During the process of capillary microcirculation, fluid diffuses out containing extremely low concentrations of protein besides lipids, nutrients, and added medicaments. Permeability of capillaries is increased by slight trauma, anoxia (lack of oxygen), and other factors so as to permit protein to leak out. Even though the fluid diffuses back into the capillaries, little protein is carried with it. Therefore, under a variety of conditions, protein can accumulate in the tissue spaces. If such fluid were allowed to accumulate unchecked, swelling would occur. Therefore, the main function of the lymphatic system is to remove this protein in addition to any high-molecular-weight molecules of drugs or macromolecular formulation excipients.

Lymphatic vessels begin as blind-ending capillaries which collect the lymph from tissue spaces. These vessels coalesce into larger channels, called lymph ducts, which eventually drain into major veins. The walls of lymphatic capillaries are very thin and highly permeable so that protein and larger foreign particles can easily enter. By definition, only when fluid enters the lymphatic system does it become lymph. Accordingly, three fluids are involved: (1) blood plasma, (2) interstitial fluid, and (3) lymph. Interstitial fluid passes from tissues to the lymph capillaries by a passive act mediated by pressure differences. Muscle movement, closely associated arteries, and their pulsation, as well as the pressure differential occurring during the breathing process, regulate the flow of lymph. Lymph returning to the venous system is filtered by a system of lymph nodes which are interposed along the chain of vessels.

The quantitative blood supply to the various organs and tissues of the body varies according to their functional requirements. Muscle can require up to or exceeding 10 times the amount of blood during vigorous contraction as during the resting stage [21]. In order to serve these requirements blood vessels supplying muscle must divide into a large number of capillaries. On the other hand, glandular tissue, which requires only a minimal blood supply, has blood vessels with only a few capillaries associated with it.

This very simplified overview of the circulatory system and its capacity should be kept in mind when examining the biopharmaceutics of injectable products. Medicaments placed in extravascular tissues must enter the capillaries of the venous and lymphatic systems in the general manner described. Once a drug enters the bloodstream it makes its way out through capillaries into the tissues, where it produces its pharmacological action. All drugs administered by injection must traverse this system before they can exert their activity either locally or at some distant organ.

2. The Intravenous Route

As stated previously, no absorption step is necessary when a drug is administered directly into the bloodstream. Therefore, there are no physiological factors affecting absorption as is the situation at extravascular sites. The rapidity of intravenous circulation times between various sites of the human body as measured by a dye dilution method is shown in Table 2. The circulation time from arm to toe in humans was shown to be approximately 25 sec. The actual onset of pharmacological effect of a drug injected intravenously will depend on the drug itself and the site of action, whether it be the smooth wall muscle of the larger blood vessels, as it is believed to be with some rapidly acting antihypertensive drugs [22], or the specific

Table 2 Circulation Times Following Intravenous Administration

Distance in body	Circulation time (sec)
Arm to ear	8 – 14
Lung to ear	3 – 5
Arm to finger	17.5 ± 4.4
Arm to toe	24.8 ± 4.4
Right ventricle to left ventricle	2 – 4

Source: Adapted from Ref. 5.

structures controlling replication of bacteria in systemic infections [23], where on-set of action is slower.

3. The Extravascular Route

In contrast to the rapidity of intravenous circulation time, the speed with which drugs enter the bloodstream via extravascular injection can vary greatly and is in-fluenced by a number of physiological factors. For absorption to occur, that fraction of drug that exists in solution must undergo eventual transfer through the capillary wall membrane, since it is believed that it is only through this mechanism that drugs are absorbed. No evidence has been reported indicating the ability for drugs to be-come absorbed directly through the walls of the larger blood vessels.

The capillary cell membrane is a very thin [75 to 100 Å (1 Å = 1 × 10^{-8} cm)] elastic material composed of approximately 55% protein, 40% lipid, and 5% polysac-charide substances [24]. Although its precise molecular structure is uncertain, it is considered to be a central layer of lipids covered by protein layers and a thin mucopolysaccharide layer on the outside surface. The lipid central region is res-ponsible for making it impervious to lipid–insoluble substances, a significant factor for the diffusion of extravascularly injected drugs. However, very small lipid-insoluble substances such as water and urea are believed to pass through the capil-lary membrane through pores by a process of filtration. The driving force is a con-centration gradient, but since the drug does not leave the aqueous solution during filtration, physicochemical factors such as pK_a and partition coefficient do not in-fluence the transport rate. Since pores are only about 30 Å in radius and the total area is less than 0.1% of the capillary wall area, this process is considered insignif-icant to the overall membrane transfer process because of its small size specificity.

The major physiological factors affecting passive diffusion through capillary cell membranes and blood flow at extravascular injection sites are: anatomical site, muscle movement, tissue condition of health, body temperature, patient age, general disease state, presence of mediators, and the concomitant use of vasoconstrictors.

Anatomical Site The anatomical characteristics of the extravascular injection site significantly influences the rate of absorption of a drug. The greater the number of capillaries at the site, the larger will be the surface area available for absorption, and consequently more absorption occurs. An example of the rate of absorption from different sites, reflected by rates of onset of tachycardia as measured by elevation in pulse rate, was demonstrated by injecting a solution of atropine into different

Table 3 Effect of Injection Site on the Rate of Onset
of Action of Atropine

	Onset of action tachycardia (min)
Intravenous	<5
Broad ligament	5-10
Subcutaneous	40
Intramuscular	40

Source: Adapted from Ref. 25.

anatomical regions. These data are shown in Table 3. Broad ligament injection
exhibited unexpectedly rapid rates that closely resemble those of intravenous injection, with 19 of 36 patients (53%) having measurable tachycardia within 5 min.
The utility of broad ligament injection was examined because of its application to
paracervical block anesthesia used during child delivery.

Other studies [26] have shown that resting blood flow is greater in the deltoid, intermediate in the thigh, and least in the buttock. This difference is considered sufficient to affect the rate of absorption of intramuscular injections from
these regions.

Muscle Movement The rate of flow through lymphatic vessels is increased
greatly with increasing muscle movement. This was demonstrated by injecting
rabbits subcutaneously with Black Tiger snake venum (molecular weight 20,000).
It took up to 8 hr for the venum to cause death in rabbits with immobilized limbs,
whereas unrestrained rabbits died in 2.5 hr [27].

Increased drug absorption resulting from increased activity or increased
blood flow as a result of activity was demonstrated in rats treated with procaine
penicillin G implants. Penicillin G absorption was 50% greater in rats placed in
activity cages and rotated at approximately 4 rpm, as opposed to nonrotated control
animals [28]. Muscular contraction occurring during exercise increases both dispersion of the drug and local blood flow. Muscle is more vascular than subcutaneous tissue; hence uptake is usually faster.

Tissue Condition Changes in tissue vascularity caused by scarring will affect
drug absorption. The clearance rate of [I^{131}] hippuran in rabbits was slower when
injection was made at a site previously mechanically traumatized by injection of
saline twice a day for a week [29]. Scar tissue can readily form by repeated injections at one site.

Injection into "insulin wheals" causes absorption to be delayed and efficacy
reduced [30]. This can be of particular importance to the diabetic patient, where
good absorption is required but where one to three injections per day must be given
for an entire lifetime. Rotation of injection sites, in addition to using sites that
provide more favorable absorption (midsection versus arm or thigh), is important
in maintaining good absorption of this lifesaving drug.

Body Temperature Rate of drug absorption changes in direct proportion to
body temperature, as does the rate of metabolism and most other physical and

chemical reactions. There is a good physical basis to consider that diffusion and blood flow, together with other physiological activities, would be affected by changes in body temperature. In general, colder external temperatures cause peripheral vasoconstriction, which is the body's way of reducing heat loss through surface vessels, whereas warmer temperatures cause vasodilation. However, the amount of body temperature change from the norm is usually not great enough to be an important or controllable factor for consideration during the design of a dosage form. On the other hand, application of heat to an injection site should result in faster absorption due to resultant local vasodilation.

Patient Age   Age and its effects on the absorption of drugs from injection sites is not well known. Although such factors as reduced adipose tissue and lowered renal clearance are known to exist with age, whether these factors play a definitive role is uncertain. Reduced adipose tissue results in a greater availability of drug to the systemic circulation since the retention of drug by such tissue is reduced, particularly if the drug has a high partition coefficient. Neonates and children usually exhibit lower drug blood levels than adults after dosing on a mg/kg basis. This is generally ascribed to high volumes of distribution, which relates to the drug's distribution into body tissues other than blood. This is because of greater relative amounts of total body water per kilogram of body weight in neonates compared to adults [31].

Ballard [3] suggested a possible increase in subcutaneous tissue thickness with age which might explain findings of increased LD_{50} values for drugs whose acute toxicity could be correlated with drug blood levels. In addition, he suggested that chemical composition of subcutaneous adipose tissue might change with age. If such were the case, the partition coefficient in younger and older tissues would be expected to change and variations in absorption could be expected. Bondrup et al. [32] showed that relative percentages of C_{12} to C_{18} triglycerides between adults and children showed pronounced differences, supporting possible change in subcutaneous adipose tissue with age.

Disease State   Absorption at the intramuscular injection site of an aqueous suspension of penicillin G seemed to be reduced in patients who suffered heart failure [33]. This can be rationalized by considering that damaged heart muscle cannot pump blood as efficiently as a healthy heart, thus affecting blood flow throughout the circulatory system. In cancer patients, instantaneous intravenous or intra-articular injections of methotrexate resulted in lower tissue levels of the drug than did prolonged continuous intravenous administration [34]. In another study the opposite was found in normal subjects receiving continuous intravenous aspirin [35]. A possible explanation for the difference in absorption rate not cited by the author is that metabolic functions of cancer cells are highly accelerated, favoring rapid drug metabolism and therefore lower drug tissue levels.

Presence of Mediator Enzymes   The enzyme hyaluronidase is known to increase the onset of drug absorption when given together with an intramuscular injection [36]. This enzyme hydrolizes hyaluronic acid, a component of tissue ground substance, which limits the spread of fluids at the injection site. After hydrolysis, the area of drug distribution in the tissue is increased and as a result, the absorption rate is also increased [37]. In a less definitive example, chymotrypsin was shown to increase the excretion of tetracyline from 13% to 37%; however, the mechanism for this effect was not elucidated [38].

Effect of Vasoactive Agents Epinephrine was shown to influence the rate of absorption of radioactive ^{24}Na given subcutaneously [15]. The drug constricts the local blood vessels in the absorption area, resulting in a reduced blood flow and therefore in reduced drug absorption. When epinephrine was coadministered with a solution of benzylpenicillin, absorption was significantly reduced over the control. This principle has been used particularly with the administration of local anesthetics. Conversely, the same investigator found that when prostaglandin E_2 was coadministered, its vasodilating effect increased blood flow and hence enhanced benzylpenicillin absorption [39].

II. APPLICATION OF PHARMACOKINETICS TO BIOPHARMECEUTIC INVESTIGATIONS: PHARMACOKINETIC MODELS

Pharmacokinetic analysis deals with the fitting of observed drug-blood level concentration versus time data to mathematical models as a means of interpreting the resulting kinetic phenomena. When plotted on semilogarithmic graph paper the data often exhibit characteristic profiles which have become attributed to processes involving absorption, distribution, metabolism, and excretion (ADME) of drugs from blood to the excreta (urine and feces). The models are simplifications of complex reactions and merely provide a handle for the treatment of such data. They help in the investigation and identification of important quantitative parameters which describe the gross kinetic processes observed following drug administration.

The profile and model fit for a particular drug will be the result of factors including mode of administration (oral, intravascular, extravascular, etc.), the mechanism of drug release from the formulation, as described earlier, and the physicochemical characteristics of the drug. Data from such investigations are very important to the formulator in assessing the performance of specifically designed dosage forms or what has become more popularly known as drug delivery systems. In summary, pharmacokinetics is an essential discipline when performing biopharmaceutic investigations, as it provides a means of quantitating the measurable drug concentration changes occurring in the body, as a result of conditions chosen in the experimental design.

This section provides examples of the simplest pharmacokinetic models, emphasizing administration by injection. Examples of how important data can be obtained directly from pharmacokinetic profiles will be illustrated. The application of pharmacokinetics to biopharmaceutics should become obvious; pharmacokinetic analysis is a means of determining the effects of variables in dosage form design and/or drug molecule on ADME processes, particularly absorption.

The simplest pharmacokinetic models are termed the one-compartment model and the two-compartment model. These models are basically characterized by drug-blood level versus time profiles exhibiting one or two exponential (logarithmic) elimination phases, respectively. In each model, variations exist depending on whether a measurable absorption phase occurs into the blood (body compartment), in addition to the rates at which drug equilibrates with compartments other than the blood, referred to as the peripheral or tissue compartment. In addition to these basic models, factors such as extent and site of metabolism often lead to more complex profiles requiring multicompartmental analysis. This treatment describes only the simplest cases where one- and two-compartmental model characteristics are involved as the result of single-dose injections, where the drug is excreted unchanged. In addition, the one-compartment model will be examined for an intravenous infusion.

A. Intravascular Injections

  1. Intravenous Injection: One-Compartment Model with
     First-Order Elimination

The one-compartment model is described as follows:

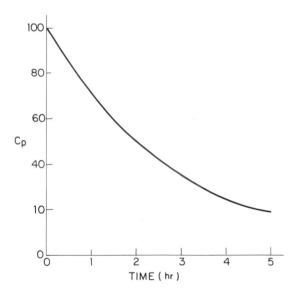

$$\text{DOSE} \xrightarrow{} \boxed{\begin{array}{c} \textbf{Body} \\ \textbf{Compartment} \\ \textbf{V}_d \ \textbf{C}_p \end{array}} \xrightarrow{k_{el}} \begin{array}{c} \textbf{DRUG} \\ \textit{in excreta} \end{array} \qquad (23)$$

A rapid (bolus) intravenous injection places drug directly into the bloodstream, C_p, and, as previously stated, there is no absorptive phase. For the case where the drug imparts the characteristics of a one-compartment model on the body, drug distributes instantaneously between the blood of volume V_d and other body fluids. The model makes the following assumptions; (1) any changes in drug blood concentration quantitatively reflects changes occurring in the tissue drug levels, and (2) the rate of elimination from the body is by a first-order process (i.e., the rate is proportional to the amount of drug in the body at that time). Following the rapid intravenous administration of a drug in solution, there is an instantaneous establishment of a drug-blood level concentration followed by a monoexponential reduction in drug concentration with time. This is shown graphically in Figure 4.

Figure 4 Hypothetical drug-blood level concentration versus time profile following rapid intravenous administration for a drug conferring the characteristics of a one-compartment model on the body.

This model is further described by the following equation:

$$C_p \xrightarrow{k_{el}} C_x \tag{24}$$

where

C_p = drug concentration in the blood (or plasma)

C_x = drug concentration in the excreta

Following first-order kinetics, the change in drug-blood level concentration with time is expressed as

$$\frac{dC_p}{dt} = -k_{el}C_p \tag{25}$$

where

dC_p/dt = instantaneous decrease in drug-blood level concentration with time

k_{el} = elimination rate constant in units of time^{-1}

The solution to this differential equation is

$$C_p = C_p^\circ e^{-k_{el}t} \tag{26}$$

Taking the logarithim of each side yields

$$\log C_p = \log C_p^\circ - \frac{k_{el}t}{2.303} \tag{27}$$

A plot of Equation (27) yields a straight line of negative slope $(-k_{el}/2.303)$ with a y-axis intercept $(\log C_p^\circ)$, as shown in Figure 5.

Determination of Important Pharmacokinetics Parameters

Elimination Rate Constant, k_{el}. From Equation (27), the slope of the line is equal to $-k_{el}/2.303$; therefore,

$$\text{Slope} = \frac{\log C_2 - \log C_1}{t_2 - t_1} = -\frac{k_{el}}{2.303} \tag{28}$$

where

C_1 = concentration of drug at time t_1

C_2 = concentration of drug at time t_2

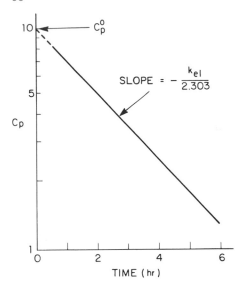

Figure 5 Semilogarithmic plot of a hypothetical drug-blood level concentration versus time following rapid intravenous administration.

Solving for k_{el} yields

$$k_{el} = -\frac{2.303(\log C_2 - \log C_1)}{t_2 - t_1} \qquad (29)$$

Values of C_1 and C_2 are chosen from actual data measurements which fall precisely on the line drawn. Hence the precision in determining k_{el} is dependent on the precision of the analytical measurements obtained. Time points t_1 and t_2 are those of the interval $C_2 - C_1$.

Half-Life, $t_{1/2}$. For a first-order process, the half-life $t_{1/2}$ is defined as the time it takes for a substance in solution to be reduced to one-half of its concentration. When referring to the biological process of drug elimination, it is the time required for the drug-blood level concentration to be reduced by 50%. The half-life of a first-order process can be determined by at least two different methods.

Graphic method. This parameter can be obtained graphically be inspection of a log concentration versus time profile, as shown in Figure 6. In this hypothetical example, the half-life is equal to 2 hr (i.e., the time it took for C_p to go from 5 concentration units to 2.5 units). As is evident from inspection, the value of 2 hr ($t_2 - t_1$) is obtained for any $C_p - C_p/2$ chosen. The accurary of this method is limited to the ability to estimate t_2 values from the graph. Usually, $C_p/2$ values do not fall at discrete t_2 values.

Calculation method. A more precise means of determining $t_{1/2}$ is by using the value for k_{el} obtained in Equation (29) as follows: Rearranging Equation (27) to

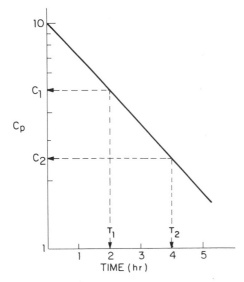

Figure 6 Graphic method of estimating $t_{1/2}$ by inspection of the plot of first-order elimination of drug from the blood. Blood concentration of drug, C_p, at any time t_1 is reduced by 50% to $C_p/2$ at time t_2. The difference $t_2 - t_1$ is equal to the biological half-life.

$$2.303 \log \frac{C_p^\circ}{C_p} = k_{el} t \tag{30}$$

and substituting

$$C_p = \frac{C_p^\circ}{2} \quad \text{and} \quad t = t_{1/2}$$

yields

$$2.303 \log \frac{C_p^\circ}{C_p^\circ/2} = k_{el} t_{1/2} \tag{31}$$

Cancelling C_p° yields

$$2.303 \log 2 = k_{el} t_{1/2} \tag{32}$$

Finally, solving for $t_{1/2}$, we have

$$t_{1/2} = \frac{0.693}{k_{el}} \tag{33}$$

Area Under the Curve (AUC) and Bioavailability. The area under the drug-blood level concentration versus time curve from $t_0 - t_\infty$ represents the amount of the administered dose found in the blood. This parameter can be calculated by several methods, such as by computer analysis or by mathematical integration of Equation (26) as follows:

$$AUC = \int_0^\infty C_p \, dt = C_p^\circ \int_0^\infty e^{-k_{el}t} \, dt = \frac{C_p^\circ}{k_{el}} \tag{34}$$

For drugs administered intravenously, the area under the curve is considered to reflect the entire intravenous dose, thus signifying 100% bioavailability. The relative bioavailability of a drug administered by other than the intravenous route is calculated as follows:

$$\%\text{Bioavailability} = \frac{AUC_{\text{extravascular}}}{AUC_{\text{intravenous}}} \times 100 \tag{35}$$

There may or may not be a significant difference in bioavailability of a drug solution injected intravenously versus intramuscularly. On the other hand, large differences can exist when drugs are administered orally since dosage forms such as capsules and tablets must undergo disintegration, dissolution, and absorption, and in some cases metabolism, prior to entry into the central blood circulation. This phenomenon is commonly referred to as first-pass metabolism since orally administered drugs must first pass through the liver, where they may become metabolized to a varying extent.

Volume of Distribution, V_d. The volume of distribution is not a true physiological volume, but it describes the volume the body would theoretically contain in order to account for the drug-blood level concentration following the administration of a dose of drug. This value is determined for a drug conferring the characteristics of a one-compartment model on the body by back extrapolation of the monoexponential line to the y axis as shown in Figure 5. The value obtained, C_p°, represents the concentration of drug found in the body at the initial phase of drug administration. Since

$$\text{Concentration} = \frac{\text{amount}}{\text{volume}} \tag{36}$$

substituting

$$\text{Concentration} = C_p^\circ$$

$$\text{Amount (of drug in the body)} = D \text{ (dose)}$$

$$\text{Volume of distribution (containing D)} = V_d$$

and solving for V_d, we get

$$V_d = \frac{D}{C_p^\circ} \tag{37}$$

By way of simple illustration, consider the following case:

$$\text{Intravenous dose} = 100 \text{ mg}$$

$$C_P^\circ = 20 \; \mu g \; ml^{-1}$$

Therefore,

$$V_d = \frac{100 \; mg}{20 \; \mu g \; ml^{-1}} \times 10^3 \; \mu g \; mg^{-1} = 5 \times 10^3 \; ml$$

$$= 5 \; liters$$

The volume of distribution reflects the distribution ratio of a drug between the blood and other fluids or tissues. If, as in the example given, V_d is found to be 5 liters, the approximate blood volume of a human adult, one can conclude that the drug was essentially all in the general blood circulation. Alternatively, a volume of distribution of several hundred liters indicates that drug is being held outside the central blood circulation compartment by a number of mechanisms, such as tissue binding and extensive metabolism and/or excretion. The value of several hundred liters obviously does not relate to a real blood volume in humans.

Example 1. The following data are obtained from the intravenous administration of a solution containing 90 mg of drug.

Time (min)	Drug blood level ($\mu g \; ml^{-1}$)
0.5	14
1.0	9.5
2.0	5.9
3.0	3.7

Determine the following parameters:

1. C_p: The data are plotted on semilogarthmic paper as shown in Figure 7. The straight line drawn through the points is extrapolated to the y axis to obtain the value of $C_p^\circ = 15.0 \; \mu g \; ml^{-1}$.
2. k_{el}: Using Equation (29):

$$k_{el} = \frac{2.303(\log C_2 - \log C_1)}{t_2 - t_1}$$

$$= \frac{2.303(\log 3.7 - \log 9.5)}{3.0 - 1.0}$$

$$= 0.47 \; min^{-1}$$

3. $t_{1/2}$: Using Equation (33):

$$t_{1/2} = \frac{0.693}{k_{el}} = \frac{0.693}{0.47} = 1.5 \; min$$

4. AUC: Using Equation (34):

$$\text{AUC} = \frac{C_p^\circ}{k_{el}} = \frac{15\ \mu g\ ml^{-1}}{0.47\ min^{-1}} = 32\ \mu g\ ml^{-1}\ min^{-1}$$

5. V_d: Using Equation (37):

$$V_d = \frac{D}{C_p^\circ} = \frac{90\ mg}{15\ \mu g\ ml^{-1}} = 6.0\ \text{liters}$$

2. Intravenous Injection: Two-Compartment Model with Rapid Distribution and First-Order Elimination

The two-compartment model is described as follows:

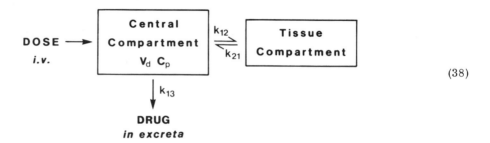

(38)

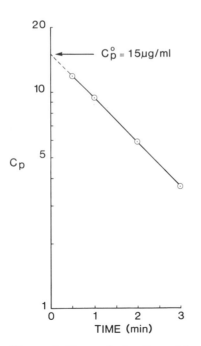

Figure 7 Example 1. Drug-blood level concentration versus time profile constructed from data for intravenous injection of a solution containing 90 mg of drug.

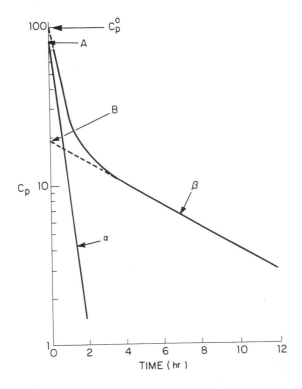

Figure 8 Hypothetical drug-blood level concentration versus time profile following rapid intravenous administration for a drug conferring the characteristics of a two-compartment model on the body.

A drug conforming to a two-compartment model following intravenous administration exhibits a profile with two distinct slopes, referred to as a biexponential curve. A typical example is shown in Figure 8. Again there is no absorption phase; however, in this case the drug does not get equilibrated instantaneously between the blood and other body fluids and tissues as in the one-compartment model. Distribution takes place at different rates until equilibrium is reached. The blood or central compartment can be monitored by sampling. The tissue compartment is comprised of those blood fluids or tissues in which drug equilibrates slowly and is inherently not easily accessible for sampling.

The initial exponential drop in the drug-blood level concentration curve shown in Figure 8 relates to the equilibrium established between the central and tissue compartment, k_{12}/k_{21}, followed then by the slower second exponential decrease with time relating to elimination from the central compartment, described by rate constant k_{13}. The solution of the differential resulting from such a model is the integrated double exponential equation:

$$C_p = Be^{-\beta t} + Ae^{-\alpha t} \qquad (39)$$

where

C_p = concentration of drug in the blood at time t

A = y-axis intercept from the α phase extrapolated

B = y-axis intercept from the β phase extrapolated

α, β = hybrid rate constants comprised of individual rate constants k_{12}, k_{21}, and k_{13}

where

$$\alpha = \frac{C_1 + \sqrt{C_1^2 - 4C_2}}{2} \tag{40}$$

$$\beta = \frac{C_1 - \sqrt{C_1^2 - 4C_2}}{2} \tag{41}$$

and

$$C_1 = k_{12} + k_{21} + k_{13} \tag{42}$$

$$C_2 = k_{21}k_{13} \tag{43}$$

Determination of Important Pharmacokinetic Parameters.

Distribution and Elimination Rate Constants. Although Equations (40) and (41) appear complex, the individual rate constants k_{12}, k_{21}, and k_{13} can be calculated from the values A, B, C_p°, α, and β obtained graphically from Figure 8 as follows:

$$C_p^\circ = A + B \tag{44}$$

$$k_{12} = \frac{AB (\beta - \alpha)^2}{C_p^\circ (A\beta + B\alpha)} \tag{45}$$

$$k_{21} = \frac{A\beta + B\alpha}{C_p^\circ} \tag{46}$$

$$k_{13} = \frac{C_p^\circ}{A/\alpha + B/\beta} \tag{47}$$

Half-life.

$$t_{1/2\alpha} = \frac{0.693}{\alpha} \quad \text{(distribution phase } k_{12}/k_{21}) \tag{48}$$

$$t_{1/2\beta} = \frac{0.693}{\beta} \quad \text{(elimination step } k_{13}) \tag{49}$$

Area Under the Curve (AUC). Integration of Equation (39) from t = 0 to t = ∞ yields

$$AUC = \int_0^\infty C_p \, dt = \left(A \int_0^\infty e^{-\alpha t} + B \int_0^\infty e^{-\beta t} \right) dt \tag{50}$$

$$AUC = \frac{A}{\alpha} + \frac{B}{\beta} \tag{51}$$

Volume of Distribution

$$(V_d)_\beta = \frac{dose}{\beta AUC} = \frac{dose}{\beta(A/\alpha + B/\beta)} = \frac{dose}{B\alpha + A\beta} \tag{52}$$

As is evident, the expression $(V_d)_\beta$ is more complex than that for the one-compartment model because the drug is distributed between the two compartments.

B. Extravascular Injections

Extravascular injections yield drug-blood level concentration versus time profiles which also conform to one- and two-compartment models. However, because of the requirement for a defined absorption phase from the site of injection [such as intramuscular (IM), subcutaneous (SQ)], different profiles result and new differential equations are required to describe the kinetics for these cases.

1. Extravascular Injection: One-Compartment Model with First-Order Absorption and Elimination

$$\begin{array}{ccc} & k_a & & k_{el} \\ \textbf{DOSE} & \longrightarrow & \boxed{\begin{array}{c} \textbf{Body} \\ \textbf{Compartment} \\ \textbf{V}_d \ \textbf{C}_p \end{array}} & \longrightarrow & \textbf{DRUG} \\ \textit{i.m., s.q.} & & & & \textit{in excreta} \end{array} \tag{53}$$

In this case absorption takes place from the site of administration at a rate depending on the drug release mechanism from the injection site. As described previously, the physicochemical properties of the drug and formulation are influencing factors. At the initial time of injection, the blood level of drug in the main circulation is zero. Absorption proceeds and drug concentration increases to a maximum followed by a decrease due to elimination by excretion, metabolism, or a combination of both. The drug-blood level concentration versus time profile for a typical drug conforming to this model and eliminated in unchanged form is shown in Figure 9.

The equation describing the kinetics of this system is

$$C_s \xrightarrow{\ k_a\ } C_p \xrightarrow{\ k_{el}\ } C_x \tag{54}$$

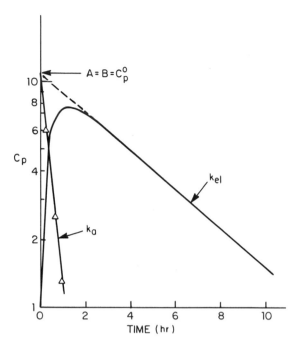

Figure 9 Hypothetical drug-blood level concentration versus time profile following extravascular administration for a drug conferring the characteristics of a one-compartment model on the body.

where

C_S = concentration of drug at the site of injection

C_p = concentration of drug in the blood

C_x = concentration of drug in the excreta

k_a = first-order absorption rate constant in units of time^{-1}

k_{el} = first-order elimination rate constant in units of time^{-1}

Assuming first-order absorption and elimination as well as rapid tissue and fluid distribution (absence of a tissue compartment), the integrated equation describing the system is

$$C_p = \frac{C_p^\circ k_a}{k_a - k_{el}} (e^{-k_{el}t} - e^{-k_a t}) \tag{55}$$

which becomes the general equation

$$C_p = Be^{-k_{el}t} - Ae^{-k_a t} \tag{56}$$

where, in addition to the parameters defined previously,

C_p° = hypothetical drug concentration at t = 0, obtained by back extrapolation of the monoexponential declining line

B = y-axis intercept of the back-extrapolated monoexponential elimination slope, equal to $-k_{el}/2.303$

A = y-axis intercept of the monoexponential absorption slope obtained by the method of residuals, also known as feathering

This technique is used for resolving a curve into its various exponential parts. The process can be described as follows. The differences between the line extrapolated to the y axis from the elimination slope and the points that lie on the blood level curve are plotted semilogarithmically at each time point. This yields a straight line with a steeper slope representing the rapid absorption phase. The slope of this line is equal to $-k_a/2.303$. The parameters C_p°, B, and A with respective slopes from which k_{el} and k_a can be determined are shown in Figure 9.

The slope of the line characterizing the absorption rate constant k_a is steeper than that of the elimination rate constant k_{el}. This is the case for most drugs administered in a dosage form from which it is readily available, thus allowing rapid absorption.

However, when the rate of absorption is significantly slower than the rate of elimination (i.e., $k_a \ll k_{el}$), the so-called flip-flop model results. As shown in Figure 10, the same type of profile will result as that shown in Figure 9; however, in this instance the absorption rate constant, k_a, is now characterized by the slower monoexponential line, whereas k_{el} is now characterized by the more rapid elimination slope, thus the term flip-flop model.

To determine whether a flip-flop model is occurring for a particular set of data that may not be known a priori, one compares the extravascular administration curves with that of intravenous administration as shown in Figure 10. The slope of the extravascular concentration-time plot, which is comparable to the elimination phase of the intravenous plot, is the elimination process. Thus, in this case, the flip-flop model characterizes this set of data.

Determination of Important Pharmacokinetic Parameters

Absorption and Elimination Rate Constants. These are determined graphically from Figure 9 for the general case or from Figure 10 for the flip-flop model.

Half-Life, $t_{1/2}$. This value can be obtained for both the absorption and elimination phases either by inspection (the graphic method) or by the use of determined k_a and k_{el} values for the general and flip-flop cases:

$$t_{1/2} = \frac{0.693}{k_a} \qquad \text{(absorption phase)} \qquad\qquad (57)$$

$$t_{1/2} = \frac{0.693}{k_{el}} \qquad \text{(elimination phase)} \qquad\qquad (58)$$

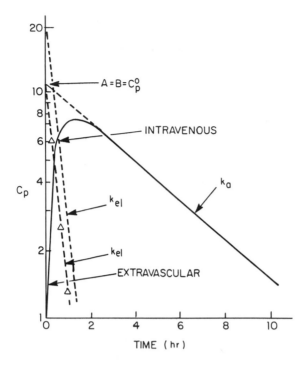

Figure 10 Schematic diagram of the flip-flop model, where an intravenous injection drug-blood level curve has been used to determine whether the ascending or descending portion of the curve following extravascular injection represents the elimination phase.

Area Under the Curve (AUC). Integration of Equation (56) from t = 0 to t = ∞ yields

$$\text{AUC} = \int_0^\infty C_p \, dt = \left(B \int_0^\infty e^{-k_{el}t} - A \int_0^\infty e^{-k_a t} \right) dt \tag{59}$$

$$\text{AUC} = \frac{B}{k_{el}} - \frac{A}{k_a} \tag{60}$$

Volume of Distribution

$$V_d = \frac{Df}{C_p^\circ} \tag{61}$$

An assumption is made that not all of the drug is available for absorption by the extravascular route. The fraction of dose absorbed, f, can be calculated from a comparison of the areas under the curves for both the extravascular and intravenous injection of the same drug as described by Equation (35).

Example 2. The following data are reported [40] from a study in which 7.5 mg kg^{-1} (an average of 539 mg per subject) of kanamycin is injected intramuscularly into 10 normal volunteers. All the drug is absorbed from this route (i.e., f = 1).

Time (hr)	Mean serum level (μg ml^{-1})
0.5	16
1	22
1.5	22
2	19
4	11
6	5.6
8	3.2

Determine the following:

1. Compartmental model: A plot of the data on semilogarithmic paper is shown in Figure 11. By inspection, the smooth curve drawn from the points provides a

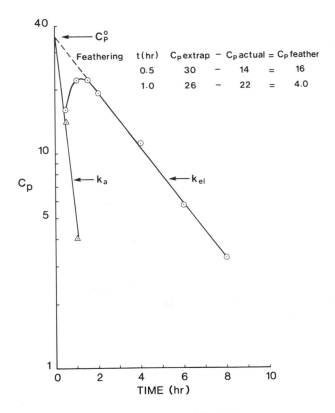

Figure 11 Example 2. Drug-blood level concentration versus time profile constructed from data for intramuscular injection of kanamycin into 10 normal volunteers. (Adapted from Ref. 40.)

typical profile for an intramuscular injection following the <u>one-compartment</u> model.

2. C_p: The initial drug concentration is determined as shown in Figure 11 by back extrapolation of the slower slope to the log concentration axis. From these data $C_p^{\circ} = 35\ \mu g\ ml^{-1}$.

3. k_{el}: The elimination rate constant k_{el} is determined from the slope of the elimination curve, which is the slower of the two reactions. From these data,

$$k_{el} = \frac{2.303(\log C_2 - \log C_1)}{t_2 - t_1}$$

$$= \frac{2.303(\log 4 - \log 19)}{7.2 - 2.0}$$

$$= 0.30\ hr^{-1}$$

4. k_a: The absorption rate constant k_a is determined by evaluating the slope of the line generated by the feathering technique. In this instance the data point 16 μg ml^{-1} at 0.5 hr is subtracted from the value 30 $\mu g\ ml^{-1}$ found directly above on the extrapolated line at the 0.5 hr time point. The difference, 30 - 16 = 14, is plotted (triangle) at the 0.5 hr time point. The same operation is performed using the data point 22 $\mu g\ ml^{-1}$ at 1 hr and the value 26 $\mu g\ ml^{-1}$ from the extrapolated line. The difference, 4 $\mu g\ ml^{-1}$, is in turn plotted at the 1 hr point. These two new points are connected using the value $C_p^{\circ} = 35\ \mu g\ ml^{-1}$ as the point of conversion since in the model developed, $A = B = C_p^{\circ}$. Using the same approach, we have

$$k_a = \frac{-2.30(\log C_2 - \log C_1)}{t_2 - t_1}$$

$$= \frac{-2.303(\log 4.0 - \log 14)}{1.0 - 0.50}$$

$$= 2.5\ hr^{-1}$$

5. V_d (68% of the drug is excreted unchanged): The volume of distribution V_d based on the totally model-dependent assumption can be calculated by using Equation (61). However, this model assumes that 100% of the drug is excreted unchanged. In this experiment only 68% of the drug is excreted unchanged; therefore, a correction must be made in the dose. Thus

$$V_d\ corrected = \frac{dose/\%\ excreted\ unchanged}{C_p^{\circ}}$$

$$= \frac{539}{35(0.68)} = 22.6\ liters$$

6. AUC: Using Equation (60) gives us

$$AUC = \frac{B}{k_{el}} - \frac{A}{k_a} = \frac{C_p^\circ}{k_{el}} - \frac{C_p^\circ}{k_a}$$

$$= \frac{35 \ \mu g \ ml^{-1}}{0.30 \ hr^{-1}} - \frac{35 \ \mu g \ ml^{-1}}{2.5 \ hr^{-1}}$$

$$= 100 \ \mu g \ ml^{-1} \ hr^{-1}$$

2. Extravascular Injection: Two-Compartment Model with First-Order Absorption But with Slow Distribution

This model is described as follows:

(62)

In this case a defined absorption step takes place depending on the means of drug liberation from the dosage form. At the initial time of injection, there is no drug in the central compartment. Absorption proceeds to a maximum followed by a sharp fall (due to slow distribution) until equilibrium is attained. The slope of the mono-exponential declining line depends on the rate of back distribution of drug from the tissue to blood described by rate constant k_{21}. Drugs conforming to this model following extravascular injection exhibit profiles similar to those shown in Figure 12.

The line with slope α is determined by the difference in actual blood level points of the elimination phase above the dashed line and corresponding value on the extrapolated dotted line at the same time points. Points lying on the line with slope k_a are obtained by the difference in points on the line with slope α and the actual blood level absorptive phase.

The overall general integrated equation that can be derived from this model is given by

$$C_p = Ae^{-\alpha t} + Be^{-\beta t} - C_p^\circ e^{-k_a t} \tag{63}$$

where

$$C_p^\circ = A + B \tag{44}$$

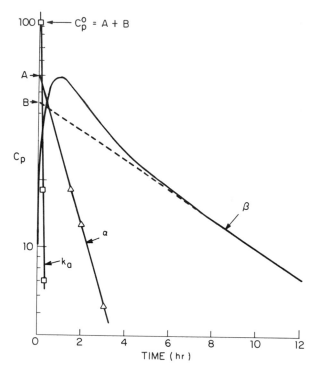

Figure 12 Hypothetical drug-blood level concentration versus time profile following extravascular administration for a drug conferring the characteristics of a two-compartment model on the body.

Determination of Important Pharmacokinetic Parameters

Absorption, Distribution, and Elimination Rate Constants. These rate constants can be calculated after determining the values of α, β, and C_p^o from Figure 12, as follows:

k_a = obtained from the slope of the absorption curve as shown in Figure 10

$$k_{12} = \frac{AB(\beta - \alpha)^2}{C_p^o(A\beta + B\alpha)} \tag{45}$$

$$k_{21} = \frac{A\beta + B\alpha}{C_p^o} \tag{46}$$

$$k_{13} = \frac{C_p^o}{A/\alpha + B/\beta} \tag{47}$$

Half-Life. The half-life $t_{1/2}$ of each of the distribution and elimination slopes is determined as shown in Equations (48) and (49). The half-life for the absorption phase is shown in Equation (64).

$$t_{1/2\alpha} = \frac{0.693}{\alpha} \text{ (distribution phase } k_{12}/k_{21}) \tag{48}$$

$$t_{1/2\beta} = \frac{0.693}{\beta} \text{ (elimination step } k_{13}) \tag{49}$$

$$t_{1/2} = \frac{0.693}{k_a} \text{ (absorption phase)} \tag{64}$$

Area Under the Curve (AUC). Integration of Equation (68) from t = 0 to t = ∞ yields

$$AUC = \int_0^\infty C_p \, dt = \left(A \int_0^\infty e^{-\alpha t} + B \int_0^\infty e^{-\beta t} - C_p^\circ \int_0^\infty e^{-k_a t} \right) dt \tag{65}$$

$$AUC = \frac{A}{\alpha} + \frac{B}{\beta} - \frac{C_p^\circ}{k_a} \tag{66}$$

Volume of Distribution of the Central Compartment

$$V_c = \frac{Df}{C_p^\circ} \tag{67}$$

However, dealing with both the central and tissue compartment, the volume of distribution at equilibrium or steady state becomes

$$V_{dss} = V_c + V_t \tag{68}$$

and

$$V_{dss} = \frac{k_{12} + k_{21}}{k_{21}} V_c \tag{69}$$

which can be calculated once k_{12} and k_{21} are determined.

C. Intravenous Infusion: One-Compartment Model

Thus far the examples described have been for rapid single-dose intravascular and extravascular injections. An important and vital mode of therapy is where the drug is administered intravenously at a constant rate. Such administration is limited to dilute solutions of drugs admixed with electrolytes or nutrients. A drug introduced into the systemic circulation at a constant rate gives rise to a drug-blood level concentration versus time profile distinctive of this mode of administration.

The differential equation describing the change in amount of drug with time is written as

$$\frac{dA}{dt} = k_0 - k_{el}A \tag{70}$$

where

k_0 = zero-order rate constant describing the rate of drug infusion expressed in amount per unit time

A = amount of drug

k_{el} = first-order elimination rate constant

By solving Equation (70), the amount of drug in the body at any time t is determined as follows:

$$A = \frac{k_0}{k_{el}} (1 - e^{-k_{el}t}) \tag{71}$$

The amount of drug A administered is determined using the relationship

$$A = \text{volume administered (ml)} \times \text{concentration (amount} \times ml^{-1}) \tag{72}$$

Therefore, substituting for A in Equation (71) and solving for concentration C yields

$$C = \frac{k_0}{k_{el}V_d} (1 - e^{-k_{el}t}) \tag{73}$$

The drug-blood level concentration rises directly after the start of an intravenous infusion and will approach a constant level when the rate of drug being delivered is equal to the rate of drug elimination. A profile for the ideal case of a hypothetical drug being administered by intravenous infusion is shown in Figure 13.

The steady-state concentration C_{ss} can be determined from Equation (73) by setting $t = \infty$. When this is done, $e^{-k_{el}t}$ approaches zero and can be dropped from the equation, yielding

$$C_{ss} = \frac{k_o}{k_{el}V_d} \tag{74}$$

This equation indicates that the steady-state concentration is directly proportional to the rate of infusion. Once infusion is stopped, the rate of change in drug-blood level concentration with time is

$$\frac{dC}{dt} = -k_{el}C_{ss} \tag{75}$$

or in the integrated form,

$$C = C_{ss}e^{-k_{el}t} \tag{76}$$

where t = t + infusion time. This equation is simply the elimination of the drug from the body following first-order kinetics where the slope of the line is equal to $-k_{el}/$ 2.303 as given originally in Equation (28).

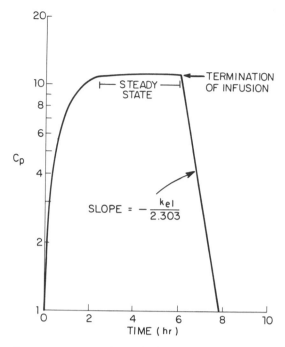

Figure 13 Hypothetical drug-blood level concentration versus time profile of a drug administered by slow intravenous infusion which establishes a steady-state concentration C_{ss}, followed by a first-order elimination phase upon termination of dosing.

There are far more complexities involved with the science of pharmacokinetics that were obviously not intended to be described in a chapter of this length. Complex metabolism, excretion, and distribution together with the effects of disease state and age are some that have a marked influence on the ADME processes. It is important to note that being able to affect the release profile of a drug through formulation design, and being able to measure such changes by pharmacokinetic experiments, provides the formulator with an invaluable technique for product development. For a more in-depth study of pharmacokinetics and the underlying mathematical justification of the equations presented herein, the reader is referred to textbooks devoted to this subject [41-45].

III. SUMMARY

The aim of this chapter has been to develop the subject of biopharmaceutics as applied to injectable medication. The sequence of events leading to absorption of drug from an injection has been described, taking into account the dynamics at the injection site, the means of ultimate entry of a drug into the complex circulatory system, the influencing physicochemical and physiological processes, and the role played by dosage form design in influencing the rate of absorption. Examination has been made of basic examples of pharmacokinetics dealing with typical drug-blood level concentration versus time profiles for rapid single intravenous and intramuscular injections as well as for slow intravenous infusion. The single one- and two-compartment models were developed for drugs excreted unchanged. Integration and utiliza-

utilization of all these factors is important toward a scientific approach to the development of injectable dosage forms.

REFERENCES

1. Schou, J., Pharmacol. Rev., 13:441(1961).
2. Wagner, J. G., J. Pharm. Sci., 50:539 (1961).
3. Ballard, B. E., J. Pharm. Sci., 57:357 (1968).
4. Simonelli, A. P., and Dresback, D. S., in Perspectives in Clinical Pharmacy (D. E. Francke and H. A. K. Whitney, Jr., eds.), Drug Intelligence Publications, Hamilton, Ill., 1972, pp. 390-420.
5. Ritschel, W. A., Pharm. Ind., 35:273 (1973).
6. Feldman, S., Bull. Parenter. Drug Assoc., 28:53 (1974).
7. Tse, F. L., and Welling, P. G., J. Parenter. Drug Assoc., 34:409 (1980).
8. Dam, M., and Olsen, V., Neurology, 16:228 (1966).
9. Serrano, E. E., Roye, D. B., Hammer, R. H., and Wilder, B. J., Neurology, 23:311 (1973).
10. Kostenbauder, H. B., Rapp, R. P., McGovren, J. P., Foster, T. S., Perrier, D. G., Blacker, H. M., Hulon, W. C., and Kinkel, A. W., Clin. Pharmacol. Ther., 18:449 (1975).
11. Assaf, R. A. E., Dundee, J. W., and Gamble, J. A. S., Anesthesia, 30:152 (1975).
12. Greenblatt, D. J., Shader, R. I., and Koch-Weser, J., N. Engl. J. Med., 291:1116 (1974).
13. Greenblatt, D. J., Duhme, D. W., Koch-Weser, J., and Smith, T. W., N. Engl. J. Med., 289:651 (1973).
14. Kakemi, K., Sezaki, H., Okumura, K., and Ashida, S., Chem. Pharm. Bull., 17:1332 (1969).
15. Kety, S., Am. Heart J., 39:321 (1949).
16. Sund, R., and Schou, J., Acta Pharmacol. Toxicol., 21:331 (1964).
17. Sidell, F. R., Clin. Pharmacol. Ther., 16:711 (1974).
18. Schriftman, H., and Kondritzer, A. A., Am. J. Physiol., 191:591 (1957).
19. Edin, J. W., Sci. Am., 28:86 (1968).
20. Langley, L. L., Telford, I. R., and Christensen, J. B., Dynamic Anatomy and Physiology, 4th ed., McGraw-Hill, New York, 1974, p. 481.
21. Langley, L. L., Telford, I. R., and Christensen, J. B., Dynamic Anatomy and Physiology, 4th ed., McGraw-Hill, New York, 1974, p. 518.
22. Goodman, L. S., and Gilman, A., eds., The Pharmacological Basis of Therapeutics, 5th ed., Macmillan, New York, 1975, pp. 705, 707, 710.
23. Goodman, L. S., and Gilman, A., eds., The Pharmacological Basis of Therapeutics, 5th ed., Macmillan, New York, 1975, p. 1091.
24. Thomas, J., Aust. J. Pharm., 54:479 (1973).
25. Burchell, R. C., and Swasdio, K., Obstet. Gynecol., 27:714 (1966).
26. Evans, E. F., Proctor, J. D., Fratkin, M. J., Velandia, J., and Wasserman, A. J., Clin. Pharmacol. Ther., 17:44 (1975).
27. Barnes, B. E., and Trueta, J., Lancet, 1:623 (1941).
28. Ballard, B. E., J. Pharm. Sci., 55:515 (1966).
29. Chezem, J. L., Nurs. Res., 22:138 (1973).
30. Root, H. F., Irvine, J. W., Evans, R. D., Reiner, L., and Carpenter, T. M., JAMA, 124:84-90 (1944).
31. Wagner, J. G., Drug Intell., 2:144 (1968).

32. Bondrup, K., Koster, N., Quaade, F., and Rosenven, H., J. Clin. Lab. Invest., 18:588 (1966).

33. Irons, E. N., JAMA, 142:97 (1950).

34. Anderson, L. L., Collins, G. J., Ojima, Y., and Sullivan, R. D., Cancer Res., 30:1344 (1970).

35. Gibaldi, M., J. Pharm. Sci., 58:327 (1969).

36. Keawn, K. K., Fisher, S. M., Downing, D. F., and Hitchcock, P., Anesthesiology, 18:270 (1957).

37. Underkofler, L. A., in Remington's Pharmaceutical Sciences, 13th ed., Mack, Easton, Pa., 1965, p. 1114.

38. Seneca, H., and Peer, P., J. Am. Geriatr. Soc., 13:708 (1965).

39. Bederka, J., Takemori, A. E., and Miller, J. W., Eur. J. Pharmacol., 15:132 (1971).

40. Doluisio, J. T., Dittert, L. W., and La Piana, J. C., J. Pharmacokinet. Biopharm., 3:25 (1975).

41. Gibaldi, M., and Perrier, D., Pharmacokinetics, Marcel Dekker, New York, 1975.

42. Wagner, J. G., Biopharmaceutics and Relevant Pharmacokinetics, Drug Intelligence Publications, Hamilton, Ill., 1971.

43. Notari, R. E., Biopharmaceutics and Clinical Pharmacokinetics: An Introduction, 3rd ed., Marcel Dekker, New York, 1980.

44. Benet, L. Z., ed., The Effect of Disease States on Drug Pharmacokinetics, American Pharmaceutical Association, Academy of Pharmaceutical Sciences, Washington, D.C., 1976.

45. Ritschel, W. A., Handbook of Basic Pharmacokinetics, 2nd ed., Hamilton Press, Hamilton, Ill., 1980.

4

Preformulation Research of Parenteral Medications

SOL MOTOLA

Merck Frosst Canada, Inc.
Pointe Claire-Dorval,
Quebec, Canada

SHREERAM AGHARKAR

Schering Corporation
Bloomfield, New Jersey

Preformulation research relates to pharmaceutical and analytical investigations carried out preceding and supporting formulation development efforts for all dosage forms. Experiments are designed to generate data characterizing specific, pharmaceutically important, physicochemical properties of the drug substance and its combination with selected solvents, excipients, and packaging components. These studies are carried out under stressed conditions of temperature, light, humidity, and oxygen in order to accelerate and detect potential reactions. Taking into account early pharmacological and biopharmaceutical data, preformulation studies yield key information necessary to guide the formulator and analyst toward the development of an elegant, stable dosage form with good bioavailability. Prior to development of the clinical and marketed dosage form, preformulation studies yield basic knowledge necessary to develop suitable formulations for toxicological use.

Due to important research leads in a highly competitive field, it is essential to rapidly progress a drug and initiate clinical studies as soon as possible. Thus an expeditious preformulation program (i.e., one typically taking 6 to 10 weeks to complete) is generally required. If clinical program acceleration is desired, it may be necessary to streamline studies and develop crucial decision-making data in shorter time periods. Should interim results indicate that a more stable or more soluble drug form is needed, expansion of the original program will be necessary. Additionally, areas of particular interest may arise, such as the elucidation of a reaction mechanism or the investigation of unusual solubility phenomena. Such studies may be of prime importance and are often addressed either initially or as second-phase preformulation studies, depending on their potential impact on the overall program.

The general subject of preformulation research has been described in detail by several investigators [1-5] and is in wide use throughout the pharmaceutical industry. These presentations have dealt mainly with studies designed for solid dosage forms. Some specific applications have been made to certain areas of parenteral interest [6, 7]. The objective of this chapter is to outline methods used in developing preformulation data necessary to characterize significant physicochemical properties of new drugs important to a parenteral formulation development program.

I. DRUG SUBSTANCE PHYSICOCHEMICAL PROPERTIES

Typical physicochemical properties of drug substances that either characterize or may exert significant influence on the development of a parenteral formulation are listed in Table 1.

A. Molecular Structure and Weight

These are the most basic characteristics of a drug substance and are among the first items to be known. From the molecular structure the investigator can make initial judgments regarding potential properties and functional group reactivities, as described in Section III.

B. Color

Color is generally a function of a drug's inherent chemical structure relating to a certain level of unsaturation. Color intensity relates to the extent of conjugated unsaturation as well as the presence of chromophores such as $-NH_2$ $-NO_2$, and $-CO-$ (ketone) which intensify color. Some compounds may appear to have color although structurally saturated. Such a phenomenon can often be due to the presence of minute traces of highly unsaturated, intensely colored impurities and/or degradation products. These substances may be prone to increased color formation under stress conditions of heat, oxygen, and light. A significant color change can become a limiting factor to the shelf life of a parenteral product even before a significant change in chemical stability is noted.

The drug substance's color should be recorded by a subjective description, as well as by an objective means such as by comparison with standard color chips [8], or by spectrophotometric analysis if the compound's color intensity in solution is proportional to concentration. The American Public Health Association (APHA) color standards [9] can be used effectively to quantitate changes in solution color with time. Visible absorbance of APHA color standards (diluted appropriately) can be measured spectrophotometrically [10] to monitor more accurately the color of solution test samples. An example plot is shown in Figure 1.

Table 1 Physicochemical Properties of Drug Substances

Molecular structure and weight	Solubility
Color	pH solubility profile
Odor	Polymorphism potential
Melting point	Solvate formation
Thermal analytical profile	Absorbance spectra
Particle size and shape	Light stability
Hygroscopicity potential	Thermal stability
Ionization constant	pH stability profile
Optical activity	

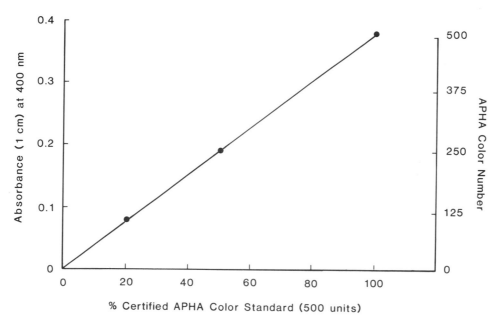

Figure 1 Typical visible absorbance readings at 400 nm for certified APHA color standard (500 units) at various dilutions versus APHA color number.

C. Odor

The odor of a new drug substance should be examined by cautiously smelling the headspace of the drug container which has been previously closed to allow volatiles to concentrate. The presence and description of any odor should be recorded. The substance may exhibit an inherent odor characteristic of major functional groups present (i.e., sulfurous or garliclike for sulfides, sulfoxides, or sulfhydryl-containing compounds, or ammoniacal as for amines). Alternatively, a drug may be void of characteristic odor or it may have an odor of residual solvent. The presence of a solvent odor should be reviewed with the synthesis chemist to determine whether the sample has been adequately dried.

D. Particle Size, Shape, and Crystallinity

The particle size of a water-soluble drug is not of concern unless it exists in large aggregates and an increase in rate of solution is desired to reduce manufacturing time. Under such circumstances milling through an appropriate size sieve [11] may be sufficient.

Particle size and shape characteristics can be determined by microscopic evaluation using either an optical microscope, preferably with polarizing attachments, or by a scanning electron microscope. The morphological characteristics of the drug substance should be recorded either by a sketch or, more accurately, by a photomicrograph which acts as a permanent record for comparison with future batches. A good estimate of particle size and particle size range can be obtained by viewing several fields of a representative sample of drug substance.

A polarizing microscope is also used to determine whether a compound is crystalline or amorphous. Crystalline materials refract polarized light and are thus visible when polarization attachments in the ocular and objective are crossed at a 90° angle (crossed polars), whereas amorphous or glassy substances become invisible.

Optical microscopes usually operate at useful magnifications of up to 1000X with a resolution limit in the vicinity of 1 μm. The scanning electron microscope provides magnifications up to 200, 000X with a resolution of approximately 25 Å to determine detailed particle surface morphology as well as individual particle surface characteristics. Whereas the optical microscope provides only a two-dimensional view, the scanning electron microscope adds the dimension of depth by tilting the stage to several angles of view during operation. Thus what may appear to be a combination of acicular and plate-shaped structures under a polarizing microscope could in reality only be a field of flat plates of various sizes with some on edge, as shown in Figure 2. This ability to resolve various shapes helps the investigator determine whether a sample is morphologically homogeneous. Mixtures of morphological forms either within a sample or between samples could indicate the existence of hydrates, solvates, or polymorphic forms which could later significantly affect properties such as solubility, stability, and bioavailability.

E. Melting Point

The melting point of a substance is thermodynamically defined as the temperature at which the solid and liquid phases are in equilibrium as described in Equation (1).

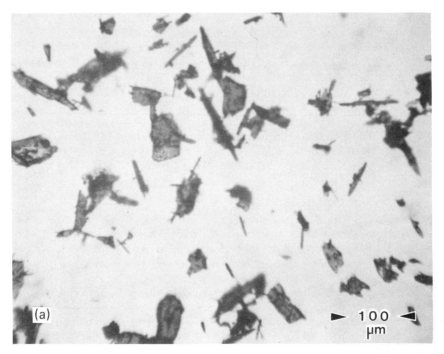

Figure 2 Microscopic examination of an experimental drug. Views through an optical microscope (a) and a scanning electron microscope (b) at various stage angles as noted. (Courtesy of E. B. Vadas, Merck Frosst Canada, Inc., Pointe Claire-Dorval, Quebec, Canada.)

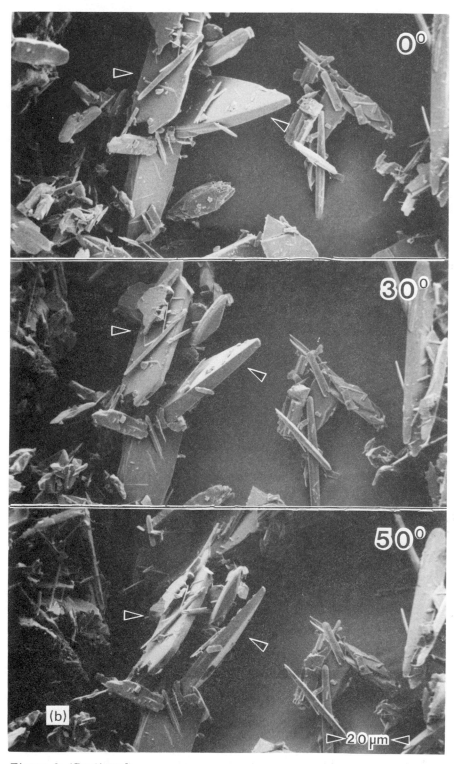

Figure 2 (Continued)

$$S_{solid} \rightleftharpoons S_{liquid} \tag{1}$$

A melting-point determination is a good first indication of purity since the presence of relatively small amounts of impurity can be detected by a lowering as well as widening in the melting-point range. Methods for determining the melting range or temperature are described in detail for various compounds [12]. Any peculiar behavior of a substance undergoing melting, such as dramatic change in volume, melting and recrystallization, gas evolution, color change, or other physical change, should be recorded and investigated further. Such behavior could be indicative of significant changes, such as a polymorphic transition, desolvation, oxidation, or decarboxylation.

F. Thermal Analytical Profile

During synthesis and isolation, a sample may have been exposed to changes in the temperature environment which may be exhibited as a thermal profile when the sample is heated between ambient temperature and its melting point. When no thermal history exists, the sample will neither absorb nor give off heat prior to its melting point. The basic technique used to study this phenomenon is called differential thermal analysis (DTA). Essentially, the sample is heated in the presence of a sensitive thermocouple while a second, balanced thermocouple electrically

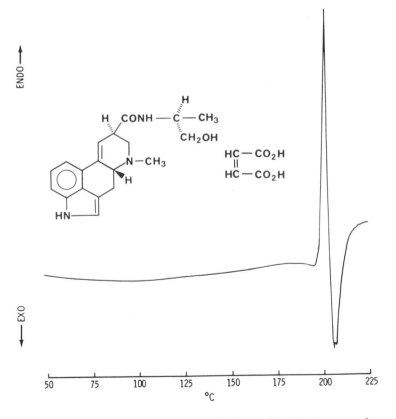

Figure 3 Structure and differential thermal analysis scan of ergonovine maleate with decomposition (USP reference standard, lot L). (From Ref. 13.)

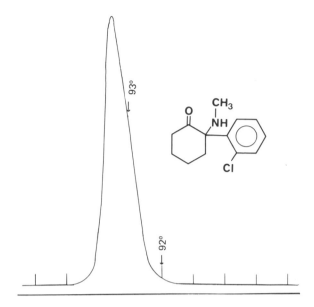

Figure 4 Structure and differential thermal analysis scan of ketamine. (From Ref. 14.)

connected in series opposition is heated at the same rate in the presence of an inert reference material. The reference substance is one that does not undergo thermal transition within the range of temperatures to be used. The data are plotted on rectilinear paper with the ordinate equal to the difference in temperature between sample and reference, ΔT, and the abscissa equal to the temperature T. Although differences in convention exist, this treatment will indicate exothermic reactions above and endothermic reactions below the baseline. If a flat signal results, no differential change in temperature (ΔT) occurred between sample and reference. When a sample shows a defined exotherm (heat liberation) or endotherm (heat absorption) resulting from physical or chemical changes as a function of temperature, these phenomena are indicative of phase transitions. Examples of characteristic endothermic transitions that can be detected by this technique are: fusion or melting, crystalline structural changes such as polymorphic transitions, sublimation, boiling, and desolvation. An exothermic effect is seen when crystallization occurs. Examples of thermal analysis profiles of melts with and without decomposition are shown in Figures 3 and 4. Decomposition upon melting is noted when the signal drops below the original baseline following the melting endotherm.

A similar process which examines this phenomena is called differential scanning calorimetry (DSC). With this technique, the area under the output curve is directly proportional to the total amount of energy (q) absorbed or liberated from the sample. The abscissa is proportional to the rate of heat transfer (dq/dt) at any given time. The loss of surface moisture and a decomposition melt is evident in the DSC curve shown in Figure 5.

The thermal analytical method used to detect the existence and stability of solvated drug molecules is called thermogravimetric analysis (TGA). In this technique relative weight loss is studied between the sample and a reference during the heating cycle. The reference chosen is one known not to undergo weight loss over the temperature range desired. Weight loss can occur as a result of the loss of sample surface moisture or by molecular desolvation or decomposition. Combined

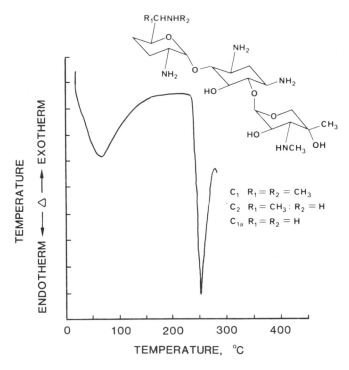

Figure 5 Structure and differential scanning calorimetry scan of gentamicin sulfate (USP reference standard). (From Ref. 15.)

DTA and TGA curves for amphotericin B showing intermediate phase transitions (DTA), weight loss, and decomposition (TGA) are shown in Figure 6. An overview of thermal analytical methods described above is available for further information [17].

G. Hygroscopicity

A compound is hygroscopic if it picks up a significant amount of moisture under a specific condition of temperature and humidity. A high degree of hygroscopicity may adversely affect the physical and chemical properties of a drug substance, making it either pharmaceutically difficult or unsatisfactory to work with.

Hygroscopicity studies are usually carried out over a range of humidity conditions relevant to the general laboratory and manufacturing areas as well as uncontrolled storage environment. A low-humidity condition can be used to determine whether a hydrate will lose water under such storage. Saturated solutions of certain salts stored in sealed containers, such as desiccators, are used to establish well-defined humidity conditions; examples are shown in Table 2.

To carry out a study, samples of compound are accurately weighed into tared containers and placed at various humidity conditions for periods up to 2 weeks. Weight gain or loss is measured at predetermined intervals until equilibrium is reached. An assessment is made regarding the relative weight gain as well as color and general flowability. Chemical analysis is often performed should physical change indicate possible chemical degradation. A hygroscopicity classification is shown in

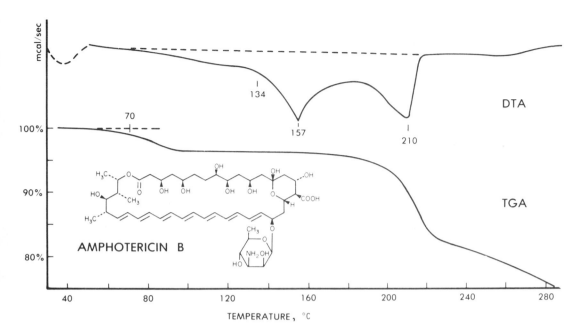

Figure 6 Structure, differential thermal analysis, and thermogravimetric analysis scan of amphotericin B. (From Ref. 16.)

Table 3. Thus from hygroscopicity studies the investigator can determine environmental humidity conditions necessary to maintain initial properties. If the drug is very hygroscopic or determined to be unstable in the presence of moisture, the drug would have to be stored under dry conditons and worked with under low humidity. Close examination of the quantity of moisture gained during these experiments is important in determining whether hydrate formation is occurring.

Table 2 Saturated Salt Solutions for Humidity Control

	% Relative humidity	Temperature (°C)
Potassium acetate, $Kc_2H_3O_2$	20	20
Calcium chloride, $CaCl_2 \cdot 6H_2O$	31	24.5
Potassium thiocyanate, KSCN	47	20
Sodium nitrite, $NaNO_2$	66	20
Sodium acetate, $NaC_2H_3O_2 \cdot 3H_2O$	76	20
Zinc sulfate, $ZnSO_4 \cdot 7H_2O$	90	20

Source: Ref 18.

Table 3 Hygroscopicity Classification

Class I—Nonhygroscopic: Essentially no moisture increases occur at relative humidities below 90%. Furthermore, the increase in moisture content after storage for 1 week above 90% relative humidity (RH) is less than 20%.

Class II—Slightly hygroscopic: Essentially no moisture increases occur at relative humidities below 80%. The increase in moisture content after storage for 1 week above 80% RH is less than 40%.

Class III—Moderately hygroscopic: Moisture content does not increase above 5% after storage at relative humidities below 60%. The increase in moisture content after storage for 1 week above 80% RH is less than 50%.

Class IV—Very hygroscopic: Moisture increase may occur at relative humidities as low as 40 to 50%. The increase in moisture content after storage for 1 week above 90% RH may exceed 30%.

Source: Ref. 19.

H. Absorbance Spectra

Molecules with structural unsaturation are able to absorb light within a specific frequency range. As mentioned previously, the degree of unsaturation coupled with the presence of chromophores will influence the extent of absorption and whether ultraviolet (400 to 190 nm) or visible (800 to 400 nm) light will be absorbed. The ultraviolet and visible spectra of compounds in solution are not highly specific; however, they are very suitable for quantitative analytical work and serve as additional information for compound identification. The ultraviolet or visible spectrum can be determined by placing approximately a 10 to 20 μg ml^{-1} solution of the compound in a 1 cm cell, and recording the spectrum versus the appropriate solvent blank in the spectral range 190 to 800 nm. An example of the ultraviolet spectrum of chlorothiazide is shown in Figure 7. Absorbance maxima are evident at 228, 292, and 310 nm.

   Relationships used to compare and quantitate ultraviolet and visible absorbance of compounds in solution are shown in Equations (2) and (3).

$$a = \frac{A}{bc} \tag{2}$$

$$\epsilon = \frac{A}{bc} \tag{3}$$

In equation (2), the quantity a, called absorptivity, is related to the absorption of a compound of concentration c (in grams per 1000 ml) through a sample cell of b centimeters and thus has the units liters per gram–centimeter. When the concentration is expressed in moles per liter, the absorptivity becomes molar absorptivity e, and is expressed in liters per mole centimeter.

   Both values should be recorded for each solvent system of interest. For quantitative use, either a or ϵ is determined. For a compound in solution the molar concentration of an unknown quantity of the same drug can be determined by knowing the absorbance at the wavelength and the cell path length. Rearranging Equation (3) yields Equation (4).

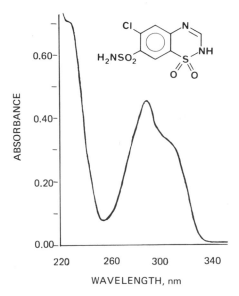

Figure 7 Structure and ultraviolet absorbance spectrum of chlorothazide. (From Ref. 21.)

$$c = \frac{A}{b\epsilon} \tag{4}$$

The infrared (IR) spectrum (run between 2.5 and 15 μm) is highly specific for each chemical structure, with small structural differences resulting in significant

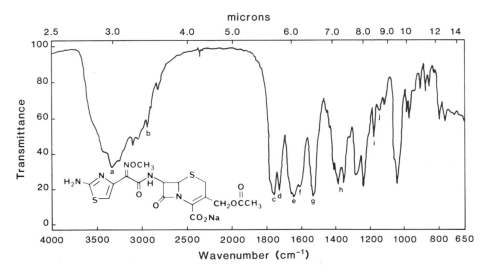

Figure 8 Structure and infrared spectrum of cefotaxime in KBr with peaks of several functional groups identified. (Adapted from Ref. 22.)

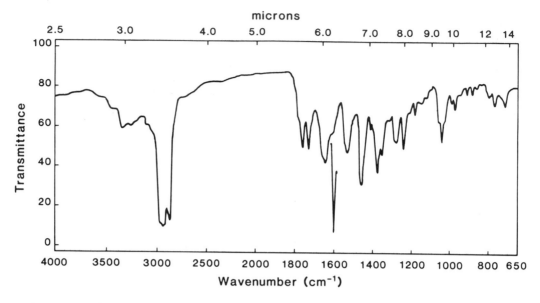

Figure 9 Infrared spectrum of cefotaxime in Nujol mull. (Adapted from Ref. 22.)

Table 4 Infrared Frequency Assignments for Cefotaxime

Frequency (cm^{-1})		Assignment
a	3420	$-NH_2$
	3340 (broad)	$-NH$, $-NH_2$
b	2940	$-S-CH_2$
c	1760	$-C{=}O$ lactam
d	1730	$-C{=}O$ carboxylic, $O-\overset{\overset{\displaystyle O}{\|}}{C}-CH_3$
e	1650	$-\overset{\overset{\displaystyle O}{\|}}{C}-NH_2$
f	1620	$-\overset{\overset{\displaystyle O}{\|}}{C}-NH$, $-C{=}N-$, $-C{=}C-$
g	1540	$-\overset{\overset{\displaystyle O}{\|}}{C}-N-$
h	1385–1355	$-O-CO-CH_3$
i	1180	$C{=}O$ in ester
j	1050	$C-O$ stretching

Adapted from Ref. 22.

Table 5 Examples of Nonaqueous
Solvents Used in the Parenteral
Product Formulation

Polyethylene glycol 400 and 600

Propylene glycol

Glycerin

Ethyl alcohol

Fixed oils

Ethyl oleate

Benzyl benzoate

Source: Ref. 20.

spectral changes. Samples can be prepared as a solution, as a dispersion in mineral oil (Nujol mull), or as a potassium bromide (KBr) pellet. After running a spectrum, significant peaks relating to major functional groups are identified; spectra
of subsequent samples of the same compound are compared with the original. If IR
spectral differences are found, the reason for and source of change should be investigated. This technique is used to detect batch-to-batch variations, as an identity
test, and for the detection of polymorphs and solvates. KBr and Nujol mull spectra

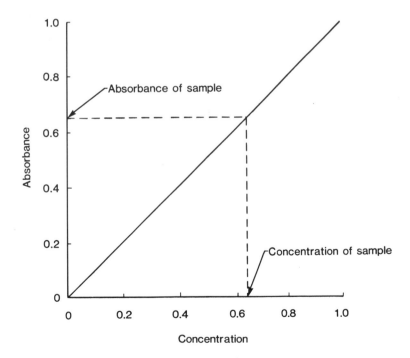

Figure 10 Hypothetical Beer's law curve relating absorbance and concentration.

of cefotaxime acid are shown in Figures 8 and 9, respectively. Peaks corresponding to various functional groups are identified by letters a-j on the KBr spectrum with assigned frequencies listed in Table 4.

I. Solubility

Solubility is of prime importance for developing solutions that can be injected either intravenously or intramuscularly. In general, solubility is a function of chemical structure; salts of acids or bases represent the class of drugs having the best chance of attaining the degree of water solubility desired. Other compound classes, either neutral molecules or very weak acid and bases which cannot be solubilized in water within the desired pH range, may require the use of nonaqueous solvents. A list of such solvents used for solubility studies as well as eventual use in products is shown in Table 5.

1. Solubility Measurement

The analytical method used in obtaining solubility measurements may vary according to the drug moiety. If the drug's structure has unsaturated conjugation, enabling it to absorb visible or ultraviolet light, spectrophotometric analysis can be performed. A predetermined excess of drug is placed into suitable ampuls (or flasks) containing a small volume (2 to 5 ml) for each solvent tested. The ampuls are sealed and placed on a suitable shaker or rotator at a controlled temperature, (e.g., 25 or 37°C) for several days to attain equilibrium. At selected time intervals samples are withdrawn by an appropriate means (syringe, pipet), filtered through a small micrometer-size (example, 0.2 to 0.45 μm) filter, and analyzed for drug in solution using the appropriate ultraviolet or visible assay methodology. For example, the absorbance is read versus a solvent blank at a predetermined wavelength. Using the appropriate Beer's law reference curve as shown in Figure 10, the concentration is either estimated from the curve or can be calculated using a previously determined molecular absorptivity.

Solubility determination of compounds that do not absorb ultraviolet or visible light can be attempted by transferring filtered aliquot solutions onto previously tared weighing pans, evaporating the solvent, and drying to constant weight under low-temperature conditions.

Due to limits in the amount of new drugs available at the first stages of pre-formulation studies, it is sufficient to determine approximate solubility values for highly soluble compounds. In such cases a minimal volume of solvent is used and fixed amounts of drug added (i.e., 150 mg to 1 ml of solvent). Should this still yield an unsaturated solution, a value (e.g., >15%) will be sufficient to denote high solubility at this stage. Equilibrium solubility can be determined when more compound is available, if important for a particular solvent.

It is also very important to run solubility determinations at refrigeration temperature (2 to 8°C) using solvents demonstrating a high potential for use in formulation studies. This is done to establish the range of concentration usable within the range 2 to 25°C without risking saturation and crystal growth during stability studies.

2. pH-Solubility Profile

Compounds with either acidic or basic functionality will show differences in solubility characteristics with changes in solution pH in accord with their ionization constants. These differences are often large and important in attaining the concentrations desired for formulations. pH-Solubility profiles can be established by running equilibrium solubility experiments within the range 3 to 4 pH units on both sides of the pK_a or pK_a'.

The relationship between solubility of an acidic drug and pH can be defined with respect to its pK_a using Equation (5):

$$pH = pK_a + \log \frac{[C_s]}{[C_a]} \tag{5}$$

where

pK_a = negative logarithm of the ionization constant of the acid

$[C_s]$ = molar concentration of salt form in water

$[C_a]$ = molar concentration of free acid in water

Knowing the pK_a, $[C_a]$, and pH, the total amount of drug that can be solubilized in water at that pH can be calculated.

Thus total solubility S_t of a weak acid is given by Equation (6).

$$S_t = [C_a] + [C_s] \tag{6}$$

The analogous equation can be developed for weak bases, as shown in Equation (7).

$$St = [C_b] + [C_s] \tag{7}$$

Using a related approach [23], excess drug is added to a beaker of distilled water and the resulting suspension stirred continuously at constant temperature. At selected time intervals small increments of acid or base are added. After a constant pH is attained, an aliquot of the suspension is filtered, assayed, and the pH recorded. This is repeated until the pH range desired is covered. The data are presented in the form of solubility as a function of pH. This procedure is particularly useful with relatively insoluble acids or bases that do not undergo rapid hydrolysis and when very limited amounts of drug are available.

3. Methods of Improving Inherent Solubility

Occasions often arise when a drug's inherently low water solubility does not meet the solution concentration desired. Various approaches used to address this problem include salt formation, prodrug design, complexation, particle size reduction, addition of a cosolvent, and use of surface-active agents. Several of these approaches will be reviewed using illustrative examples.

Salt Formation. The compound α-(2-piperidyl)β-3, 6-bis(trifluoromethyl)-9-phenanthrenemethanol(I), an antimalarial agent, and its hydrochloride salt are both only slightly soluble in water, as shown in Table 6. To improve the aqueous solubility of the base, various organic acid salts were prepared. Results presented indicate that a significant increase in solubility can be achieved with a proper choice of the salt form (e.g., the lactate salt is approximately 200 times as soluble as the hydrochloride salt). This enhanced aqueous solubility was attributed in part to the decrease in crystal lattice energy as indicated by a reduction in melting point be-

I

tween the hydrochloride salt and the lactate salt. If a particular salt form cannot
be isolated due to its very high solubility, the same end result (i.e., desired aqueous solubility) can be achieved by in situ salt formation. This is accomplished by
using an appropriate acid or base to adjust the pH while formulating the drug product
solution. Various salt forms of use in pharmaceuticals, including parenterals, has
been reviewed [24].

Cosolvents. Cosolvents are used to solubilize a drug substance when its aqueous
solubility alone is insufficient to achieve the desired level. Cosolvents used in some
commercially available products are listed in Table 7. Phenobarbital is a classical
example of a case where a cosolvent approach has been used to achieve a significant
increase in solubility [27]. These investigators studied the solubility of phenobarbital
in water, alcohol, glycerin, and various combinations. Phenobarbital was found to
be relatively insoluble in water and glycerin but has good solubility in 100% alcohol.
Solubility in alcohol is further increased by addition of glycerin; solubility in 100%
alcohol is 12.3%, whereas solubility in an 80:20 alcohol-glycerin mixture is 16.3%.
A summary of these investigators' results is presented in graphic form in Figure 11.

Table 6 Apparent Solubilities and Melting Points of the Salt Form of I

Salt form	Melting point ($^\circ$C)	Apparent solubility[a]
Hydrochloride	331	12-15 mg liter^{-1}
Free base (I)	215	7-8 mg liter^{-1}
dl-Lactate	172 dec.	1.8-1.9 g liter^{-1}
l-Lactate	192-193 dec.	0.9-0.95 g liter^{-1}
2-Hydroxyethane-1-sulfonate	250-252 dec.	0.62 g liter^{-1}
Methanesulfonate	290 dec.	0.3 g liter^{-1}
Sulfate	270 dec.	20 mg liter^{-1}

[a]At 25°C in water.
Source: Ref. 24

Table 7 Some Parenteral Products Containing Cosolvents

Trade name	Manufacturer	General name	Cosolvent composition
Dramamine	Searle	Dimenhydrinate	50% propylene glycol
Apresoline	Ciba	Hydralazine HCl	10% propylene glycol
MVI	USV	Multivitamin infusion	30% propylene glycol
Nembutal	Abbott	Phenobarbital sodium	10% ethanol, 40% propylene glycol
Luminal	Winthrop	Pentobarbital sodium	67.8% propylene glycol
Dilantin	Parke-Davis	Phenytoin sodium	10% ethanol, 40% propylene glycol
DHE 45	Sandoz	Dihydroergotamine mesylate	6.1% ethanol, 15% glycerin
Cedilanid	Sandoz	Deslanoside	9.8% ethanol, 15% glycerin
Robaxin	Robbins	Methocarbamol	50% polyethylene glycol
Serpasil	Ciba	Reserpine	10% dimethylacetamide, 50% polyethylene glycol
Ativan	Wyeth	Lorazepam	80% propylene glycol, 20% polyethylene glycol
Librium	Roche	Chlordiazepoxide	20% propylene glycol
Valium	Roche	Diazepam	10% ethanol, 40% propylene glycol
Lanoxin	Burroughs Wellcome	Digoxin	10% ethanol, 40% propylene glycol

Source: Ref. 26

In another example, solubilization of a salt of the antimalarial agent (I), cited previously, was also accomplished using cosolvents [25], as shown in Table 8.

Complexation. Complexation is another means of improving the aqueous solubility of insoluble compounds. It can be described as shown in Equation (8).

$$n[D]_s + m[L]_s \rightleftharpoons [D_n:L_m]_s \tag{8}$$

where

$[D]_s$ = concentration of drug in solution

$[L]_s$ = concentration of ligand in solution

$[D_n:L_m]_s$ = concentration of (drug:ligand) complex in solution

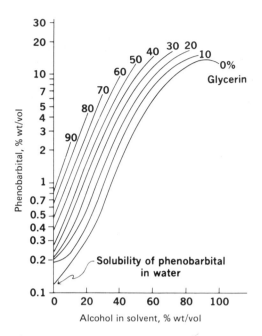

Figure 11 Solubility (g/100 ml) phenobarbitol in mixtures of water, alcohol, and glycerin. Adapted by Ref. 28 from original data of Ref. 27.

A complex is an entity formed when two molecules, such as a drug and a solubilizing agent (ligand), are held together by weak forces (e.g., dipole-dipole interaction or hydrogen bonding). For complex formation to occur, drug and ligand molecules should be able to donate or accept a pair of electrons. Complex formation between the drug benzocaine and ligand caffeine can be attributed to the dipole-dipole interaction between a partial negative charge on carboxyl oxygen of benzocaine and a

Table 8 Apparent Solubility of 2-Hydroxyethane-1-sulfonate Salt of Antimalarial Agent I at 25°C in Commonly Used Parenteral Vehicles

Vehicle	Apparent solubility (g liter^{-1})
20% Ethanol-20% glycerin in water	1.9
20% Propylene glycol-5% ethanol in water	0.6
10% Dextrose in Water	0.75

Source: Ref. 24

partial positive charge on nitrogen of caffeine, as shown in the following structures:

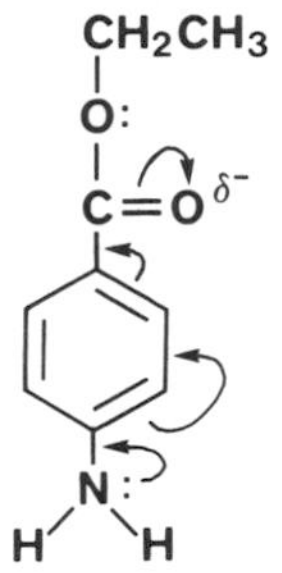

Benzocaine 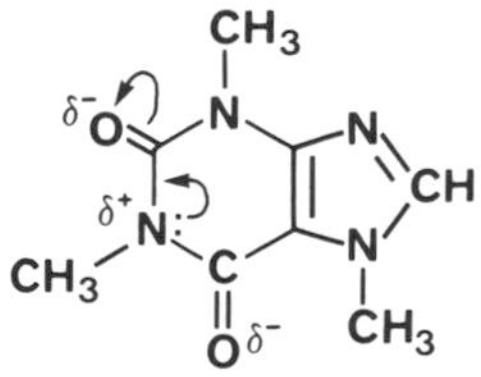   Caffeine

Complex formation between drug substrate and potential ligand can be studied using the phase solubility technique [29]. A constant amount of drug substance is placed into various screw-cap vials. The vials are numbered and increasing volumes of a stock solution of complexing agent are added. All vials are brought to constant final volume with the solvent. The vials are sealed and shaken in a water bath at a constant temperature. Following equilibration, the contents of the vials are filtered and the total concentration of the drug in solution is determined using an appropriate assay procedure. The data are plotted as concentration of drug in solution versus the concentration of complexing agent in solution.

Application to a parenteral formulation was demonstrated when the apparent solubility of hexamethylmelamine (an anticancer agent) was increased as much as 90-fold via complexation with gentisate ion [30]. This increased solubility allowed evaluation of the anticancer agent as an injectable product at a desired pH. The solubility of hexamethylmelamine as a function of gentisate ion concentration is shown in Figure 12. When the complexation approach is used, identification of a pharmaceutically and physicologically acceptable ligand may not be a simple task.

Prodrug Approach. The solubility characteristics of a drug can be altered via chemical modification. This has been referred to as a prodrug approach. The term prodrug was first used by Albert [31] and was defined as a compound that undergoes biotransformation prior to eliciting a pharmacological response. The antiviral agent ara-A (see structure below) has a low aqueous solubility (approxi-

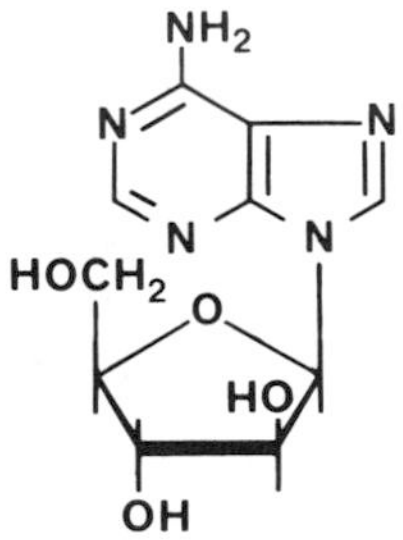

ara-A 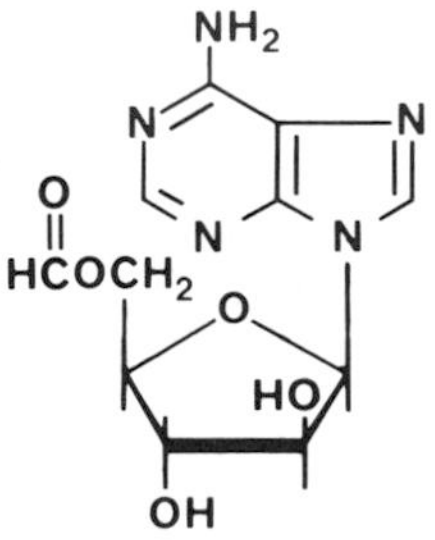   ara-A-5'-formate mately 0.002 M) at 25°C. The formate ester of ara-A (see structure below) was reported to be 66 times more soluble in water than was ara-A [32].

In another example [33] the compound metronidazole, with only 10 mg ml^{-1} solubility in water, was solubilized to the order of approximately 500 mg ml^{-1} under similar conditions by synthesizing the water-soluble prodrug metronidazole phosphate, enabling parenteral administration of this compound (structures shown below). Additional examples of this approach to enhance aqueous solubility of various medicinal agents are presented in Table 9.

J. Partition Coefficient

The partition coefficient P is a measure of lipophilicity of a compound. It is measured by determining the equilibrium concentration of a drug in an aqueous phase (generally water) and an oil phase (generally octanol or chloroform) held in contact with each other at a constant temperature and is expressed as shown in Equation (9).

$$P = \frac{[C_{oil}]}{[C_{water}]} \qquad (9)$$

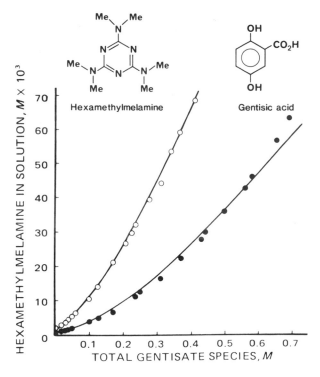

Figure 12 Solubility of hexamethylmelamine in aqueous solution at pH 4.5 (○, actual) and pH 5.0 (●, calculated) at 25°C as a function of gentisic acid species added.

Metronidazole

Metronidazole Phosphate
Dipotassium Salt

Since biological membranes are lipoidal in nature, they play a major role in drug transport. The ability of a drug molecule to cross a membrane at an absorption site can be related to the oil-water partition coefficient of the drug.

In case of parenteral emulsions, P values may provide an indication of the duration of activity that a drug is likely to achieve. If the partition coefficient is high (in favor of the lipid phase), a depot effect can be expected for the drug dissolved in the oil phase. Partition coefficient data are also useful for analytical separations required for drug assay.

Table 9 Water-Soluble Prodrugs of Sparingly Soluble Drugs

Prodrug	Parent drug
Oxazepam sodium succinate	Oxazepam
Prednisolone sodium succinate	Prednisolone
Prednisolone disodium phosphate	Prednisolone
Prednisolone N, N-dimethyl-glycinate	Prednisolone
Prednisolone m-benzoylsulfonic acid	Prednisolone
Hydrocortisone	
Bethamethasone	
Methylprednisole	Parent corticosteroids
Dexamethasone (all as their sodium succinates or disodium phosphates)	
Δ'-Tetrahydrocanabinol as various amino acid esters	Δ'-Tetrahydrocanabinol
Δ'-Tetrahydrocanabinol disodium phosphate	Δ'-Tetrahydrocanabinol

Source: Modified from Ref. 34.

K. Ionization Constant

The ionization constant provides information about the solubility dependence of the compound on the pH of the formulation, as discussed previously. The pK_a is generally determined by potentiometric pH titration or by pH-solubility analysis using Equation (2). An example of the potentiometric titration of tris(hydroxymethyl) aminomethane (TRIS), a buffer used as an analytical reference standard as well as a pharmaceutical salt-former, is shown in Figure 13. As shown by the dashed line, end-point detection can be made by inspection or more objectively by a first derivative plot. Both the partition coefficient and ionization constant are discussed in greater detail in Chapter 3.

L. Optical Activity

Molecules capable of rotating a beam of plane-polarized light are termed optically active. When a substance turns the beam of light to the right or clockwise by an angle α, the substance is said to be dextrorotatory. Conversely, a substance that

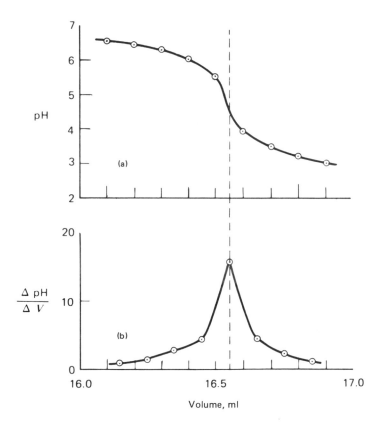

Figure 13 (a) Potentiometric titration plot of 1.816 meq TRIS with HCl at 20°C. (b) First derivative plot. (From Ref. 35.)

rotates plane-polarized light counterclockwise is levorotatory. Other designations, d or (+) and l or (-), are used to indicate dextrorotatory and levorotatory, respectively. The intensity of optical rotation of a compound can be expressed in two different but related ways. One is by the specific rotation $[\alpha]$ given by Equation (10).

$$[\alpha]_{\lambda}^{t} = \frac{100\,\alpha}{l\,c} \tag{10}$$

where

α = observed rotation, deg

c = solute concentration, g/100 ml

l = path length,

t = temperature

λ = wavelength

Alternatively, to compare optical rotation on a molecular basis, Equation (11) is used:

$$[M]_{\lambda}^{t} = \frac{\alpha \times mol\ wt}{l\ c} \tag{11}$$

where $[M]^{t}$ is the molecular rotation. Optical rotation is measured either using a light of fixed wavelength, such as the sodium D line (589.2 nm) with polarimeters, or by varying the wavelength as done with units measuring optical rotatory dispersion (ORD).

An asymmetric carbon atom is one that has four different atoms or groups bonded to it. An example is shown below for epinephrine. During chemical synthesis a 50:50 mixture of both the d and l forms is obtained and since they have the same specific optical rotation $[\alpha]$, the resulting molecule may show a zero specific rotation. The form that is more biologically active is selected for development. In the case of epinephrine, only the l form is an active vasoconstrictor. Because of this, an equal mixture of d and l would be 50% as potent and the d form, which in this example is totally inactive.

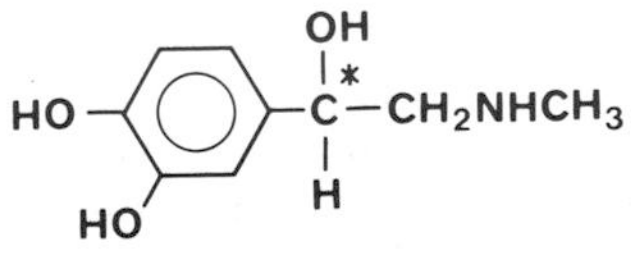

HO—⟨◯⟩—$\overset{\displaystyle OH}{\underset{\displaystyle H}{\overset{|}{\underset{|}{C}}}}$*—CH₂NHCH₃

Epinephrine

Considering the above, when working with an optically active compound during preformulation studies, it is essential to monitor optical rotation since chemical assay alone will not always coincide with biological activity. Examples of optically active pharmaceutical compounds used in parenterals are listed in Table 10.

Table 10 Specific Rotations of Some Optically Active Compounds
Used in Parenterals

Compound	$[\alpha]D$	Temp. (°C)	c	Solvent
L-Ascorbic acid	+48	23	1	Methanol
Benzylpenicillin	+269	20	0.6	Methanol
Codeine	-112	15	2	Chloroform
Epinephrine	-52	25	5	0.5 N HCl
Kanamycin	+121	23	1	Water
Morphine	+132	25	1	Methanol

Source: Adapted from Ref. 36.

II. ACCELERATED STABILITY EVALUATION

A. Drug Substance

Various stress tests are performed on solid and solution samples to establish the
effect of heat, light, oxygen, and pH on drug substance stability.

1. Heat Stability

Heat stability of a drug substance in solution will have a major influence on the
marketable physical form of the injectable product as well as processing parameters
allowable. Drugs that are not stable in solution require refrigerated storage or lyophilization. Lyophilized products are limited to constitution and use within a short
period of time, whereas the need for refrigerated storage is economically undesirable and a marketing disadvantage unless completely justifiable.

A typical drug substance heat-stability program may be carried out as follows.
Accurately weighed samples of the drug substance are placed into appropriate containers such as glass ampuls. The following are typical variations studied; (1) drug
substance as is, (2) drug substance with approximately 5% moisture added as water,
(3) drug equilibrated at 75% relative humidity, and (4) overlaying the headspace of
the ampul with nitrogen or argon versus air prior to sealing.

The ampuls are sealed and placed at several temperature conditions and tested
according to a typical scheme shown in Table 11. The investigator must select times
and conditions so as best to utilize available information (if any) concerning projected
stability. Refrigeration and room-temperature samples serve as controls for the
assay procedure and are often tested only if losses are observed at higher temperatures.

2. Light Stability

The effect of light on the physical and chemical stability of a drug is examined
to determine whether light protection is required for the drug substance alone as
well as in the final dosage formulation. Stability changes can occur in the form of

Table 11 Typical Short-Term Accelerated Stability Program

Temperature (°C)	Duration[a] (weeks)			
	1	2	4	8
Refrigeration	(x)	(x)	(x)	(x)
Room temperature	(x)	(x)	(x)	(x)
55	x	x	x	x
75	x	x	x	x
95	x	x		

[a]Parentheses indicate samples pulled but not assayed.

color change, precipitation, pH shift, or decomposition. Although there are no proven methods for extrapolating accelerated light stability data to normal lighting conditions, the detrimental effect of light can usually be observed during such studies, particularly when a compound is very light sensitive.

Samples of drug substance are placed in an open petri dish to expose a large surface. Controls are placed in a light-resistant container such as amber glass, foil wrapped, or in a cardboard box. A solution or suspension of drug is packaged in both clear and light-protected ampuls. These samples are placed into a well-vented temperature-monitored light cabinet of specified lumens (e.g., 500 footcandles) and exposed for 4 weeks, with weekly examinations. If a perceptible color change, pH shift, or precipitation occurs in solid or solution in clear ampuls, the compound can be considered potentially light sensitive and should be handled accordingly. Significant changes may become a limitation to the physical stability of the drug in the dry state or in the formulation even if chemical stability is not significantly affected.

3. Effect of Oxygen

To study the effect of oxygen on a drug substance as well as a solution of drug substance, appropriate samples are placed into ampuls. Prior to sealing, the headspace is evacuated and purged with an inert gas such as argon or nitrogen. Air headspace samples are used as positive controls. Samples are placed at 75°C for 1 week and analyzed. The effect of oxidation is most noticable when using smaller amounts of drug. Significant oxidation may be evident by potency loss, color change, or both.

Following are general methods used to reduce or eliminate oxidation of parenterals during preformulation experiments:

1. Purging the solution or suspension and container headspace with an inert gas such as nitrogen or argon
2. Use of antioxidants such as sodium bisulfite, sodium sulfite, and sodium formaldehyde sulfoxylate
3. Use of complexing agents such as edetate disodium, which is known to complex trace metal ions capable of accelerating oxidative reactions
4. Use of well-sealed containers such as ampuls and avoiding the use of multiple-dose vials

4. pH–Stability Profile

A pH–stability profile experiment is performed with solution samples between pH 2 and 12 at a selected elevated temperature. Analytically prepared solutions, close to the desired product concentration (should it be known), are prepared using buffer solutions within the selected pH range and filled into ampuls. The samples are placed into a constant–temperature bath or oven and maintained at specific temperatures between 55 and 95°C for 2 weeks. Here again the air headspace of ampuls is replaced with nitrogen or argon to avoid any oxidative effects.

At preselected preset intervals, samples are quenched and assayed by a procedure that separates the parent drug from degradation product(s). The data are plotted on rectilinear paper as shown in Figure 14. The pH range of maximum stability is usually evident by inspection. This would be the range recommended for formulation development.

This procedure may be used for samples remaining in solution over the pH range studied. An accurate assessment of pH stability for suspensions that may form within the pH range studied is not possible since only the fraction of drug in solution is able to undergo reaction. If the fraction of drug in solution is very small and the approach to equilibrium solubility is slow, the compound could appear more stable than expected. For example, an amine hydrochloride with a pk_a value of 5 in a pH 8 solution would have only 1 part in solution as the more soluble protonated species, whereas 999 parts would exist as the less soluble free base.

5. Autoclaving Studies

Since autoclaving is a preferred means of achieving the sterility of solutions, an early determination of stability to autoclaving should be made. Ampuls containing solutions at the optimum pH range previously established are exposed to autoclaving conditions of 121°C at 30 psig for 20, 30, 45, and 90 min. The higher time points are used in an attempt to force degradation. Assay data are recorded together with evaluation of change in color, pH, and particulate matter content.

6. General Analysis Methods

Thin–layer chromatography (TLC) has been classically used for analysis of preformulation experiments. A more rapid technique, high–performance liquid chromatography (HPLC), has become popular, particularly with large numbers of samples because of the capability of automatic sampling. With TLC, the spot representing starting substance is quantitatively removed from the plate and eluted with the appropriate solvent. If the compound absorbs ultraviolet or visible light, an absorbance reading is taken versus the standard at the appropriate wavelength.

B. Drug–Excipient Compatibility

One of the objectives of a preformulation study is to identify compatible, potentially useful pharmaceutical excipients so that a stable formulation can be developed quickly. Generally, several binary mixtures of a drug and various excipients, such as buffering agents, antioxidants, chelating agents, and preservatives, are prepared and subjected to accelerated studies. Excipients exhibiting physical and chemical compatibility are subsequently recommended for formulation development. A major drawback of this approach is that it does not take into account interactions among several excipients that may constitute the final formulation. Two statistical designs

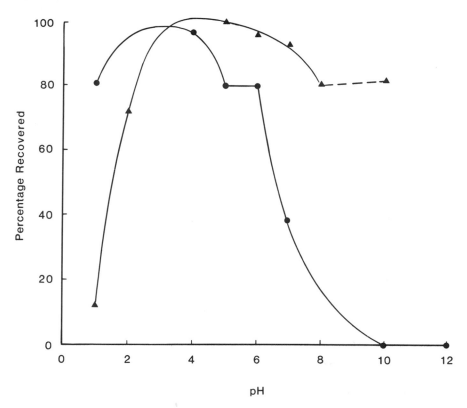

Figure 14 Typical accelerated pH stability profile for solutions of two experimental compounds. Conditions: ●, 1 week at 75°C; ▲, 8 days at 95°C. The dashed line indicates the drug was partially in suspension between pH 8 and 10.

described in this section are particularly useful for screening various excipients and conditions prior to selection of a formulation.

1. Plackett-Burman Design

A Plackett-Burman design is composed of a specific fraction of the 2^p factorial design. These designs allow determination of the effect of variables with a minimum number of experiments (e.g., the effects of up to 12 variables can be determined with only 20 experiments). However, these designs do not yield estimates of the extent or type of interaction between variables. Several advantages of utilizing factorial designs in preformulation studies are:

1. Efficiency increases.
2. Each variable is screened at two levels.
3. Each variable is screened in the presence of all other variables, as opposed to conventional binary mixtures.
4. Experiments are self-contained and provide enough data to include an estimate of variability.
5. The number of experiments usually gets larger and larger when working with one variable at a time, whereas factorial design treatment results in narrowing the field.

Table 12   Twelve-Run Plackett-Burman Design

Trial	X_1	X_2	X_3	X_4	X_5	X_6	X_7	X_8	X_9	X_{10}	X_{11}	Response, Y
1	+	+	−	+	+	+	−	−	−	+	−	
2	+	−	+	+	+	−	−	−	+	−	+	
3	−	+	+	+	−	−	−	+	−	+	+	
4	+	+	+	−	−	−	+	−	+	+	−	
5	+	+	−	−	−	+	−	+	+	−	+	
6	+	−	−	−	+	−	+	+	−	+	+	
7	−	−	−	+	−	+	+	−	+	+	+	
8	−	−	+	−	+	+	−	+	+	+	−	
9	−	+	−	+	+	−	+	+	+	−	−	
10	+	−	+	+	−	+	+	+	−	−	−	
11	−	+	+	−	+	+	+	−	−	−	+	
12	−	−	−	−	−	−	−	−	−	−	−	

[a]See the text for an explanation of + and −.
Source: Ref. 37.

The effect of variables such as light, oxygen, buffering agents, tonicity adjusting agents, antioxidants, chelating agents, surface-active agents, and various rubber closure formulations, among others, on the chemical stability of a drug solution or suspension can be quickly screened using factorial design. Tables 12 and 13 provide Plackett-Burman designs for up to 6 and 12 variable screening studies, respectively. X_1, X_2, X_3, ..., X_n are the variables under investigation. Y is the measured response (e.g., solubility or percent potency assay). A + sign represents the presence of a variable at the high level, and - sign represents the presence of a variable at the low level [e.g., + could be 0.06 mg ml^{-1} ethylenediaminetetraacetic acid (EDTA) and - could be 0.01 mg ml^{-1} EDTA]. Alternatively, + could designate a sample exposed to light and - could be the sample protected from light. Thus, for a six-variable screening experiment, any six columns are chosen as six variables (e.g., X_1 to X_6) (see Table 12).

Twelve mixtures are prepared as described in Table 12, containing high and low levels of six variables plus a constant amount of drug. These samples (generally in ampuls) are sealed and then exposed to a reasonably high temperature for a specific period of time (e.g., 2 weeks at 75°C). At the end of the experiment all 12 samples are analyzed for the drug remaining, using an appropriate assay procedure that can separate drug from the mixture. It is desirable to use the entire sample for assay to reduce experimental error.

After 12 samples are analyzed, Y values (percent parent compound remaining, in this case) for each sample are recorded as "percent recovery," as in Table 14. The Y values for each column when the variable was + are added and recorded as "sum +." Similarly, Y values for each column when the variable was - are added and recorded as "sum -." If the variable has no effect on measured Y, then sum + must equal sum -. To measure the average effect of each variable X on the response Y, the difference between sum + and sum - is divided by the number of times each variable was + (six in this case). Thus the average effect of variable X_2 on response Y is calculated to be

$$\frac{502 - 486}{6} = \frac{16}{6} = 2.7$$

The effect of unassigned variables X_7 through X_{11} (in this case) are used to calculate experimental error. This experimental error estimate is then used to calculate a minimum significant factor effect E_{ms}. In this instance, any effect having an absolute value greater than the minimum significant effect is considered to be statistically significant on the stability of drug.

To calculate the minimum significant factor effect E_{ms}, square each of the unassigned effects (i.e., for variables X_7 to X_{11} in this case), add them together, divide by the number of unassigned variables (i.e., 5 in this case), and take the square root. This value is called the standard deviation of the factor effect, S_{FE}. Finally, $E_{ms} = t \cdot S_{FE}$. As t has degrees of freedom equal to the number of unused variables (five in this example), with 5 degrees of freedom it is desirable to choose a t value at the 90% confidence level. Any effect value greater than E_{ms} is statistically significant. Thus by calculation,

$$S_{FE}^2 = \frac{(-3.7)^2 + (-2.0)^2 + (0.33)^2 + (2.7)^2 + (5)^2}{5}$$

$$S_{FE} = \sqrt{10.02} = 3.16$$

$$E_{ms} = t \cdot S_{FE} = (2.02)(3.16) = 6.4$$

Where the t value has been obtained from Student's t tables at 90% confidence limits.

As shown in Table 14, variable X_6 (oxygen in this case) has a significant destablizing effect on the drug under investigation, whereas X_1, X_2, X_3, X_4, and X_5 have no significant effect on drug stability. Thus, using a 12-mixture experiment for 2 weeks at 75°C, variables affecting stability of the drug were determined. This was identified in the presence of all other variables under investigation, as opposed to studies of binary mixtures. Additionally, this was carried out in a well-designed experiment, the results of which can be supported with statistical significance.

2. 2 X 3 Factorial Design

When only three variables are to be evaluated, (e.g., two buffers, two pH values, and two antioxidants), an experimental design that can screen these variables as well as detect possible interactions among these variables is more useful. Such a design is often referred to as a 2 X 3 factorial design and is shown in Table 15.

Thus, by preparing eight solutions as described in Table 15 and subjecting these eight solutions to appropriate testing (e.g., 4 weeks at 55°C, etc.), followed by analysis for drug concentration, this three-variable system would be thoroughly evaluated while answering all stability questions related to these three variables.

Table 13 Twenty-Run Plackett-Burman Design

Trial	X_1	X_2	X_3	X_4	X_5	X_6	X_7	X_8	X_9	X_{10}	X_{11}	X_{12}	X_{13}	X_{14}	X_{15}	X_{16}	X_{17}	X_{18}	X_{19}
										Variable[a]									
1	+	+	−	−	+	+	+	+	−	+	−	+	−	−	−	−	+	+	−
2	+	−	−	+	+	+	+	−	+	−	+	−	−	−	−	+	+	−	+
3	−	−	+	+	+	+	−	+	−	+	−	−	−	−	+	+	−	+	+
4	−	+	+	+	+	−	+	−	+	−	−	−	−	+	+	−	+	+	−
5	+	+	+	−	−	+	−	+	−	−	−	−	+	+	−	+	+	−	−
6	+	+	+	+	+	−	+	−	−	−	−	+	+	−	+	+	−	−	+
7	+	+	−	+	−	+	−	−	−	−	+	+	−	+	+	−	−	+	+
8	+	−	+	−	+	−	−	−	−	+	+	−	+	+	−	−	+	+	+
9	−	+	−	+	−	−	−	−	+	+	−	+	+	−	−	+	+	+	+

10	11	12	13	14	15	16	17	18	19	20
–	+	–	+	–	–	–	–	+	+	–
+	–	+	–	+	–	–	–	–	+	–
+	+	–	+	–	+	–	–	–	–	–
+	+	+	–	+	–	+	–	–	–	–
+	+	+	+	–	+	–	+	–	–	–
–	+	+	+	+	–	+	–	+	–	–
–	–	+	+	+	+	–	+	–	+	–
+	–	–	+	+	+	+	–	+	–	–
+	+	–	–	+	+	+	+	–	+	–
–	+	+	–	–	+	+	+	+	–	–
+	–	+	+	–	–	+	+	+	+	–
+	+	–	+	+	–	–	+	+	+	–
–	+	+	–	+	+	–	–	+	+	–
–	–	+	+	–	+	+	–	–	+	–
–	–	–	+	+	–	+	+	–	–	–
–	–	–	–	+	+	–	+	+	–	–
+	–	–	–	–	+	+	–	+	+	–
–	+	–	–	–	–	+	+	–	+	–
+	–	+	–	–	–	–	+	+	–	–

aSee the text for an explanation of + and –.
Source: Ref. 37.

Table 14 Plackett–Burman Design to Study Effects of Excipients on the Stability of Compound X after 2 Weeks of Storage at 75°C

Trial	Amount of mixture drug (mg)	X_1	X_2	X_3	X_4	X_5	X_6	X_7	X_8	X_9	X_{10}	X_{11}	Percent Recovery
						Variable[a]							
1	50	+	+	−	+	+	+	−	−	−	+	−	83
2	50	+	−	+	+	+	−	−	−	+	−	+	87
3	50	−	+	+	+	−	−	−	+	−	+	+	89
4	50	+	+	+	−	−	−	+	−	+	+	−	84
5	50	+	+	−	−	+	+	−	+	+	−	+	84
6	50	+	−	−	+	−	−	+	+	−	+	+	91
7	50	−	−	+	−	+	+	+	−	+	+	+	81
8	50	−	−	−	+	+	+	−	+	+	+	−	74
9	50	−	+	−	+	+	−	+	+	+	−	−	85
10	50	+	−	+	+	−	+	+	+	−	−	−	65
11	50	−	+	+	−	+	+	+	−	−	−	+	77
12	50	−	−	−	−	−	−	−	−	−	−	−	88
Sum +:		494	502	476	490	497	464	483	488	495	502	509	
Sum −:		494	486	512	498	491	524	505	500	493	486	479	
Average effect:		0.0	2.7	−6.0[c]	−1.3	1.0	−10.0[b]	−3.7	−2.0	0.33	2.7	5.0	

[a] See the text for an explanation of + and −.
[b] Significant effect.
[c] Borderline effect.

Table 15 2 X 3 Factorial Design

	pH = a		pH = b	
	Buffer A	Buffer B	Buffer A	Buffer B
Antioxidant 1	x	x	x	x
Antioxidant 2	x	x	x	x

Such a study design and results should increase the level of confidence in selecting appropriate components for a formulation.

III. GENERAL MODES OF DRUG DEGRADATION

Various functional groups within a molecule may be prone to a specific type of reactivity under appropriate conditions. Although not limited to parenteral drug moieties, the conditions necessary for degradation are generally more pronounced when drugs are in solution or in suspension. Developing an astute knowledge of basic organic chemical reactions will help the preformulation investigator to anticipate, avoid, or at least minimize potential reactions for the particular molecule under investigation. Described next are examples of reactions that are commonly encountered.

A. Hydrolysis

This form of degradation is one of the most common to occur in pharmaceuticals, probably because of the numerous types of structures capable of undergoing hydrolysis. Amongst these are esters, sugars, amides, lactones, nitriles, salts of weak acids or weak bases, thioesters, polymeric materials, and thiolhalides. Typical examples of well-known drugs capable of undergoing hydrolysis are cefoxitin sodium, procaine hydrochloride, chlorothiazide, sodium phenobarbital, and benzylpenicillin G. Stabilization of such systems must be approached by determining conditions of optimum stability, such as pH, ionic strength, noncatalyzing buffer species selection, and complexing agents. In a classical example, the hydrolysis of procaine hydrochloride was studied [38] and found to be catalyzed by hydroxyl ion. The general hydrolysis reaction for procaine is shown in Equation (12).

$$(12)$$

B. Oxidation

This mode of degradation can be considered of equal importance to hydrolysis for parenteral solutions. Significant oxidative discoloration can take place without major detectable chemical loss [4]. Oxidation that takes place under mild conditions and is basically due to molecular oxygen is called autoxidation.

Several types of oxidation are possible. The electrochemical definition of oxidation is the loss of electrons. Thus the conversion of ferrous to ferric ion is an oxidation reaction as shown in Equation (13).

$$Fe^{2+} \rightleftharpoons Fe^{3+} + e^-$$

(13)

The more common form of oxidation of organic molecules is the addition of an oxygen atom to the molecule such as the oxidation of phenol, a colorless, commonly used preservative agent to p-benzoquinone, a bright yellow compound. Furthermore, p-benzoquinone forms a brilliant red addition product with phenol known as phenoquinone [39]. These reactions are shown in Equations (14) and (15).

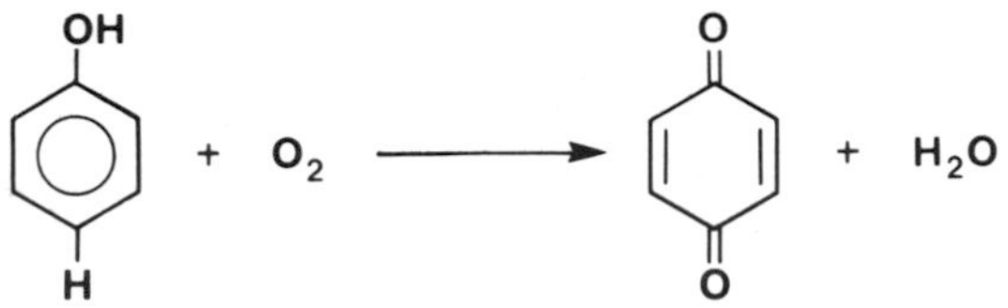

(14)

$$C_6H_4O_2 + 2C_6H_5OH \longrightarrow C_6H_4O_2 \cdot 2C_6H_5OH$$

(15)

Oxidation occurs in aqueous and nonaqueous media. The most common functional groups involved are aldehydes, amines, sulfur-containing compounds, alcohols, phenols, unsaturated compounds, fatty acids, and sugars. Other representative examples of drugs that undergo oxidation are ascorbic acid, epinephrine, and benzyl alcohol.

C. Decarboxylation

This refers to the loss of carbon dioxide from a chemical substance such as a carboxylic acid. Decarboxylation of an acid RCOOH should occur most readily if within the R group there is a strongly electron attracting substituent such as —phenyl, —NO_2, —CCl_3, —$C\equiv N$, or —$\overset{|}{C}=O$ [40]. This type of reaction is not as common as those discussed and though a large percentage of decarboxylations occur under high-temperature conditions near or above their melting points, some do occur in dilute solution under mild conditions. A classical example is the decarboxylation of p-aminosalicylic acid [40] shown in Equation (16). In this case decarboxylation was shown to occur in dilute acid solution at 40°C.

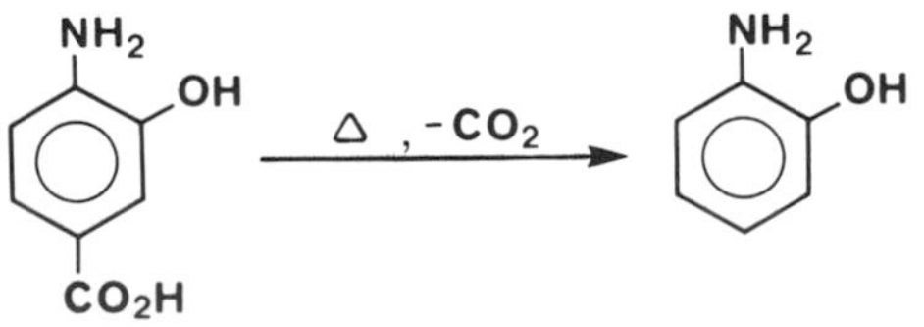

(16)

D. Racemization

An optically active compound undergoes racemization when its optical rotation changes without structural change. The optical pairs or enantiomorphs [i.e., dextrorotatory (+) or levorotatory (-) forms] may possess different degrees of physiologic action and a change can result in reduced or lost therapeutic effect. An example of such situations is the acid-catalyzed racemization of epinephrine [42]. The general equation for racemization of 1-epinephrine is shown in Equation (17).

$$\text{levo } (-)\text{ form} \qquad\qquad\qquad \text{racemic } (\pm)\text{ form} \tag{17}$$

E. Acylation

Reversible acylation of primary amines such as aniline by anhydride forms of dicarboxylic acids such as citric, succinic, and tartaric acid have been reported [43,44]. Under conditions of high temperature (i.e., 95°C and at solution pH values of 4 to 5, aniline was acylated by the anhydride species of tartaric acid, which have been shown to exist as reactive intermediates by recovery of significant amounts of acylated aniline [45]. A general case reaction is shown in Equation (18).

$$\tag{18}$$

The potential for this type of reaction to occur should be considered when using buffers of dicarboxylic acids during high-temperature pH profile studies. Any unexpected loss occurring at a pH utilizing a dicarboxylic acid buffer should be checked by repeating the experiment using an alternative buffer under the same conditions of pH and temperature.

F. Polymorphism

A substance capable of existing in more than one crystalline form is said to exhibit polymorphism. The form isolated at any given time may be influenced by the nature of the crystallizing solvent(s), as well as the process parameters of crystallization. A classical example of polymorphism found in nature, which highlights the physical and chemical differences that can exist between polymorphs, is that observed between hexagonal carbon graphite and cubic diamond.

The importance of polymorphism in pharmaceuticals is that each polymorph of a compound has a distinct crystalline structure and properties such as melting point, solubility, stability, density, hardness, and optical and electrical properties as well as vapor pressure [46]. The polymorphic forms possess higher potential energy with respect to the thermodynamically stable or lowest energy form. This potential energy can be released by several means. For pharmaceuticals, one important way is by going into solution. In some cases the potential energy may be sufficient for the compound to exhibit an apparent solubility greater than the more stable form. This is a nonequilibrium condition and eventually the drug in solution will revert to the less soluble or stable form [47].

If a suspension contains two polymorphs, the higher-energy form will have a tendency to go into solution and the lower-energy form may undergo crystal growth and agglomeration such as with cortisone acetate. The means of manufacturing one of five polymorphic forms of this compound led to a stable product [48]. Drug substance stability may also be different for amorphous and crystalline forms. The amorphous form of sodium and potassium penicillin G was shown to be unstable to dry heat, whereas the crystalline form was stable to heat for several hours [49].

The existence of polymorphs can be determined by several methods; among the most popular are the detection of differences in infrared spectra, differential thermal analysis, microscopy, and most explicitly by x-ray powder diffraction. In the latter case different crystal lattice forms yield distinctly different x-ray diffraction scattering patterns. Amorphous substances exhibit nondescript x-ray patterns. Such forms are generally more rapidly soluble since there are no crystal lattice forces required to be overcome by the solvent.

Polymorphic changes can play a significant role in development of a lyophilized product. The freeze-drying cycle selected may play a role in producing a particular type of crystal form. When lyophilizing cefazolin sodium [50] an amorphous product is produced when a standard lyophilization cycle is used followed by warming to remove the aqueous phase. If the frozen solution is warmed to its eutectic temperature and refrozen prior to final warm-up, a crystalline product results. It is likely that this freeze-warm-freeze cycle initiates crystal formation in the originally frozen amorphous form. Here again, amorphous form of the drug may not be as stable as the crystalline form [51, 52].

G. Solvate Formation

A drug may incorporate molecules of crystallization solvent within its crystal lattice, significantly altering physical and chemical properties important for development of an injectable dosage form. Thus it is important to determine at an early stage whether the drug substance exists as an anhydrous or solvated form. This is generally done by infrared analysis as well as weight-loss studies such as by thermogravimetric analysis described previously. The most important and prevalent class of solvates from a pharmaceutical point of view are hydrates. The hydrate form of a drug is more thermodynamically stable and commonly exhibits lower solubility [53] than the anhydrous form. Potential problems can therefore arise should an amorphous form in solution revert to a less soluble hydrate and precipitate. Similarly, the suspension of an anhydrous form could undergo transformation to the hydrate, causing a change in particle size characteristics.

In order to predict such phenomena it is useful to attempt recrystallization from hot water and allowing the saturated solution to cool gradually, whereas another solution is chilled rapidly. The crystals are then analyzed to determine whether a hydrate form exists. Organic solvates such as the pentanol solvate of succinylsulfathiazole [54] exhibits an eightfold increase in solubility compared to the stable hydrate. This increase in solubility could also cause problems if an aqueous solution is made at a concentration higher than that based on the solubility of the stable hydrate. In such a case, precipitation of the hydrate could occur.

Although the various functional group reactivities and physicochemical phenomena cited are not meant to be a complete listing of all possible reactions, they do represent a large percentage of those which may occur during preformulation investigations of new compounds. The important factor is that the preformulation investigator must consider all possible reactions based on those known for structurally similar compounds.

IV. PREFORMULATION SCREENING OF PARENTERAL PACKAGING COMPONENTS

One of the more difficult and often time-consuming requirements during parenteral product development is the selection of compatible packaging components, generally comprised of glass, elastomeric closures, and plastics. Although the dividing line between where preformulation stops and where formulation and package development studies begin may be defined differently among industrial organizations, preformulation work done toward package selection is often critical to the early smooth development and progression of a parenteral product. In many cases extension of expiration dates of parenteral products are limited to a physical incompatibility involving elastomeric closure and/or glass interaction with the formulation.

For example, the investigation for a compatible elastomeric closure and multiple-dose vial can be approached by screening studies initiated at a later stage of preformulation or, if need be, initially for those requiring the use of multiple-dose vials throughout the development program.

A. Closure Selection Process

Basic considerations for the selection of a compatible closure formulation are based on numerous factors. Those of high importance at the preformulation stage are physical and chemical compatibility of the closure with the formulation as well as the rate of water vapor permeability, oxygen permeability (if oxidation is a problem), sorption of active and preservative, level and type of extractives, pH change, color change, and particulate matter formation. These criteria as well as others have been reviewed [55] and presented as guidelines [56] for closure selection. The reactivity of the formulation and presence of certain excipients, such as preservatives, buffers, antioxidants, and chelating agents may influence the general type of elastomer required.

Several general properties of elastomeric closures useful for initial closure screening studies are:

1. Oxygen permeation through butyl rubber is almost 20 times less than natural rubber [55], and is therefore of choice in circumstances where oxidation is likely to cause color formation, color change, or chemical loss.
2. Swelling characteristics of neoprene in oil at 160°C is 7 to 10 times less than for natural rubber or butyl [57], therefore making neoprene a prime choice for oil products.
3. Butyl closures have been shown not to absorb the preservatives benzyl alcohol and methylparaben from solution, whereas natural rubber and neoprene absorbed approximately 10% after 12 weeks of storage at 60°C [58]. Significant loss of preservative in a multiple-dose vial could result in serious microbial contamination following multiple entries.

4. Elastomeric closures contain metallic salts which may be incompatible with certain excipients in a formulation. The presence or absence of closure-derived incompatible ions should be determined by an extraction procedure [59] using distilled water or the formulation vehicle. Should certain metallic ions be present that appear to be incompatible with the product, such as zinc for a phosphate-buffered product, procedures can be designed to remove the surface excess zinc and other group II ions by an appropriate washing and autoclaving procedure using edetate disodium [60].

5. Other tests relating to performance and identity characteristics as well as a list of potential elastomeric closures in use for various product applications is available [61].

B. Closure Screening Experiment

Assuming that the investigator has developed general information as described above and has previous experience with a similar drug product, a series of closures can be identified for screening with appropriate input by the closure manufacturer. For example, if five closure formulations are identified for trial with a solution of drug in water at the appropriate pH, the following types of tests can be run:

1. Place 400 ml of formulation into each of five 1 liter type I glass bottles or flasks. Into each flask place a sufficient number of whole closures to provide a total exposed surface area of approximately 200 cm^2. The closures should have been previously washed and an example procedure is to wash the closures in a detergent solution such as benzalkonium chloride followed by adequate rinsing and autoclaving for 30 min at 121°C with an appropriate vacuum drying cycle. This will ensure an equal pretreatment for all closures. A blank using the formulation alone is prepared similarly. The flasks are appropriately sealed with either Teflon-lined screw caps or ground-glass stoppers.

2. The containers are placed at room temperature and 35°C on a shaker set at a low rpm rate so that the solution movement is obtained with minimum discernible closure movement to avoid abrasion. Samples are examined at 1- and 2- week intervals for the following:

    a. pH change from initial reading.
    b. Visual comparison of color: Each flask should stand for at least 5 min to allow for settling. A 10 ml sample is withdrawn from the top portion of the sample and placed into an appropriately sized test tube. These tubes are then placed onto a white background and viewed from the top of the test tube down onto the paper. A color ranking is then recorded for each closure formulation versus the water, such as: no change from initial, slight color, pronounced color, and so on. If appropriate, APHA color can be determined as described previously.
    c. Solution clarity: Visual solution clarity is determined from the supernatant liquid of each flask using descriptions such as: clear with no precipitate, clear with precipitate, cloudy without precipitate, cloudy with precipitate, very cloudy. Samples are ranked in accordance to degree of clarity.
    d. Particulate matter: A determination is made by shaking each flask and quickly withdrawing a 50 ml aliquot by pipet and transferring onto a prewashed, preweighed 0.45 μm membrane. The precipitate is washed with 10 ml of fresh distilled water and dried to constant weight. Each membrane is weighed and viewed under a stereoscopic microscope at a 10X magnifica-

tion. A rank order of sample cleanliness and weight of precipitate is determined.

e. Physical dimensions: Physical dimensions of the closures are checked
versus untreated samples to detect swelling, color change, and so on, and
hardness.

f. Chemical assay: The chemical assay for active and preservative is determined by the appropriate procedure.

Test parameters are checked at weekly intervals for at least 2 weeks, at which time
each closure is ranked and selection of the best two performing candidates is made.
If all closures are judged unsatisfactory, additional selections must be made. Experiments using two or more closure manufacturers at the same time may increase
chances of success since factors involved in closure product compatibility are still
unpredictable. Alternatively, a more rigorous extraction procedure [59] can be employed where closures contained in extraction flasks covered by beakers are autoclaved for 2 hr at 121°C. Following this procedure, tests are run on the extract
after cooling to room temperature.

The goal of the screening process should be to identify at least two closures
that can be recommended to the formulator for long-term product evaluation.

C. Glass Selection

When possible, glass ampuls should be used during preformulation studies. The
work necessary to identify suitable vial and closure systems usually takes much
more time than available at this stage. Studies done in ampuls can usually be directly carried over to the formulation stage for use in toxicological and early clinical
trials. Ampuls provide the best seal to either exclude oxygen or retain an inert atmosphere if required, and their reactivity with formulations is relatively low compared to glass vials and elastomeric closures, particularly over a wide pH range.

Type I glass, as defined in USP XX, refers to borosilicate glass, which is
generally used for preparations intended for parenteral administration. Type II
glass, soda-lime glass that is treated with an agent such as ammonium bisulfite to
remove surface alkalinity, is usually used for packaging acidic and neutral preparations. To be classified as such, type I and type II glass must pass a test related
to alkalinity of an aqueous extract.

Although such a test defines type I glass, there are subtle differences in the
manufacture of type I glass which may affect compatibility [62, 63]. Some type I
glass is made without added barium ions, and is highly preferred for use with drug
solutions containing sulfate ions since leaching of barium from the glass matrix can
often result in microprecipitates in the form of very insoluble $BaSO_4$. In such a
case, barium-free glass is desirable and should be recommended.

Large volume containers as well as small vials and ampuls must be scrupu-
lously washed using a production-type washing procedure before carrying out preformulation studies, especially if examination of particulate matter is to be made
and results are to be predictive of product manufactured during the development
program.

D. Inspection for Particulate Matter

The inspection of small and large volume parenteral containers for particulate
matter can be done by several methods, all of which provide important information.

1. General visual inspection of each unit can be made using a fluorescent light source against a light and dark background with or without the aid of magnifying lens. Such inspection is useful in determining the presence of visual particulate matter in each unit tested.
2. A particle counting device can be used to determine the number of particles generated within specific particle size ranges. Quantitative data are obtainable and can be used to rank accurately numbers of particles among samples [63].
3. Samples can be filtered onto retentive membranes and examined using a stereoscopic microscope, or by an electron probe, should particulate analysis be desired. This method provides x-ray diffraction data and can be used to determine the qualitative composition of a crystal, particularly if it is inorganic in nature [59].
4. Particles can be examined directly in the vial or ampul by use of a specially constructed inverted microscope. This instrument is able to focus through the glass wall of the container where the particulate matter has settled. Although this method provides only visual analysis, it can serve to identify specific particles in the container and therefore aid the analyst in their recovery by the membrane filtration technique.

V. SUMMARY

This chapter presented various parameters that are considered important to preformulation research of parenteral products. With a good knowledge of physical and organic chemistry and the techniques described, the preformulation investigator can gather significant data to determine key properties of a new compound and guide the formulator toward the next stage of product development.

The following are typical preformulation worksheets that can be used to summarize all data during the progress of experiments.

V. PREFORMULATION WORKSHEET

                                                    Investigator(s):

                                                    Start Date:

1. Compound Name or Designation: _____

2. Batch Number: _____

3. Molecular Weight: _____

4. Molecular Structure

5. Color:

            a. Description   _____

            b. APHA value in solution: _____

                        solvent: _____

                        wavelength: _____

6. Odor: _____

7. Particle Size Range: _____ Method: _____

                Shape: _____ Photomicrograph:_____

            Crystallinity: _____

8. Melting Point: _____

            Special characteristics on melting _____

9. Thermal Analysis Profile

            DTA characteristics: scan ref. no.:_____

            DSC characteristics: scan ref. no.:_____

            TGA characteristics: scan ref. no.:_____

10. Hygroscopicity:

% R.H.	Init. wt.	% Wt. Gain	Temp.	Exposure Time
40	_____	_____	_____	_____
79	_____	_____	_____	_____
90	_____	_____	_____	_____

11. Absorbance Spectra

a) Ultraviolet: spectra ref. no.: _____

    conc., solvent & pH: _____

        λ max: _____

        ε =   _____

b) Infrared:

    KBr: spectra ref. no.:_____

    Nujol: spectra ref. no.:_____

Characteristic Frequencies	Functional Groups
_____	_____
_____	_____
_____	_____
_____	_____
_____	_____

12.

a) Solubility: Temperature _____

Solvents	mg/ml
_____	_____
_____	_____
_____	_____
_____	_____
_____	_____
_____	_____

b) pH-Solubility Profile

Buffer	pH	Solubility (mg/ml)
_____	_____	_____
_____	_____	_____
_____	_____	_____
_____	_____	_____
_____	_____	_____
_____	_____	_____
_____	_____	_____
_____	_____	_____

c) Salt forms examined:

Salt	Solubility mg/ml
_____	_____
_____	_____
_____	_____
_____	_____
_____	_____

d) Cosolvents examined:

Cosolvent	Solubility (mg/ml)
_____	_____
_____	_____
_____	_____

e) Complexation studies:

Added ligand	Solubility (mg/ml)
_____	_____
_____	_____
_____	_____
_____	_____

f) Prodrug considered: _____

        Repeat items 1-12 for each candidate.

13. Partition Coefficient:

$$\frac{Octanol}{Water} \ = \ \underline{\hspace{4cm}}$$

14. Ionization Constant:

Solvent: _____

Method: _____

pKa   =   _____

pKa'   =   _____

15. Optical activity:

$[\alpha]_{\lambda}^{t}$ =   _____

$[M]_{\lambda}^{t}$ =   _____

Solvent: _____

16. Accelerated Stability Evaluation

a) Heat

Temp	Exposure Time	% Recovery	Appearance
55°	_____	_____	_____
75°	_____	_____	_____
95°	_____	_____	_____

b) Light Stability:

	Solid	Solution
Lumens:	_____	_____
Exposure Time:	_____	_____
Appearance:	_____	_____
% Recovery:	_____	_____

c) Effect of Oxygen:

Exposure Time _____

Temperature   _____

	Substance		Solution	
	O_2	N_2	O_2	N_2
Color	_____	_____	_____	_____
pH	_____	_____	_____	_____
% Recovery	_____	_____	_____	_____
Solution Clarity	_____	_____	_____	_____

d) pH-Stability Profile

Temp: _____

Conc. _____

pH	Buffer	% Recovery	pH	Buffer	% Recovery
_____	_____	_____	_____	_____	_____
_____	_____	_____	_____	_____	_____
_____	_____	_____	_____	_____	_____
_____	_____	_____	_____	_____	_____
_____	_____	_____	_____	_____	_____
_____	_____	_____	_____	_____	_____
_____	_____	_____	_____	_____	_____
_____	_____	_____	_____	_____	_____
_____	_____	_____	_____	_____	_____
_____	_____	_____	_____	_____	_____

e) Autoclaving Study
       Initial pH   _____
       Buffer   _____
       Packaging   _____

Exposure Time (min) 121° and 30 psig	Color	Clarity	pH	Assay
20	_____	_____	_____	_____
30	_____	_____	_____	_____
45	_____	_____	_____	_____
90	_____	_____	_____	_____

III. Excipient Compatibility

a) Plackett Burman Design

Excipients	Interaction	No Interaction
_____	_____	_____
_____	_____	_____
_____	_____	_____

b) 2 x 3 Design

	Variable 2		Variable 2a	
	Variable 3	Variable 3a	Variable 3	Variable 3a
Variable 1	_____	_____	_____	_____
Variable 1a	_____	_____	_____	_____

IV Closure Screening:

Test vehicle _____   Initial pH _____

Exposure Time _____   Color _____

Conditions   _____   Dimensions_____

Closure	Phys.Dimen.	Soln. Appearance	pH	Color	Particulate Matter wt.
_____	_____	_____	___	_____	_____
_____	_____	_____	___	_____	_____
_____	_____	_____	___	_____	_____
_____	_____	_____	___	_____	_____
_____	_____	_____	___	_____	_____
_____	_____	_____	___	_____	_____
_____	_____	_____	___	_____	_____

REFERENCES

1. Simon, T. H., Ind. Pharm. Tech. Div., Am. Pharm. Assoc. 114th Meet.,
    Las Vegas, Apr. 9-14, 1967.
2. Shami, E. G., Dudzinski, J. R., and Lantz, J., Jr., in The Theory and
    Practice of Industrial Pharmacy (L. Lachman, H. A. Lieberman, and J. L.
    Kanig, eds.), Lea & Febiger, Philadelphia, 1976, p. 1.

3. Greene, D. G., in Modern Pharmaceutics (G. S. Banker and C. T. Rhodes, eds.), Marcel Dekker, New York, 1979, p. 211.
4. Wadke, D. A., and Jacobson, H., in Pharmaceutical Dosage Forms: Tablets (H. A. Lieberman and L. Lachman, eds.), Vol. 1, Marcel Dekker, New York, 1980, p. 1.
5. Akers, M. J., Can. J. Pharm. Sci., 11:1 (1976).
6. Patel, R. M., and Hurwitz, A., J. Pharm. Sci., 61:1806 (1972).
7. Akers, M. J., J. Parenter. Drug Assoc., 33:346 (1979).
8. Munsell Color, Macbeth Division of Kollmorgen Corp., 2441 North Calvert Street, Baltimore, MD 21218.
9. Rand, M. C., Greenberg, A. E., and Taras, M. J., eds., in Standard Methods for the Examination of Water and Wastewater 14th ed. American Public Health Association, Washington, D.C., 1975, p. 64.
10. Yuen, P. C., Taddei, C. R., Wyka, B. E., and Chaudry, I. A., Am. J. Hosp. Pharm., 40:1007 (1983).
11. Macek, T. J., in Remington's Practice of Pharmacy, 15th ed., Mack, Easton, Pa., 1975, p. 1357.
12. The United States Pharmacopeia, The United States Pharmacopeial Convention, Inc., Rockville, MD., 1980, p. 961.
13. Reif, V. D. in Analytical Profiles of Drug Substances (K. Florey, ed.), Vol. 11, Academic Press, New York, 1982, p. 273.
14. Sass, W. C., and Fusari, S. A., in Analytical Profiles of Drug Substances (K. Florey, ed.), Vol. 6, Academic Press, New York, 1977, p. 297.
15. Rosenkrantz, B. E., Greco, J. R., Hoogerhdeide, J. G., and Oden, E. M., in Analytical Profiles of Drug Substances (K. Florey, ed.) Vol. 9, Academic Press, New York, 1980, p. 295.
16. Asher, I. M., and Schwartzman, G., in Analytical Profiles of Drug Substances (K. Florey, ed.), Vol. 6, Academic Press, New York, 1977, p. 1.
17. Levy, P. R., Am. Lab., E. I. Du Pont De Nemours and Co., Inc. (1970).
18. Windholz, M., ed., The Merck Index, 9th ed., Merck and Co., Rahway, N.J.,
19. Callahan, J. C., Cleary, G. W., Elefant, M., Kaplan, G., Kensler, T., and Nash, R. A., Drug. Dev. Ind. Pharm., 8:355 (1982).
20. Spiegel, A. J., and Noseworthy, M. M., J. Pharm. Sci., 52:917 (1963).
21. Hayden, A. L., Sammul, O. R., Selzer, G. B., and Carol, J., J. Assoc. Off. Agric. Chem., 45:797 (1962).
22. Muhtadi, F. J., and Hassan, M. M. A., in Analytical Profiles of Drug Substances (K. Florey, ed.), Vol. 11, Academic Press, New York, 1980, p. 139.
23. Dittert, L. W., Higuchi, T., and Reese, D. R., J. Pharm. Sci., 53:1325 (1964).
24. Agharkar, S., Lindenbaum, S., and Higuchi, T., J. Pharm. Sci., 65:747 (1976).
25. Berge, S. M., Bighley, L. D., and Monkhouse, D. C., J. Pharm. Sci., 66:1 (1977).
26. Yalkowsky, S. H., and Roseman, T. J., in Techniques of Solubilization of Drugs (S. H. Yalkowsky, ed.), Marcel Dekker, New York, 1981, p. 91.
27. Krause, G. M., and Cross, J. M., J. Am. Pharm. Assoc. Sci. Ed., 40:137 (1951).
28. Martin, A. N., Swarbrick, J., and Cammarata, A., Physical Pharmacy, 2nd ed., Lea & Febiger, Philadelphia, 1969, p. 312.
29. Higuchi, T., and Connors, K. A., in Advances in Analytical Chemistry and Instrumentation (C. N. Reilley, ed.), Vol. 4, Wiley-Interscience, New York, 1965, p. 117.

30. Kreilgard, B., Higuchi, T., and Repta, A. J., J. Pharm. Sci., 64:1850 (1975).
31. Albert, A., Nature, 182:421 (1958).
32. Repta, A. J., in Pro-drugs as Novel Drug Delivery Systems (T. Higuchi and V. Stella, eds.), American Chemical Society, Washington, D.C., 1975, p. 196.
33. Cho, M. J., Kurtz, R. R., Lewis, C., Machkovech, S. M., and Houser, D. J., J. Pharm. Sci., 71:510 (1982).
34. Stella, V. J., Mikkelson, T. J., and Pipkin, J. D., Drug Delivery Systems: Characteristics and Biomedical Applications (R. L. Juliano, ed.), Oxford University Press, London, 1980.
35. Connors, K. A., A Textbook of Pharmaceutical Chemistry, 3rd ed., Wiley, New York, 1982, p. 141.
36. Connors, K. A., A Textbook of Pharmaceutical Chemistry, 3rd ed., Wiley, New York, 1982, p. 274.
37. Strategy of Experimentation, E. I. Du Pont de Nemours and Co., Inc., Applied Technology Division, Wilmington, Del.
38. Higuchi, T., Havinga, A., and Busse, L. W., J. Am. Pharm. Assoc. Sci. Ed., 39:405 (1950).
39. Noller, C. A., Chemistry of Organic Compounds, 2nd ed., W. B. Saunders, Philadelphia, 1957, p. 505.
40. Gould, E. S., Mechanism and Structure in Organic Chemistry, Holt, Rinehart and Winston, New York, 1959, p. 346.
41. Rekker, R. F., and Nanta, W. Th., J. Med. Pharm. Chem., 2:281 (1960).
42. Schroeter, L. C., and Higuchi, T., J. Pharm. Sci., 47:426 (1958).
43. Higuchi, T., and Miki, T., J. Am. Chem. Soc., 83:3899 (1961).
44. Higuchi, T., Miki, T., Shah, A. C., and Herd, A. K., J. Am. Chem. Soc., 85:3665 (1963).
45. Higuchi, T., Uno, H., and Shunada, I., J. Pharm. Sci., 54:302 (1965).
46. Halebian, J., and McCrone, W., J. Pharm. Sci., 58:011 (1969).
47. Flynn, G., Meeting, American Pharmaceutical Association, Academy of Pharmaceutical Sciences, Washington, D.C., Nov. 1967.
48. Macek, T. J., U.S. Pat. 2,671,750 (Mar. 9, 1954).
49. Macek, T. J., Am. J. Pharm., 137:217 (1965).
50. Gatlin, L., and DeLuca, P., J. Parenter. Drug Assoc., 34:398 (1980).
51. Pikal, M. J., Lukes, A. L., Lang, J. E., and Gaines, K., J. Pharm. Sci., 67:767 (1978).
52. Pikal, M. J., Lukes, A. L., and Lang, J. E., J. Pharm. Sci., 66:1312 (1977).
53. Shefter, E., in Techniques of Solubilization of Drugs (S. H. Yalkowsky, ed.) Marcel Dekker, New York, 1981, p. 159.
54. Shefter, E., and Higuchi, T., J. Pharm. Sci., 54:781 (1963).
55. Hopkins, G., J. Pharm. Sci., 54:138 (1965).
56. Anschel, J., Bull. Parenter. Drug Assoc., 31:47 (1977).
57. Le Bras, J., Rubber, Chemical Publishing Company, New York, 1957.
58. Lachman, L., Urbanyi, T., and Weinstein, S., J. Pharm. Sci., 52:244 (1963).
59. Extractables from Elastomeric Closures: Analytical Procedures for Characterization/Identification, Parenteral Drug Association, Tech. Methods Bull. (1980).
60. Motola, S., and Clawans, C., Bull. Parenter. Drug Assoc., 26:163 (1972).
61. Elastomeric Closures: Evaluation of Significant Performance and Identity Characteristics, Parenteral Drug Association, Tech. Methods Bull. (1981).

62. Adams, P. B., J. Parenter. Drug. Assoc., 31:213 (1977).

63. Glass Containers for Small Volume Parenteral Products: Factors for Selection and Test Methods for Identification, Parenteral Drug Association, Tech. Methods Bull. 3 (1982).

64. Lantz, R. J. Jr., Shami, E. G., and Lachman, L., Bull. Parenter. Drug Assoc., 30:234 (1976).

5

Formulation of Small Volume Parenterals

PATRICK P. DeLUCA

College of Pharmacy
University of Kentucky
Lexington, Kentucky

JAMES C. BOYLAN*

G.D. Searle & Company
Skokie, Illinois

Whereas a parenteral can be defined as a sterile drug, solution, or suspension that is packaged in a manner suitable for administration by hypodermic injection, either in the form prepared, or following the addition of a suitable solvent or suspending agent [1], the term small volume parenteral (SVP) has not yet officially received the distinction of a definition. However, the official compendium [2] categorizes "sterile preparations for parenteral use" according to the physical state of the product into distinct classes as follows:

1. Solutions or emulsions of medicaments suitable for injection
2. Dry solids or liquid concentrates containing no additives which, upon the addition of suitable solvents, yield solutions conforming in all respects to requirements for injections
3. Preparations the same as described in class 2 but containing one or more additional substances
4. Suspensions of solids in a suitable medium which are not to be injected intravenously or into the spinal column
5. Dry solids which, upon the addition of suitable vehicles, become sterile suspensions.

Although the term sterile pharmaceuticals is applicable to all injections (radiopharmaceuticals included), ophthalmic preparations, and irrigating solutions, this chapter emphasizes the formulation of injectable dosage forms.

The successful formulation of an injectable preparation requires a broad knowledge of physical, chemical, and biological principles and expertise in the application of these principles. Such knowledge and expertise are required to effect rational decisions regarding the selection of (1) a suitable vehicle (aqueous, nonaqueous, or cosolvent), (2) added substances (antimicrobial agents antioxidants, buffers, chelating agents, and tonicity contributors), and (3) the appropriate container and container components. Inherent in all of the decisions above is the obligatory concern for product safety, effectiveness, stability, and reliability.

---

*Present affiliation: Hospital Products Division, Abbott Laboratories, North Chicago, Illinois

This chapter focuses on the physical-chemical aspects of preparing a stable product in a suitable container recognizing that safety must be established through evaluation of toxicity, tissue tolerance, pyrogenicity, sterility, and tonicity, and efficacy must be demonstrated through controlled clinical investigations.

The majority of parenteral products are aqueous solutions, preferred because of their physiologic compatibility and versatility with regard to route of administration. However, cosolvents or nonaqueous substances are often required to effect solution or stability. Furthermore, the desired properties are sometimes attained through the use of a suspension or an emulsion. Although each of these dosage forms has distinctive characteristics and formulation requirements, certain physical-chemical principles are common. Those common principles will be discussed in a general manner and the differences distinctive of each system will be emphasized.

I. FORMULATION PRINCIPLES

A. Influence of the Route of Administration

Since parenteral preparations are introduced directly into the intra-or extracellular fluid compartments, the lymphatic system, or the blood, the nature of the product and the desired pharmacological action are factors determining the particular route of administration to be employed. The desired route of administration, in turn, places certain requirements and limitations on the formulations as well as the devices used for administering the dosage forms. Consequently, a variety of routes of administration (see Chap. 2) are currently used for parenteral products.

One of the most important considerations in formulating a parenteral product is the appropriate volume into which the drug should be incorporated. The intravenous route is the only route by which large volumes (i.e., greater than 10 ml) can be administered, although the rate of administration must be carefully controlled. Volumes up to 10 ml can be administered intraspinally, while the intramuscular route is normally limited to 3 ml, subcutaneous to 2 ml, and intradermal to 0.2 ml.

The choice of the solvent system or vehicle is directly related to the intended route of administration of the product. Intravenous and intraspinal injections are generally restricted to dilute aqueous solutions, whereas oily solutions, cosolvent solutions, suspensions, and emulsions can be injected intramuscularly and subcutaneously.

Isotonicity is another factor that must be taken into consideration. Although isotonic solutions are less irritating, cause less toxicity, and eliminate the possibility of hemolysis, it is not essential that all injections be isotonic. In fact, for subcutaneous and intramuscular injections hypertonic solutions are often used to facilitate absorption of drug due to local effusion of tissue fluids. With intravenous solutions isotonicity becomes less important as long as administration is slow enough to permit dilution or adjustment in the blood. However, intraspinal injections must be isotonic because of slow circulation of the cerebrospinal fluid, in which abrupt changes of osmotic pressure can give rise to severe side affects.

B. Selection of the Vehicle

Most parenteral products are aqueous solutions. Chemically, the high dielectric constant of water makes it possible to dissolve ionizable electrolytes and its hydrogen-bonding potential facilitates the solution of alcohols, aldehydes, ketones, and amines. Water for Injection, USP, is the solvent of choice for making parenterals. It must be prepared fresh by distillation or by reverse osmosis and contain no added substance. When it is not possible to use a wholly aqueous solution, for physical or chemical reasons, the addition of solubilizing agents or cosolvents may be necessary. For instance, nonpolar substances (i.e., alkaloidal bases) possess limited solubility in water and it is necessary to add a cosolvent such as glycerin, ethanol, propylene glycol, or polyethylene glycol. In other cases, to prevent chemical degradation (i.e., hydrolysis, oxidation, decarboxylation, or racemization) water may have to be eliminated partially or totally. Consequently, parenteral product formulators should be aware not of only the nature of the solvent in parenterals but also of the method of administration.

1. Solubility and Solubilization

To enhance the solubility of drugs, in addition to using organic solvents which are miscible with water as cosolvents, other substances are used as solubilizers. Surface-active agents, by virtue of their association tendencies in solution and the ability to orient into concentrated polar and nonpolar centers (micelles), have been used to solubilize drugs and other substances, such as vitamins, hormones, sulfonamides, dyes, resins, and volatile oils. These surfactants are powerful wetting agents and form colloidal dispersions which have the appearance of a true solution. Ethylenediamine is required in aminophylline injections to maintain the theophylline in solution since aminophylline is a salt that ionizes into its constituent ions theophylline and ethylenediamine.

$$\text{Aminophylline} \longrightarrow 2 \text{ theophylline}^- + \text{ethylenediamine}^{2+}$$

Ethylenediamine, a strongly alkaline substance, is volatile and if it escapes, the pH will be lowered, causing theophylline ion to be converted to free theophylline ($pK_a \sim 8.8$), which is only slightly soluble in water (8 mg ml^{-1}).

$$\text{Theophylline}^- + \text{H}^+ \longrightarrow \text{theophylline (free)}$$

Creatinine, niacinamide, and lecithin have been used for solubilizing steroids in the free alcohol form. The use of the salt or ester of these steroids or vitamins eliminates the need to use solubilizers but requires other additives to ensure stability.

The solubility of a substance at a given temperature is defined quantitatively as the concentration of the dissolved solute in a saturated solution (i.e., the dissolved solute phase). Generally, drugs are present in solution at unsaturated or subsaturated concentrations; otherwise, crystallization of the drug can occur as a result of changes in pH or temperature or by seeding from other ingredients or particulates in the solution. A brief description of the phenomenon of solubility will be helpful to the formulator in selecting the best solvent or agent to overcome difficulties that arise in the preparation of pharmaceutical dosage forms containing poorly soluble drugs. With parenterals, the drug and other dissolved substances should remain solubilized throughout the shelf life of the product.

Solubility Expressions. Solubility of a substance can be expressed in a number of ways. Generally, the concentration is expressed as percent (w/v), that is, grams per 100 ml of solution, but molarity and molality have been used. Molarity is defined as the number of moles per 1000 ml of solution. Molality is the number of moles of solute per 1000 g of solvent and therefore, being a weight relationship, is not influenced by temperature. The United States Pharmacopeia (USP) lists solubility in terms of the number of milliliters of solvent required to dissolve 1 g of substance. If exact solubilities are not known, the USP provides general terms to describe a given range. These descriptive terms are listed in Table 1.

Table 1 USP Expressions for Approximate Solubility

Term	Relative amount of solvent to dissolve 1 part of solute
Very soluble	< 1
Freely soluble	1-10
Soluble	10-30
Sparingly soluble	30-100
Slightly soluble	100-1000
Very slightly soluble	1000-10,000
Practically insoluble, or insoluble	>10,000

Measuring Solubility. Methods for determining the solubility of drug substances in various solvents have been described [3-6]. The phase solubility technique is especially applicable to determining the solubility of pure substances and
also detecting the presence of impurities [6]. In this method, successively larger
portions of the substance are added to the same volume of solvent in suitable containers which are agitated at constant temperatures, generally $30 \pm 0.1°C$. In those
containers in which excess drug is present (undissolved), samples of the supernatant are withdrawn and assayed until the concentration is constant (i.e., the
system has reached equilibrium). For a pure compound, a phase solubility diagram is constructed as shown in Figure 1a. The solubility is readily determined
by extrapolating the line with a slope of zero to the y axis. If an impurity exists in
the substance, a phase solubility diagram as shown in Figure 1b results, which
shows an inflection in the ascending line. Extrapolation of the horizontal line
gives the solubility of the substance plus the impurity on the y axis, while extrapolation of the ascending line gives the solubility of the impurity.

Bonding Forces. For a substance to dissolve, the forces of attraction that
hold the molecules together must be overcome by the solvent. The solubility will
be determined by the relative binding forces within the substance (solute-solute
interactions) and between the substance and the vehicle (solute-solvent interactions).
If an environment similar to that of the crystal structure can be provided by the
solvent, then the greater the solubility (i.e., "like dissolves like"). Ionic compounds dissolve more readily in water by virtue of ion-dipole interactions, whereas
hydrophobic substances dissolve more easily in organic solvents as a result of
dipole or induced dipole interactions (van der Waals, London, or Debye forces).
     The solubility of the drug substance is due in large part to the polarity of the
solvent, often expressed in terms of dipole moment, which is related to the dielectric constant. Solvents with high dielectric constants dissolve ionic compounds
and are water soluble, whereas solvents with low dielectric constants are not water
soluble and do not dissolve ionic compounds. The former are classified as polar
solvents (e.g., water, glycerin, and methanol), while the latter are nonpolar
(e.g., chloroform, benzene, and the oils). Solvents with intermediate dielectric
(e.g., acetone and butanol) are classified as semipolar. The dielectric constants

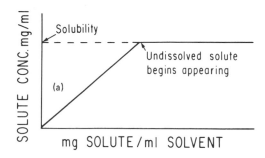

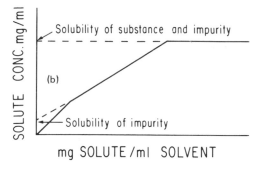

Figure 1 Phase solubility diagrams for a pure substance (a) and a substance containing an impurity (b).

of most pharmaceutical solvents are known [7, 8] and values for a number of binary and tertiary blends have been reported [9] and, if not reported, can be readily estimated [10]. Table 2 is a listing of the dielectric constants of some liquids used in pharmaceutical systems.

The solubility profiles of a number of pharmaceuticals as a function of dielectric constant have been reported by Paruta and co-workers and others [11-17]. By determining the solubility of a substance in a system at various dielectric constants, a graph such as that shown in Figure 2 can be constructed to determine

Table 2 Dielectric Constants of Some Solvents at 25°C

Solvent	Dielectric constant	Solvent	Dielectric constant
Water	78. 5	Acetone	19. 1
Glycerin	40. 1	Benzyl alcohol	13. 1
Ethylene glycol	37. 7	Polyethylene glycol 400	12. 5
Methanol	31. 5	Cottonseed oil	3. 0
Ethanol	24. 3	Benzene	2. 3
N-Propanol	20. 1	Dioxane	2. 2

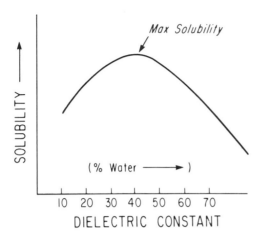

Figure 2 Hypothetical plot of solubility of a substance versus dielectric constant in various mixtures of dioxane and water.

the dielectric constant that will provide the required solubility. As can be seen from the plot, to obtain the maximum concentration a dielectric constant of around 40 is required. Not all mixtures will show a maximum, but such a plot will show the required dielectric constant to obtain the desired concentration. For example, if a dielectric constant (d.c.) of 60 were selected, a mixture of water (d.c. 80 at 20°C), polyethylene glycol (PEG) 400 (d.c. 12.5 at 20°C), and ethanol (d.c. 25.7 at 20°C) could be used. Selecting an amount of ethanol necessary to dissolve the drug (e.g., 10%), the percentages of PEG 400 and water can be calculated as follows:

$$(10)(25.7) \ + \ (X)(80) \ + \ (90 - X)(12.5) \ = \ (100)(60)$$

where X is the percentage of water required and is calculated to be 68.4%. Therefore, the vehicle to provide a dielectric constant of 60 will have the following composition:

Ethanol	10%
PEG 400	21.6%
H_2O	68.4%
	100%

Examples of drugs marketed in water-miscible systems include digitoxin, phenytoin, and diazepam. These injections are formulated in a water-miscible system containing glycols and alcohol and adjusted to a suitable pH. Although such systems are stable in individual containers, care must be exercised upon administration. For example, phenytoin is dissolved as the sodium salt in a vehicle containing 40% propylene glycol and 10% ethanol and adjusted to a pH of 12 with sodium hydroxide. However, if this solution is added to a large volume intravenous solution and the pH is lowered to a value close to the pK_a of the drug (pK_a = 8.3), precipitation of the drug can occur. This is due to the fact that in aqueous systems at pH below 11, the amount of undissociated phenytoin exceeds its solubility [18]. The dielectric constant of 60 however solvates the sodium salt by hydrogen bonding and van der

Waals forces and reduces the risk of precipitation upon addition to an infusion solution prior to intravenous administration [19]. Nevertheless, such preparations should be administered slowly into the systemic circulation because rapid injection could result in the precipitation of the drug in the blood stream [20]. The influence of pH on solubility of phenytoin will be demonstrated later.

Hydrogen bonding, the strongest type of dipole-dipole interaction, is characterized by a positive center in the hydrogen atom (proton donor). Because of its small size, the hydrogen atom can approach the negative center (electron donor) of a neighboring dipole more closely than any other atom. As a result of this spatial maneuverability, both intramolecular bonding (i.e., between groups within a single molecule) and the intermolecular type (i.e., between molecules) can occur. The latter is responsible for association in most solvents and dissolution of most drugs.

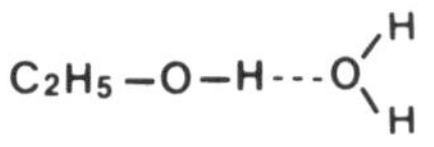

$$C_2H_5-O-H\cdots O\begin{smallmatrix}H\\\\H\end{smallmatrix}$$

intermolecular H bonding

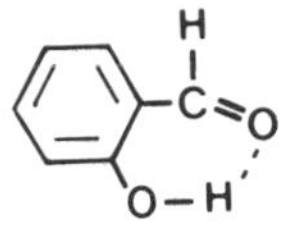

intramolecular H bonding

Generally, the proton is donated by a carboxyl, hydroxyl, amine, or amide group. The hydrogen from S-H or C-H can also form hydrogen bonds, but generally the bonds are weaker. The proton attached to a halogen is generally quite active. HF forms strong hydrogen bonds. Typical electron contributors are oxygen, nitrogen, and halogen atoms found in alcohol, ethers, aldehydes, ketones, amines, and N-heterocyclic compounds. Some examples of hydrogen bonding with water follows:

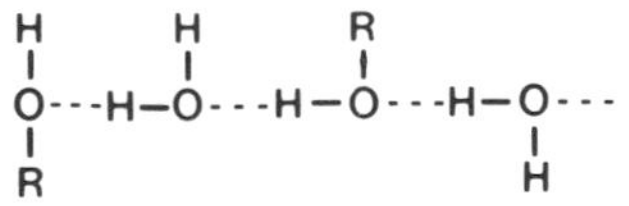

alcohol

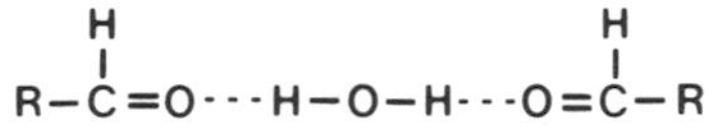

ketone

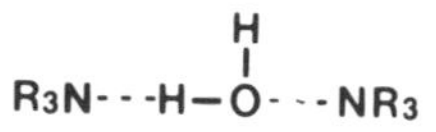

amine

Alcohols dissolve in water by hydrogen bonding up to an alkyl chain length of five carbon atoms. Phenols dissolve in water and alcohol and as the number of hydroxyl groups increase, the water solubility increases because of the increased opportunity for hydrogen bonding. Most aromatic carboxylic acids, steroids, and cardiac glycosides are not water soluble but dissolve in alcohol, glycerin, or glycols by hydrogen bonding.

Dipole-ion interactions are responsible for the dissolution of ionic crystalline substances in polar solvents (i.e., water or alcohol). Ions in aqueous solution are generally hydrated (surrounded by water molecules) by as many water molecules as can spatially fit around the ion. The attributes of a good solvent for electrolytes include (1) a high dipole moment, (2) a small molecular size, and (3) a high dielectric constant to reduce the force of attraction between the oppositely charged ions in the crystal. Water possesses all of these characteristics and is therefore a good solvent for electrolytes. The cation of the electrolyte is attracted to the negative oxygen atom, when the anion attracts the hydrogen atoms to the dipolar water molecules.

Generally, when electrolytes dissolve in water, heat is generated because the ion-dipole interaction energy exceeds the sum of the ion-ion interaction energy of the solute and the dipole-dipole interaction energy of the solvent. Examples of a negative heat of solution are anhydrous magnesium sulfate and sodium hydroxide. Where the ion-dipole energy is less than the sum of the energies holding the solute and solvent molecules together, heat is absorbed from the surrounding area to make up for the energy deficit. Electrolytes showing a positive heat of solution include potassium iodide and sodium bromide. Hydrated salts generally show a positive heat of solution. Citric acid, sorbitol, and mannitol have positive heats of solution so that during dissolution the solution becomes cool. When reconstituting dry products containing large amounts of these substances, which is quite common in freeze-dried products, it is necessary to be aware of this phenomenon and warm the solution prior to injection.

Many complexes result because of an ion-induced dipole interaction. For example, iodine is solubilized in a solution of potassium iodide in the following manner:

$$I_2 + K^+I^- \longrightarrow K^+I_3^-$$

Although the iodine molecule is electrically neutral, a temporary polarity may result from electronic movements within the molecule. Such movements induce dipoles in neighboring molecules and are responsible for maintaining benzene and carbon tetrachloride in the liquid state. The iodide complex forms because the strong electrical field of the electrolyte in solution induces a dipole in the polarizable iodine molecule. Benzene is a neutral molecule that is readily polarizable and soluble in alcohol.

Symmetrical molecules, such as benzene and carbon tetrachloride, possess a zero dipole moment and are nonpolar. Solubility of such molecules or their existence in a liquid state is due to van der Waals forces. In the manner described earlier, an induction effect occurs in these electrically neutral molecules and the molecules orient themselves with surrounding molecules so that negative and positive poles are together. Such orientation is referred to as resulting from induced dipole-induced dipole interactions. These very weak attractions are sometimes called London forces, because they were first described by London in 1930. They are responsible for dissolution of hydrophobic substances in nonpolar solvents (e.g., wax in carbon tetrachloride and paraffin in petroleum benzin). If the solute and solvent in nonpolar systems are similar in size and structure, they can be mixed without any appreciable heat of solution. If the heat of solution is zero, the solution is referred to as an ideal solution.

Another type of van der Waals force is that resulting from induced dipole-dipole interactions, also called Debye interactions. In this case, a dipolar molecule is capable of inducing an electrical dipole in a nonpolar molecule. A molecule that resonates, such as benzene, can be polarized by a dipolar substance such as methyl alcohol. Other examples of such interactions include mixtures of chloral hydrate in carbon tetrachloride and phenol in mineral oil.

Effect of pH   Most drug substances are weak electrolytes and therefore exist in solution in the dissociated and undissociated forms. The ratio of these forms is determined by the pH of the solution. As a result, properties such as solubility, partition coefficient, and chemical stability which are markedly different for the undissociated and dissociated forms will be influenced by pH.

Many of the organic electrolytes used in parenteral systems contain a basic nitrogen atom in the molecule. These include antihistamines, alkaloids, local anesthetics, and so on, which are practically insoluble in water but dissolve readily in dilute solutions of acids due to salt formation. The addition of alkali to these solutions increases the pH and causes free base to precipitate. Examples are atropine sulfate, ephedrine sulfate, lidocaine hydrochloride, and pyribenzamine hydrochloride.

ephedrine cation in dilute acid

In compounds containing an electron withdrawing group, such as oxygen, a positive center is created which in turn attracts electrons from an adjacent nitrogen, and if a hydrogen atom is attached the N-H bond is weakened. As a result, in alkaline solution, a more soluble anion is formed. This is illustrated for phenobarbital and sulfanilamide.

phenobarbital anion   sulfanilamide anion

The addition of acid to the solutions above will cause the free acid form to precipitate. Even the addition of a salt of a strong acid such as morphine sulfate will cause precipitation.

To calculate the solubility of a weak electrolyte as a function of pH, it is necessary to express the equilibrium in solution for a weak acid or weak base:

$$\mathrm{HA} \overset{\mathrm{HOH}}{\rightleftharpoons} \mathrm{H}^+ + \mathrm{A}^- \tag{1}$$

$$\mathrm{B} \rightleftharpoons \mathrm{BH}^+ + \mathrm{O\overline{H}} \tag{2}$$

In Equation (1) (HA) represents the concentration of weak acid present in undissociated form at equilibrium, and (A^-) represents the concentration of dissociated (or salt) form present at equilibrium. In Equation (2) (B) is the slightly soluble undissociated basic substance and (BH^+) is the dissociated salt form. The concentration of the undissociated forms (HA) and (B) will remain essentially constant. Therefore,

S_0, the solubility of the undissociated form, can represent the concentration of (HA) or (B) in solution. For a weak acid the dissociation constant K_a for the equilibrium between species may be written as

$$K_a = \frac{(H^+)(A^-)}{(HA)} \tag{3}$$

Rearranging yields

$$(A^-) = K_a \frac{(HA)}{(H^+)} \tag{4}$$

Total drug solubility, S, will be the sum of undissociated and dissociated forms.

$$S = (HA) + (A^-) \tag{5}$$

or

$$S = S_0 + K_a \frac{S_0}{(H^+)} \tag{6}$$

Therefore, the total solubility of a weak acid electrolyte is a function of the hydrogen ion concentration. The solubility equation may be expressed in logarithmic form by rearrangement:

$$\log (S - S_0) = \log K_a + \log S_0 - \log (H^+) \tag{7}$$

or

$$pH = pK_a + \log \frac{S - S_0}{S_0} \tag{8}$$

Considering the earlier example, phenytoin, which is formulated as the sodium salt, the following equilibria occur:

$$Na^+ \, phenytoin^- \overset{HOH}{\rightleftharpoons} Na^+ + phenytoin^- \tag{9}$$

$$Phenytoin^- + HOH \rightleftharpoons phenytoin_{(u)} + OH^- \tag{10}$$

These equilibria indicate that a high OH^- concentration is required in order to keep the reaction in the direction of the soluble dissociated species. The aqueous solubility of the undissociated phenytoin is 0.016 mg ml^{-1} [21] and at pH values below 5, phenytoin exists essentially in the practically insoluble undissociated species. Using Equation (8), in which S_0 is the aqueous solubility of undissociated phenytoin and S is the total concentration of phenytoin in solution (i.e., phenytoin$^-$ and phenytoin$_{(u)}$), the pH required to maintain a concentration of 50 mg ml^{-1} in solution can be determined:

$$pH = 8.3 + \log \frac{1.823 \times 10^{-1} - 1.34 \times 10^{-5}}{1.34 \times 10^{-5}} \tag{11}$$

$$pH = 8.3 + \log 2874 = 11.7 \tag{12}$$

Therefore, in water for injection a pH of 11.7 is required. At this pH the phenytoin is 99.97% dissociated. In the commercial preparation the hydroalcoholic solvent maintains the solution at a lower pH due to the dielectric effect discussed earlier.

For a weak base the dissociation constant K_b for the equilibrium between species may be written as

$$K_b = \frac{(BH^+)(OH^-)}{(B)} \tag{13}$$

Rearranging yeilds

$$(BH^+) = K_b \frac{(B)}{(OH^-)} \tag{14}$$

The total solubility S is the sum of the dissociated and undissociated forms:

$$S = (BH^+) + (B) \tag{15}$$

or

$$S = S_0 + K_b \frac{S_0}{(OH^-)} \tag{16}$$

Since $K_w = (OH^-)(H^+)$, the hydroxyl ion concentration can be expressed in terms of the hydrogen ion concentration:

$$S = S_0 + S_0 \frac{K_b(H^+)}{K_w} \tag{17}$$

Expressed in logarithmic form,

$$\log (S - S_0) = \log S_0 + \log K_b + \log (H^+) - \log K_w \tag{18}$$

or

$$pH = pK_w - pK_b + \log \frac{S_0}{S - S_0} \tag{19}$$

Effect of Molecular Structure. Spatial and structural relationships often play a major role in determining relative solubility. Crystals composed of unsymmetrical molecules tend to be more soluble than those of highly symmetrical molecules. For example, $\underline{N}, \underline{N}, \underline{N}^1, \underline{N}^1$-tetramethylorthophthalamide,

```
        O   CH3
        ||  |
        C—N—CH3
   /==\ |
  |    ||
   \==/ |
        C—N—CH3
        ||  |
        O   CH3
```

has a solubility of 700 g liter^{-1}, while the more symmetrical para form,

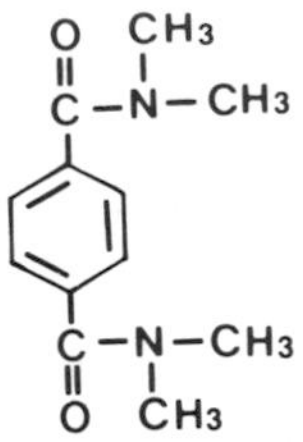

$$
\begin{array}{c}
\overset{\text{O}}{\underset{\text{C}}{\|}}-\overset{\text{CH}_3}{\underset{\text{N}}{|}}-\text{CH}_3
\end{array}
$$

is only one-seventh as soluble. Symmetrical molecules tend to fit into the crystal lattice more readily than unsymmetrical molecules, which generally have higher entropy factors (greater degree of disorder in orientation).

The tendency for atoms is to take on or discharge electrons from the outer shell in order to contain eight electrons, the most stable configuration. This stabilization is achieved either by <u>induction</u>, which arises from an unequal sharing of electrons in a bond between atoms of different kinds or is transmitted through similar atoms, or by <u>resonance</u>, where polarization results in a net electronic displacement and the existence of an open or ionic bond. Examples of induction:

In propyl chloride the charge is transmitted through the chain to the electrophilic chlorine atom and therefore a negative charge rests with the chlorine while the positive charge is distributed over the carbon chain. Examples of resonance (electromeric shift):

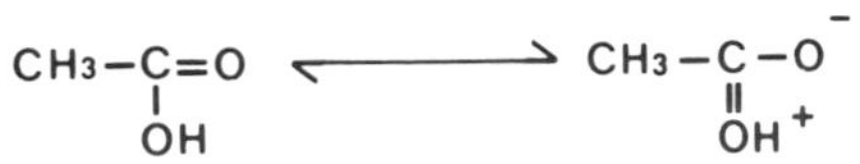

$$
\text{CH}_3-\underset{\text{OH}}{\overset{|}{\text{C}}}=\text{O} \quad \longleftarrow\quad\longrightarrow\quad \text{CH}_3-\underset{\overset{||}{\text{OH}}{}^{+}}{\text{C}}-\text{O}^{-}
$$

The above is often written

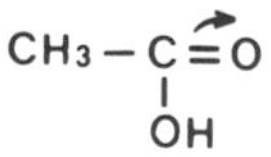

$$
\text{CH}_3-\underset{\text{OH}}{\overset{|}{\text{C}}}\overset{\nearrow}{=}\text{O}
$$

Inductive and electromeric shifts influence the strength of acids and bases by

1. Withdrawing electrons from the acidic group ($-CO_2H$ or $-OH$) and creating a positive charge on the acid group which then makes it easier for the H^+ to leave. <u>Note</u>: A shift of electrons to the acidic group would make it more difficult for the H^+ to leave.
2. Withdrawing electrons from a basic group ($-NR_2$), reducing basicity and causing a repelling of incoming protons. A shift of electrons toward the basic group will promote the attraction of protons.

The solubility of orthophthalamide,

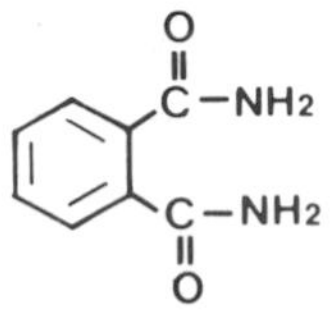

is only 5g liter^{-1} in water because of the strong dipolar nature of the amide function and the intramolecular bonding tendencies. Blocking these dipole-dipole interactions by substituting the hydrogens with methyl groups,

results in a 140-fold increase in solubility [22].

Often a substance will exist in more than one crystalline form, such as chloramphenicol, progesterone, sulfathiazole, cortisone, and prednisolone, to name a few. The polymorphs show different solubilities and rates of solution, hence different absorption (bioavailability) tendencies. Polymorphic transformations are structural differences resulting from different arrangements of molecules in the solid state. Polymorphism as it pertains to physical and chemical stability and also to therapeutic activity has been discussed by a number of researchers [23-26].

Effect of Temperature. Substances generally dissolve faster if heat is applied to the system and the solubility of most solids is increased by an increase in temperature. This is true if the substance absorbs heat during the course of dissolution. The degree to which temperature can influence solubility is determined by the heat of solution, more specifically the differential heat of solution, ΔH, which represents the rate of change of the heat of solution per mole of solute in a solution of specified concentration. The higher the heat of solution, the greater the influence of temperature on solubility. The following equation shows the influence of temperature on solubility:

$$\frac{d \ln S}{dT} = \frac{\Delta H}{RT^2} \tag{20}$$

where S is the solubility or concentration of a saturated solution, often expressed in terms of molality, molarity, or mole fraction; R is the gas constant; and T is the absolute temperature. Equation (20) can be written

$$\log S = \frac{\Delta H}{2.303R} \frac{1}{T} + \text{constant} \tag{21}$$

By plotting the logarithm of the solubility in moles per liter versus the reciprocal of the absolute temperature as shown in Figure 3, the differential heat of solution can be calculated from the slope of the line, which is equal to

$$-\frac{\Delta H}{(2.303)(1.987)}$$

A positive heat of solution indicates that the process is endothermic (i.e., the solute absorbs heat when dissolving). Therefore, an increase in temperature will increase solubility. A negative value indicates that the process is exothermic (i.e., the solute evolves heat when dissolving). In this case, an increase in temperature results in a decrease in solubility. A differential heat of solution around zero indicates that the solubility is not significantly influenced by temperature. The heats of solution for a number of substances are listed in Table 3.

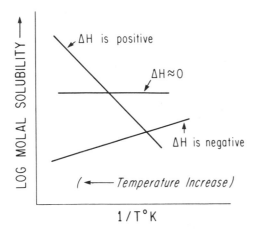

Figure 3 Effect of temperature on solubility of a substance. ΔH represents the differential heat of solution and is calculated from the slope of the line, $-\Delta H/(2.303)$ (1.987).

Effect of Other Substances. Drug solubility can be increased by the use of solubilizing agents and by nonaqueous solvents or mixed solvent systems. Examples of such materials include the surface-active agents (surfactants) sorbitan mono-oleate and polyoxyethylene sorbitan monooleate and the solvents ethanol, glycerin, propylene glycol, and polyethylene glycol. The surfactants are generally used in the range 0.05 to 0.5%, whereas the solvents mentioned may comprise up to 50 to 60% of the total vehicle.

Table 3 Heats of Solution for Some Inorganic Compounds

Compound	ΔH (kcal mol^{-1})
Endothermic process	
Sodium sulfate, decahydrate	18.8
Silver chloride	15.0
Boric acid	10.8
Potassium iodide	5.1
Cesium chloride	5.0
Potassium chloride	4.2
Sodium chloride	1.0
Calcium sulfate, dihydrate	0.3
Exothermic process	
Sodium iodide	−1.2
Lithium chloride	−10.0
Calcium chloride	−17.4
Magnesium sulfate, anhydrous	−20.3
Aluminum chloride	−76.5

Surfactants are effective solubilizing agents because by virtue of their wetting properties and association tendencies, they are able to disperse water-insoluble substances. These surfactants exist as individual molecules at low concentrations and can adsorb to the surfaces of molecules. At higher concentrations an orientated aggregation occurs and the surfactants exist as molecules. The concentration at which such association occurs is called the critical micelle concentration (CMC). Surfactants can be either ionic (i.e., the ability to lower surface tension rests with the anion or cation in the molecule) or nonionic, Figure 4 diagrammatically shows spherical orientations of a nonionic and ionic micelle. It has been proposed [27] that poorly soluble hydrophobic molecules locate in the hydrocarbon core of the micelle, while polar molecules would associate with the polar ends. Molecules that contain polar and nonpolar groups would align themselves between the chains of the micelle with the nonpolar part directed into the central region and the polar end extending out into the hydrophilic chains. These mechanisms are schematically illustrated in Figure 5.

With the exception of the nonionic type, surfactants are not generally used in parenterals because of destruction to biological membranes. When such substances as well as the nonaqueous solvents are employed, it is essential that safety (LD_{50}, tissue tolerance, hemolysis, etc.) be evaluated.

2. Types of Vehicles

Aqueous. The vast majority of injectable products are administered as aqueous solutions because of the physiological compatibility of water with body tissues. Additionally, the high dielectric constant of water makes it possible to dissolve ionizable electrolytes, and its hydrogen-bonding potential facilitates the solution of alcohols, aldehydes, ketones, and amines.

The current USP [2] has monographs for Purified Water, Water for Injection (WFI), Sterile Water for Injection, Bacteriostatic Water for Injection, and Sterile Water for Irrigation. WFI is the solvent of choice for making parenterals. It must be prepared fresh and be pyrogen-free. Other USP requirements include no more than 10 parts per million (ppm) of total solids, a pH of 5.0 and 7.0, absence of chloride, sulfate, calcium, ammonium ions, and carbon dioxide, and limits for heavy metals and organic material (tannins, lignins). Requirements for WFI are generally the same among the various pharmacopeias, although significant differences do exist. For example, only the British Pharmacopoeia and the USP have standards for particulate matter (standards not applicable to all parenteral dosage forms); only Pharmacopeé Belge has the same pH limits as the USP (5.0 to 7.0),

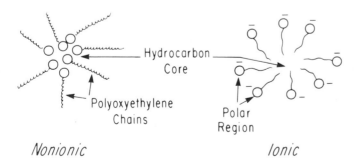

Hydrocarbon Core

Polyoxyethylene Chains

Polar Region

Nonionic   *Ionic*

Figure 4 Diagrammatic illustration of the spherical orientation of surfactant micelles.

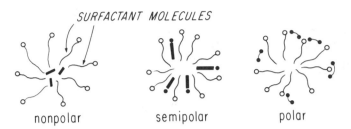

SURFACTANT MOLECULES

nonpolar   semipolar   polar

Figure 5 Schematic representation of the proposed mechanisms of micellar solubilization.

other pharmacopeias are grouped as pH 6.8 to 8.4 or 4.2 to 7.6; several pharmacopeias limit only copper, lead, and iron, not heavy metal. The specific differences among pharmacopeias have been summarized by Boylan and Fites [28].

WFI may be prepared by either distillation or reverse osmosis, but the distillation method is by far the most common and accepted method. Due to the excellent solvent properties of water, it is both difficult to purify and difficult to maintain pure. Microorganisms, dissolved gases, organic and inorganic substances, and foreign particulate matter are the most common contaminants of water.

Prior to distillation, the water used as the source for WFI is usually subjected to chlorination, carbon treatment, deionization, and sometimes, reverse osmosis treatment (forced passage through membrane materials). After distillation it is filtered and then stored in a chemically resistant tank (stainless steel, glass, or blocked tin) at a cold temperature around 5°C or at an elevated temperature between 65 and 85°C to inhibit microbial growth and prevent pyrogen formation. Generally, the water is continually circulated during storage and usually filtered again prior to use in manufacturing.

Sterile WFI and Bacteriostatic WFI are permitted to contain higher levels of solids than WFI because of the possible leaching of glass container constituents into the water during sterilization and storage. Bacteriostatic WFI should not be sold in containers larger than 30 ml to prevent injection of unacceptably larger amounts of bacteriostatic agents (such as phenol and thimerosal).

Water-Miscible. Cosolvents are employed in those systems in which a wholly aqueous solution is unsuitable for physical or chemical reasons. Although these water-miscible solvents are used in parenterals principally to enhance drug solubility, they also serve as stabilizers for those drugs that degrade by hydrolysis. The more common solvents include glycerin, ethyl alcohol, propylene glycol, and polyethylene glycol 300 and 400.

Mixed solvent systems may be irritating or increase toxicity, especially when present in large amounts or higher concentrations. A solution containing a high percentage of ethanol will produce pain on injection. It is also important to be aware that when such preparations are administered intravenously, too rapid an injection could result in the precipitation of the drug in the blood stream [20]. Excellent reviews of water-miscible solvents used in parenteral products have been published [16, 17].

Nonaqueous. Drugs that are insoluble in aqueous systems are often incorporated in metabolizable oils. Steroids, hormones, and vitamins are incorporated in vegetable oils, such as peanut, sesame, corn, olive, and cottonseed. Oil injections are only administered intramuscularly. There are strict specifications for the vegetable oils used in manufacturing intramuscular injections. Storage of these preparations is important if stability is to be maintained. For example, they should not be subjected to conditions above room temperature for extended periods of time. Although the oils used for injections are of vegetable origin, federal regulations require that the specific oil be listed on the label of a product because some patients have exhibited allergic responses to certain vegetable oils.

Sesame oil is the preferred oil for most of the compendial injections formulated with oil. It is the most stable of the vegetable oils (except to light) because it contains natural antioxidants. Sesame oil has also been used to obtain slow release of fluphenazine esters given intramuscularly [29]. Excessive unsaturation of an oil can produce tissue irritation. The use of injections in oil has diminished somewhat in preference to aqueous suspensions, which generally have less irritating and sensitizing properties. Benzyl benzoate may be used to enhance steroid solubility in oils if desired. Table 4 summarizes the oil injections official in USP XX.

C. Added Substances

Added substances such as antioxidants, buffers, bulking agents, chelating agents, antimicrobial agents, solubilizing agents, surfactants, and tonicity adjusting agents must frequently be incorporated into parenteral formulas in order to provide safe, efficacious, and elegant parenteral dosage forms. Any additive to a formulation must be justified by a clear purpose and function. Hospital pharmacists who are involved in intravenous additive programs should be aware of the types of additives present in products that are being combined.

Pharmacopeias often specify the type and amount of additive substances that may be included in injectable products. These requirements often vary from compendia to compendia, so it is important to refer to the specific pharmacoepia that applies to the product in question. Two examples are sulfite and chelating agents. The USP allows the use of up to 3.2 mg of sodium bisulfite per milliliter of solution, whereas the French Pharmacoepia allows only 1.6 mg per milliliter.

Ethylenediaminetetraacetic acid derivatives and salts are sometimes used to complex and thereby inactivate trace metals that may catalyze oxidative degradation of drugs. Japan does not allow the use of these particular chelating agents in any parenteral products. Table 5 summarizes the commonly used parenteral additives as well as their usual concentration.

1. Buffers

Changes in the pH of a preparation may occur during storage because of degradation reactions within the product, interaction with container components (i.e., glass or rubber), and dissolution of gases and vapors. To avoid these problems, buffers are added to many products to resist a change in pH. An excellent review on pH control within pharmaceutical systems by Flynn is recommended to the reader [31]. A suitable buffer system should have an adequate buffer capacity to maintain the pH of the product at a stable value during storage while permitting the body fluids to adjust the pH easily to that of the blood following administration. Therefore, the ideal pH to select would be 7.4, the pH of the blood. Extreme deviation from this pH can cause complications. Above pH 9 tissue necrosis often occurs, while below pH 3, extreme pain and phlebitis are experienced. For intravenous SVPs the acceptable range is 3.0 to 10.5, because blood itself is an excellent buffer. Parenterals administered by other routes are generally adjusted to a pH between 4 and 9.

Table 4 Official Injections in Oil

USP XX	Oil commonly used
Desoxycorticosterone acetate	Sesame
Diethylstilbestrol	Sesame, cottonseed
Dimercaprol	Peanut
Dromostanolone propionate	Sesame
Estradiol benzoate	Sesame
Estradiol cypionate	Cottonseed
Estradiol dipropionate	
Estradiol valerate	Sesame
Estrone	Sesame
Fluphenanazine enanthate	Sesame
Hydroxyprogesterone caproate	
Menadione	Sesame
Nandrolone decanoate	Sesame
Nandrolone phenpropionate	Sesame
Progesterone	Sesame
Testosterone cypionate	Cottonseed
Testosterone enanthate	Sesame
Testosterone propionate	Sesame

A suitable buffer system can be selected from knowledge of a pH profile of the drug in solution. A typical pH profile on both solubility and stability is shown in Figure 6 for procaine penicillin G. By following the degradation over a given pH range and plotting the rate constants versus pH, the pH of maximum stability (pH 6.6) can be determined. In the case of procaine penicillin G, the solubility is lowest between pH 6 and 7, which is desirable since the product is formulated as a suspension. Once the desired pH is determined, a buffer system that provides sufficient buffer capacity can be selected. The buffer capacity, β, is an indication of the resistance to change in pH upon the addition of either basic or acid substances and can be represented by the following expression:

$$\beta = \frac{dB}{dpH} = 2.303C \left[\frac{K_a H^+}{(K_a + H^{+2})} \right] \tag{22}$$

where

   dB = change in concentration of base or acid
   dpH = change in pH

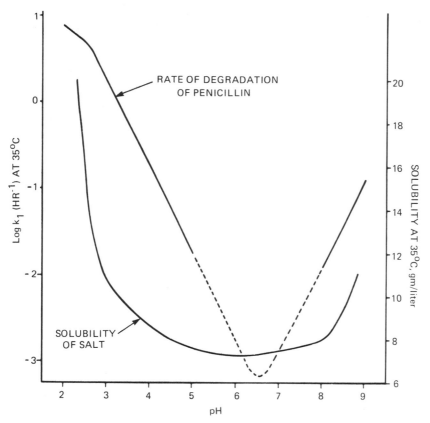

Figure 6 Solubility and rate of degradation of procaine penicillin G as a function of pH. ([From M. A. Schwartz and F. H. Buckwalter, J. Pharm. Sci., 51:1119 (1962).]

$$C = \text{molar concentration of buffer system}$$
$$K_a = \text{dissociation constant of the buffer}$$

A hypothetical plot of β versus $pH-pK_a$ is illustrated in Figure 7 for a monobasic acid. A maximum value at zero indicates that the greatest buffer capacity occurs at a pH equal to the pK_a of the buffer system and further suggests that a buffer system with a pK_a within ±1.0 unit of the desired pH should be selected. For polyfunctional groups the buffer capacities of the individual species are additive (Figure 8).

Buffer systems for parenterals generally consist of either a weak base and the salt of a weak base or a weak acid and the salt of a weak acid. Buffer systems commonly used for injectable products are acetates, citrates, phosphates, and glutamates. Figure 9 shows the effective range of typical pharmaceutical buffers. The distance indicated by the arrows represents the effective buffer range for each system and the dashed lines represent the pK_a for the system.

The Henderson-Hasselbach equation is used to calculate the quantities of buffer species required to provide a desired pH.

$$pH = pK_a + \log \frac{C \text{ salt}}{C \text{ acid}} \qquad (23)$$

Table 5 Commonly Used Substances in Parenteral Products

Substance	Usual concentrations (%)
Antimicrobial agents	
Benzalkonium chloride	0.01
Benzethonium chloride	0.01
Benzyl alcohol	2.0
Chlorobutanol	0.5
Chlorocresol	0.1-0.3
Cresol	0.3-0.5
Methyl p-hydroxybenzoate	0.18
Phenol	0.5
Phenylethyl alcohol	0.5
Phenylmercuric nitrate and acetate	0.002
Propyl p-hydroxybenzoate	0.02
Thimerosal	0.01
Antioxidants[a]	
Acetone sodium bisulfite	0.2
Ascorbic acid	0.1
Ascorbic acid esters	0.015
Butylhydroxyanisole (BHA)	0.02
Butylhydroxytoluene (BHT)	0.02
Cysteine	0.5
Nordihydroguaiaretic acid (NDGA)	0.01
Sodium bisulfite	0.15
Sodium formaldehyde sulfoxylate	0.1
Sodium metabisulfite	0.2
Tocopherols	0.5
Chelating agent	
Ethylenediaminetetraacetic acid (salt)	0.01-0.075
Buffers	
Acetic acid and a salt, pH 3.5-5.7	1-2
Citric acid and a salt, pH 2.5-6	1-3
Glutamic acid, pH 8.2-10.2	1-2
Phosphoric acid salts, pH 6-8.2	0.8-2
Tonicity adjustment	
Dextrose	5.5
Sodium chloride	0.9
Sodium sulfate[b]	1.6

[a]Concentrations represent the maximum concentrations in parenterals.
[b]Do not use in glass containers containing barium [30].

where C_{salt} and C_{acid} are the molar concentrations of the salt form and the acid form, respectively. As shown by the following calculation, an acetate buffer system ($pK_a = 4.8$) consisting of 0.1 M acetic acid and 0.05 M sodium acetate would result in a pH of 4.5.

$$pH = 4.8 + \log \frac{0.05}{0.1} \tag{24}$$

$$pH = 4.8 - 0.3 = 4.5 \tag{25}$$

The acetate system is suitable for the buffering of an injection of atropine sulfate. The pH of maximum stability is 4.0, while the maximum biological activity occurs at 6.8 to 7.2. Therefore, since it is desirable to have the solution easily adjusted to physiologic pH upon injection, as low a concentration of salt and acid as possible should be used.

Equation (23) shows that at equal molar concentrations of dissociated and undissociated species (i.e., $C_{salt} = C_{acid}$), the pH and pK_a are equal (point of maximum buffer capacity). The Henderson-Hasselbach expression is well suited for monobasic or univalent buffer systems such as acetate, diethanolamine, triethanolamine, and NH_4Cl and also for those polybasic systems where the pK_a values are sufficiently separated, such as for the phosphate and carbonate systems. However, for those systems where the buffer capacity curves overlap, such as the hypothetical illustration in Figure 8, and for example the citrate and glutamate systems (Fig. 9), all the species and pK_a values must be taken into account.

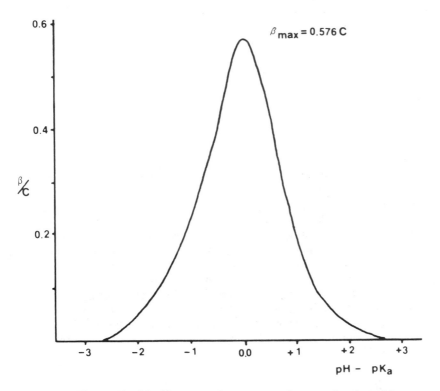

Figure 7 Theoretical buffer capacity curves of a monobasic acid.

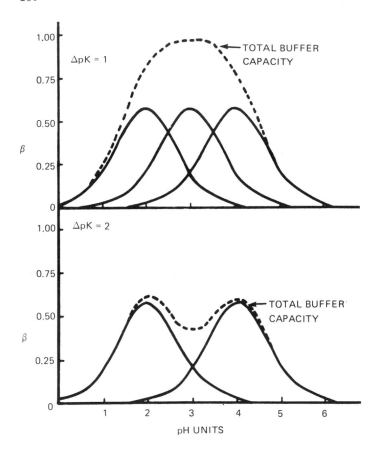

Figure 8 Hypothetical buffer capacity curves for polybasic acids. The total buffer capacity is represented by the dashed line [From J. J. Windheuser, Bull. Parenter. Drug Assoc., 17:1 (1963).]

Although buffers assure the stability of pH of solution, the buffer system itself can alter other properties such as kinetic and solubility aspects. Buffers can act as general acid or general base catalysts and cause degradation of the drug substance. Such a mechanism occurs with a number of amine and amine derivatives in systems containing polycarboxylic acids (e.g., citric, tartaric, and succinic). In such cases, as shown in Figure 10, the degradation of vitamin B_1 increases with increase in citrate buffer concentration. The degradation of chloramphenicol has been found to be pH independent below pH 7, but in the presence of buffers a pH rate profile as shown in Figure 11 occurs. The totally undissociated and ionized forms were found to be inactive, but the half-salt was highly unstable in the buffer systems.

The ionic strength contributions of the buffer system can affect both isotonicity and stability. For example, if adjustment of pH is made with sodium hydroxide, say of a solution containing monosodium phosphate, the effect of the generation of disodium salt on isotonicity and the effect of HPO_4^{2-} ion on stability as shown in Figure 12 must be taken into account.

2. Antioxidants

Many drugs in solution are subject to oxidative degradation. Such reactions are mediated either by free radicals or by molecular oxygen and often involve the

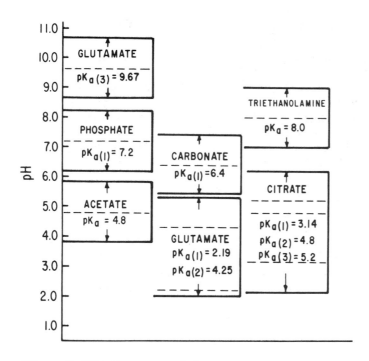

Figure 9 Effective range of pharmaceutical buffers, indicated by the arrows. The dashed line represents the pK$_a$ values.

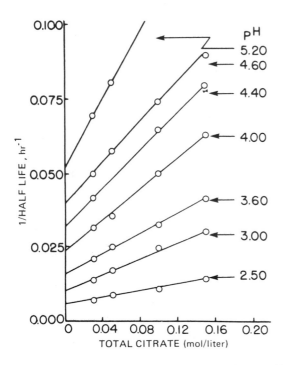

Figure 10 Effect of citrate buffer concentration on thiamine hydrolysis at 96.4°C at constant ionic strength and at different pH values. [From J. J. Windheuser and T. Higuchi, J. Pharm. Sci., 51:354 (1962).]

addition of oxygen or the removal of hydrogen. Oxidative decomposition is catalyzed by metal, hydrogen, and hydroxyl ions. Drugs possessing a favorable oxidation potential will be especially vulnerable to oxidation. For example, a great number of drugs are formulated in the reduced form (e.g., epinephrine, morphine, ascorbic acid, etc.) and are easily oxidized. By increasing the oxidation potential of the drug, oxidation can be minimized. As illustrated in Figure 13, lowering the pH of the solution will increase the oxidation potential. This occurs because according to a simplified version of the Nernst equation:

$$E = E° + \frac{RT}{2} \log \frac{[H^+] \cdot [Ox]}{[Rd]} \tag{26}$$

an increase in hydrogen ion concentration causes an increase in the actual oxidation potential, E. In this equation E° is the standard oxidation potential, R the gas constant, T the absolute temperature, and 2 represents the number of electrons taking part in the oxidation-reduction reaction. For products in which oxygen is directly involved in the degradation (i.e., autooxidation), protection can be afforded by displacing oxygen (air) from the system. This is accomplished by bubbling nitrogen or carbon dioxide through the solution prior to filling and sealing in the final container.

Agents that have a lower oxidation potential than the drug in question, and thus can be preferentially oxidized, are called antioxidants. Such agents are added to parenteral solutions either alone or in combination with a chelating agent or other antioxidant and function in at least two ways: (1) by being preferentially oxidized and thereby gradually consumed or (2) by blocking an oxidative chain reaction in which they are not usually consumed.

Morphine in aqueous solution undergoes a pH-dependent oxidative degradation. The rate is slow and constant between pH 2 and 5, where morphine exists in the protonated form as shown in Figure 14. However, above pH 5 the oxidation increases

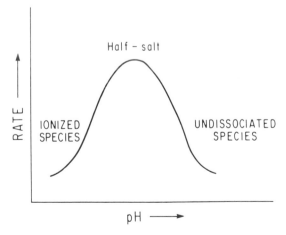

Figure 11 pH profile for the degradation of chloramphenicol in the presence of buffers showing that in the range where the species exists as the half-salt the degradation is buffer dependent.

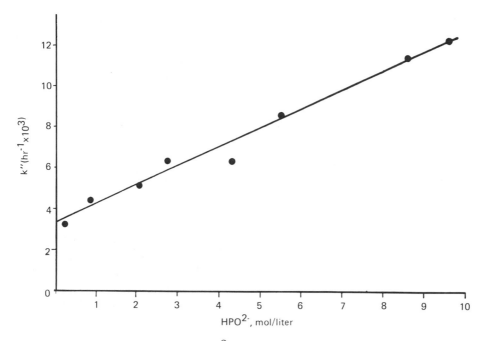

Figure 12 Catalytic effect of HPO_4^{2-} ion on the rate of hydrolysis of phenethicillin at 35°C. [From M. A. Schwartz, A. P. Granatek, and F. H. Buckwalter, J. Pharm. Sci., 51:523 (1962).]

with increase in pH [32]. Therefore, morphine can be stabilized by lowering the pH or by adding an antioxidant such as ascorbic acid which will be preferentially and reversibly oxidized between pH 5 and 7. In fact, ascorbic acid can act as an antioxidant for hydroquinone because it has a lower oxidation potential and will be preferentially oxidized. Table 6 lists some standard oxidation potentials.

Table 6 Standard Oxidation Potentials for Various Substances

Substance	$E^{\circ a}$ (V)	pH	Temp. (°C)
Riboflavin	+0.208	7.0	30
Dithiothreitol	+0.053	7.0	30
Sodium thiosulfate	+0.050	7.0	30
Thiourea	+0.029	7.0	30
Ascorbic acid	+0.003	7.0	25
	−0.115	5.2	30
	−0.136	4.58	30
Methylene blue	−0.011	7.0	30
Sodium metabisulfite	−0.114	7.0	25
Sodium bisulfite	−0.117	7.0	25
Propyl gallate	−0.199	7.0	25

Table 6 (continued)

Substance	$E°^a$ (V)	pH	Temp. (°C)
Acetylcysteine	-0.293	7.0	25
Vitamin K	-0.363	–	20
Epinephrine	-0.380	7.0	30
Hydroquinone	-0.673	–	–
Resorcinol	-1.043	–	–
Phenol	-1.089	–	–

^{a}$E°$ values correspond to the reaction (reduced) = (oxidized) + e^-.
Source: Ref. 33.

     Salts of sulfur dioxide, including bisulfite, metabisulfite, and sulfite, are the most common antioxidants in aqueous solutions. Irrespective of which salt is added to the solution, the antioxidant moiety depends on the final concentration of this compound and the final pH of the formulation [34]. The metabisulfite is used at low pH values [35]. Some drugs can be inactivated by bisulfites. For example, epinephrine is stabilized through the formation of an addition product, epinephrine sulfonate,

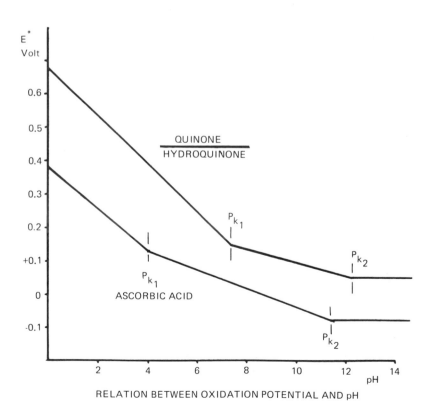

Figure 13 Relationship between oxidation potential and pH. [From G. Schell, Farm. Rev., 58:45 (1959).]

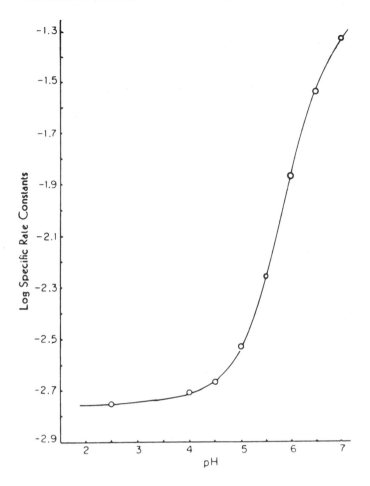

Figure 14 Reaction rate constant for the first-order oxidative degradation of morphine at 95°C as a function of pH. (From Ref. 32.)

which is inactive [36]. Ortho- or para-hydroxybenzyl alcohol derivatives react in a similar manner.

While undergoing oxidation reactions the sulfites are converted to sulfates. Since small amounts (picograms) of barium or calcium can be extracted even from type I glass, an insoluble sulfate can form [30]. Therefore, additional care must be exercised to inspect visibly preparations containing sulfite antioxidants or sulfate drugs for the presence of fine particles which will appear, upon gently shaking, as a swirl originating from the bottom of the container. Sulfite levels are determined by the reactivity of the drug, the type of container (glass seal versus rubber stopper), single- or multiple-dose use, container headspace, and the expiration dating period to be employed.

Often a single antioxidant may not be sufficient to protect the product completely. Certain compounds (e.g., ascorbic acid and citric acid) have been found to act as synergists, increasing the effectiveness of antioxidants, particularly those that block oxidative reactions. Frequently, chelating agents such as ethylenediaminetetraacetic acid derivatives and salts complex with trace amounts of heavy metals which otherwise would catalyze oxidative reactions.

3. Antimicrobials

Agents with antimicrobial activity must be added to preparations packaged in multiple-dose containers unless prohibited by the monograph or unless the drug itself is bacteriostatic (an example being methohexital sodium for injection). They are often added to unit-dose solutions which are not sterilized at the terminal stage of their manufacture. In the case of multiple-dose preparations the antimicrobial agent is required as a bacteriostat to inhibit any microbes accidentally introduced while withdrawing doses. Antimicrobial agents may also serve a role as adjuncts in aseptic processing of products (e.g., syringes), where there may be product exposure during transfer, filling, and stoppering operations. Thus, should trace contamination occur during the manufacturing process, the antimicrobial agent may render the product sterile. Also, antimicrobial agents should be present as adjuncts in intermittent heat sterilizations (i.e., tyndallization methods in which the product is subjected to two or more heat treatments at temperatures below that normally used for sterilization). Clearly, the use of antimicrobial agents is not a substitute for good manufacturing practices.

Antimicrobial agents are specifically excluded in the large volume injections which are used to provide fluids, nutrients, or electrolytes, such as Dextrose and Sodium Chloride Injection, Dextrose Injection, Ringer's Injection, Lactated Ringer's Injection, and Sodium Chloride Injection. Bacteriostatic agents may be added to Dextrose and Sodium Chloride Injection when it is labeled for use as a sclerosing agent, because the amount of injection used for such purposes is small, and the quantity of antibacterial present would not be harmful to the patient.

Consideration must be given to the stability and effectiveness of the antimicrobial agent in combination with the active ingredient and other added substances. Many papers have been published describing the incompatibilities or binding of preservatives with surfactants, pharmaceuticals, and rubber closures [37-41].

Antimicrobial activity was shown by Kostenbauder [40] to be significantly reduced in the presence of macromolecules due to binding. The activity of the antimicrobial agent was due to the concentration of the free form, as illustrated in Figure 15. These workers showed that in the presence of polysorbate 80, the concentration of free antimicrobial agent was reduced in relation to the nonionic surfactant concentration (Fig. 16). Such a plot follows the linear expression

$$\frac{\text{Total}}{\text{Free}} = 1 + kM \tag{27}$$

where k is the slope and M is the concentration of the macromolecule. Knowing the ratio of total to free preservative, the inhibitory concentration at any macromolecule concentration can be calculated from the following:

$$\frac{\text{Total}}{\text{Free}} \times \text{inhibitory preservative concentration at 0\% M} \tag{28}$$

Table 7 shows the concentrations of two quaternary ammonium compounds required to inhibit the growth of Aerobacter aerogenes in the presence of polysorbate 80.

Rubber closures and rubber extractives have been found to influence significantly preservative loss from solution and antimicrobial activity, respectively. Lachman and co-workers [39,41] studied the interaction of preservatives with various types of rubber and found significant losses of a number of preservatives (i.e., chlorobutanol, chlorophenylethyl alcohol, methylparaben, and benzyl alcohol) to natural and neoprene rubber. Table 8 shows the loss of these preservatives from

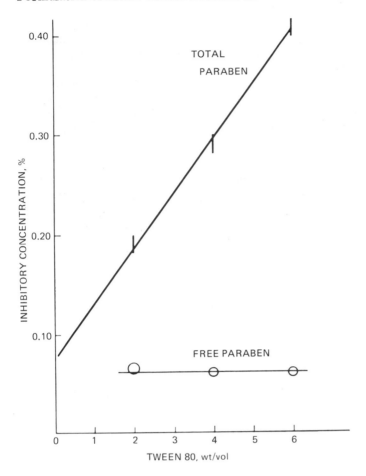

Figure 15 Comparison of the total methylparaben concentration and the free methyl-paraben concentration required to inhibit growth of <u>Aerobacter aerogenes</u> in the presence of polysorbate 80. [From F. Pisano and H. B. Kostenbauder, <u>J. Am. Pharm. Assoc. Sci. Ed.</u>, <u>48</u>:310 (1959).]

Table 7 Influence of Nonionic Surfactant on Concentrations of Cationic Agent Required to Inhibit <u>Aerobacter aerogenes</u>

| | Inhibitory concentration of: | |
Nonionic	Cetylpyridinium chloride	Benzalkonium chloride
0	1-100,000 to 1-250,000	No growth at 1-100,000
0.5% polysorbate 80	1-2500 to 1-5000	-
2.0% polysorbate 80	1-250 to 1-500	-
3.0% polysorbate 80	1-100 to 1-250	1-500 to 1-1000

Source: P. P. DeLuca and H. B. Kostenbauder, <u>J. Am. Pharm. Assoc. Sci. Ed.</u>, <u>49</u>:430 (1960).

solution in the presence of these rubber closures. On the other hand, the loss of preservative was minimal in the presence of butyl rubber.

The effectiveness of antimicrobial agents can be tested by challenging the product with selected organisms to evaluate the bacteriostatic or bactericidal activity in a formulation. This challenge test described in the USP [42] should be performed with the formulation throughout and near the end of the expiration date to ensure that adequate levels of preservative are still available. Table 9 lists the minimum inhibitory concentrations (MIC) for a number of antimicrobial agents.

4. Tonicity

Isotonic solutions exert the same osmotic pressure as blood plasma. Solutions may also exert less (hypotonic) or more (hypertonic) osmotic pressure than plasma. Red blood cells (erythrocytes) when introduced into hypotonic solutions will swell and often burst because of diffusion of water into the cell (hemolysis). If the cells are placed into hypertonic solutions, they may lose water and shrink

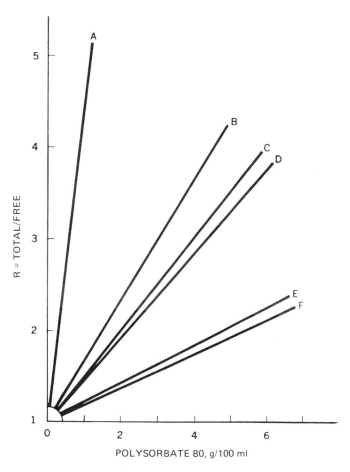

Figure 16 Binding of representative preservatives by a nonionic surface-active agent, polysorbate 80, in aqueous solution at 30°C. (A) Propylparaben, (B) methylparaben, (C) chlorobutanol, (D) benzoic acid, (E) phenylethyl alcohol, (F) benzyl alcohol. (From Ref. 40.)

Table 8 Apparent Distribution of Preservative Between Rubber and Buffer Solutions[a] After 4 Weeks of Storage

Preservative	$Kt = \dfrac{Cr}{Cb}$ Closure	Temperature (°C) 25	40
Phenylethyl alcohol	Natural	1.72	1.39
	Neoprene	4.23	4.13
Chloro-β-phenyl- ethyl alcohol	Natural	6.05	5.70
	Neoprene	16.40	21.80
Chlorobutanol	Natural	9.85	6.83
	Neoprene	14.50	14.50
Benzyl alcohol	Natural	0.63	0.63
	Neoprene	1.66	1.93
Methylparaben	Natural	1.36	1.43
	Neoprene	7.27	8.40

[a]Solutions buffered to a pH of 4.0.
Source: Ref. 41.

(crenation). In isotonic solutions (e.g., 0.9% sodium chloride) the cells maintain their "tone" and the solution is isotonic with human erythrocytes.

To minimize tissue damage and irritation, reduce hemolysis of blood cells, and prevent electrolyte imbalance upon administration of small volume parenterals, the product should be isotonic, or nearly so. This is not always feasible, as a result of the high concentrations of drug utilized and the low volumes required for some injections, the wide variety of dose regimens and methods of administration, or product stability considerations. Historically, there has been concern over the osmolarity or tonicity of intravenous infusion fluids because of the large amounts of solution administered to hospitalized patients, but in the last few years there has also been interest in the osmolarity of other parenteral dosage forms. The British Pharmacopeia [43] states that aqueous solutions for subcutaneous, intradermal, or intramuscular injection should be made isotonic if possible. As mentioned previously, sodium or potassium chloride and dextrose are commonly added to adjust hypotonic solutions.

Calculation of tonicity is illustrated by the following example. There are several methods available to calculate tonicity [44]. The sodium chloride equivalent method will be used in the present example. It is desired to make a 2 g/100 ml solution of sodium cephalothin isotonic with sodium chloride. Sodium cephalothin has a molecular weight of 238. The equation used is

$$E = 17 \frac{L_{iso}}{M} \tag{29}$$

where E is the weight of NaCl with the same freezing-point depression as 1 g of sodium cephalothin; L_{iso} is the freezing-point depression for univalent electrolytes and has a calculated value of 3.4, and M is the molecular weight of sodium cephalothin. Then

$$E = 17 \times \frac{3.4}{238} = \frac{57.8}{238} = 0.24 \text{ g-eq} \tag{30}$$

Table 9 Minimum Inhibitory Concentration (MIC) for Parenteral
Antimicrobial Agents

Agent	MIC range* (%)	Amount Most Often Used (%)
Benzalkonium chloride	0.005-0.03	0.01
Benzethonium chloride	0.005-0.03	0.01
Benzyl alcohol	1.0-10.0	1.0
Chlorobutanol	0.2-0.8	0.5
Chlorocresol	0.1-0.3	0.1-0.25
Cresol	0.1-0.6	0.3
Parabens, parasepts	0.5-0.25 methyl	0.18
(methyl, ethyl, propyl, butyl esters)	0.005-0.03 others	0.02
Phenol	0.1-0.8	0.5
Phenylmercuric nitrate	0.001-0.05	0.002
Thimerosal	0.005-0.03	0.01

*Affected by produce pH, ionic strength, storage temperature, packaging
materials, etc.

Since 2 g of drug is used in the 100 ml of fluid, $2 \times 0.24 = 0.48$ g-eq is contributed
by sodium cephalothin toward the 0.90 g of sodium chloride needed for isotonicity.
Hence 0.90 g - 0.48 g = 0.42 g of sodium chloride must be added to 2 g of sodium
cephalothin in 100 ml to achieve isotonicity of the resulting solution.

The sodium chloride equivalent method was used for determining the osmolarity of a number of infusion solutions and compared with measured values (Table
10). There is good agreement between measured and calculated values until the
concentration becomes high.

Isoosmosity, determined by physical methods, should be distinguished from
isotonicity, determined by biological methods (i.e., the hematocrit method with
human erythrocytes). This distinction is necessary because of the variable dif-
fusibility of different medicinal substances across the cell membrane, which does
not always behave as a truly semipermeable membrane. Solutions that are theoretically isoosmotic with the cells may cause hemolysis because solutes diffuse
through the cell membrane. For example, a 1.8% solution of urea has the same
osmotic pressure as 0.9% sodium chloride, but the urea solution produces hemolysis, because urea permeates the cell membrane.

If a solution is hypertonic, not much can be done with the formulation unless
it can be diluted with water prior to administration. Administration of a hypertonic
solution should be done slowly to permit dilution by the blood. In some cases, where
injection of such solutions produces pain, as in an intramuscular injection, a local
anesthetic may be added. The effect of isotonicity on reducing pain on injection
is somewhat vague, although it may at least reduce tissue irritation. Pain on injection may occur during and immediately following the injection, or it may be a
delayed or prolonged type of pain which increases in severity after subsequent

Table 10 Comparison of Measured Osmolality Values with Those Calculated from Sodium Chloride Equivalents

Solution (g/100 ml)		Measured osmolality (mean mOsm ± S.D.)	Sodium chloride equivalent method	
			Osmolality (mOsm kg^{-1})	Percent of measured
Dextrose				
5.0		262 ± 5.9	249	95.0
10.0		547 ± 6.2	499	91.2
20.0		1176 ± 14.9	998	84.9
Alanine	Glycine			
1.0	1.0	246 ± 0.5	256	104
2.0	2.0	480 ± 1.7	512	107
5.0	5.0	1245 ± 10.8	1281	103
0.2 NaCl in 5% dextrose		311 ± 5.85	312	100
0.45% NaCl in 5% dextrose		385 ± 5.48	390	98.7
Ringer's Solution, USP		294 ± 4.98	281	95.6
Lactated Ringer's, USP		264 ± 3.23	248	93.9
Travasol 5.5%		554 ± 11.4	596	107.6
67% Travasol (5.5%), 33% dextrose (50%)		1330 ± 29.6	1223	91.9

Source: Ref. 45.

injections. The actual cause of the pain is often unknown and will vary significantly among patients according to the product. In some cases pain may be reduced by minor formulation changes such as adjusting tonicity and pH or adding an anesthetic agent such as benzyl alcohol or lidocaine hydrochloride. In other cases pain is more inherent to the drug and the problem is more difficult or impossible to resolve. Pain, soreness, and tissue inflammation are often encountered in parenteral suspensions, especially those containing a high amount of solids.

D. Special Types of Parenterals

1. Suspensions

A parenteral suspension is a dispersed, multiphased, heterogeneous system of insoluble solid particles intended principally for intramuscular and subcutaneous injection. Because a delicate balance of variables is required in order to formulate a suitable product, a suspension is one of the most difficult parenteral forms to prepare. Such a product must not cake during shipping and storage and should be easy to suspend and inject through an 18 to 21 gauge needle throughout its shelf life. To achieve these goals it is necessary to control the crystallization, particle size reduction (micronization), and sterilization of the drug substance, as well as the processes involved in wetting of the drug with surfactants, aseptic dispersion and milling, and final filling into containers. Uniform distribution of the drug is required to ensure that an adequate dose is administered to the patient.

Parenteral suspensions exhibit instability in ways not applicable to solutions and dry solids. Injectable suspensions may be made with either vegetable oils or aqueous vehicles. Many contain low concentrations of solids (5% or less) whereas a few, such as procaine penicillin G, may contain up to 58% w/v solids. Therefore, properties such as resuspendibility, zeta potential, rheology, and particle size distribution become important, and often need to be monitored as a part of a stability program for these products. When particles interact to form clumps or aggregates, the process is termed flocculation or agglomeration. The process of dispersing aggregates into individual particles is called deflocculation. The size of individual particles may also change due to temperature fluctuation during storage and/or polymorphic changes. For example, if the solubility of a drug is very temperature dependent, individual crystals can dissolve or grow in size depending on the circumstances encountered. If the bioavailability or injectability of the drug depends on the particle size distribution of the dispersed insoluble drug, the intended performance of the product may be altered.

The requirements for, limitations in, and difference between the design of injectable suspensions and other suspensions have been summarized by several authors [46-49]. The requirements and limitations relate to (1) microbiological purity, (2) ingredients allowed, and (3) mechanical flow properties. The microbiological purity requirements, like all parenterals, involve sterility and freedom from pyrogens.

The wide variety of injectable suspensions can be illustrated with the following examples. Sterile Ampicillin for Suspension, USP, represents a powder to which an aqueous diluent is added to make an injectable suspension. Sterile Aurothioglucose Suspension, USP, is an example of a ready-to-use suspension in vegetable oil. Aqueous ready-to-use suspensions include Betamethasone Acetate Suspension, USP, Insulin Zinc Suspension, USP, and Tetanus Toxoid Adsorbed, USP.

A formula for an injectable suspension might consist of the active ingredient suspended in an aqueous vehicle containing an antimicrobial agent, a surfactant for wetting and preventing crystal growth (by reducing free surface energy), a dispersing or suspending agent, and perhaps a buffer or salt. Table 11 lists materials commonly used to formulate parenteral suspensions. Two basic methods are used to prepare parenteral suspensions: (1) sterile vehicle and powder are combined aseptically, or (2) sterile solutions combined and the crystals formed in situ.

In the first method, an aqueous vehicle containing the water-soluble components are heat sterilized, when possible, or filtered through a 0.22 μm sterilizing membrane filter into a presterilized mixing/filling tank. The sterile drug powder is gradually added to the sterile solution, aseptically, while mixing. The sterile drug powder is obtained by aseptically filtering a solution of the drug through a sterilizing membrane into a sterile vessel into which a presterilized solution of antisolvent is introduced, causing the drug to crystallize. The crystals or powder are separated aseptically by filtration or centrifugation, washed, dried, and sized through milling. After all tests have been completed on the bulk material, it is aseptically filled.

In the second method, the vehicle is prepared and sterilized by filtration. The drug is dissolved separately in a nonaqueous solvent and sterilized by filtration. The sterile drug solution is added, aseptically, to the sterile vehicle, causing the drug to crystallize. The resulting suspension is then diluted with sterile vehicle,

Table 11 Examples of Ingredients Used in
Parenteral Suspensions

Suspending agents

  Aluminum monsterate

  Gelatin (nonantigenic)

  Mannitol

  Povidone

  Sodium carboxymethylcellulose

  Sorbitol

Surfactants

  Lecithin (soybean)

  Polyoxyethylene-polyoxypropylene ethers

  Polyoxyethylene sorbitan monolaurate

  Polysorbate 80

  Silicone antifoam

  Sorbitan trioleate

Solubilizing agents

  Polyethylene glycol 300

  Propylene glycol

pH adjustment

  Citric acid

  Sodium citrate

---

mixed, the crystals allowed to settle, and the supernatant solution siphoned off.
The suspension is then brought to volume and filled in the normal manner.

    Rheologically, an injectable suspension can present some formidable challenges. While a suspension can usually be formulated that can be filled, shipped, and injected, it is frequently difficult to formulate a product in which these three qualities will remain relatively unchanged throughout its shelf life [48]. Rheological evaluation should be done with a recording viscometer that continuously measures the shear throughout the hysteresis loop.

    The critical nature of the flow properties of parenteral suspensions becomes apparent when one remembers that those products are frequently administered through 1 1/2 in. or longer needles, having internal diameters in the range of only 300 to 600 μm. In addition, microscopic examination shows a very rough interior needle surface, further hindering flow. The flow properties of parenteral suspensions are usually characterized on the basis of syringeability or injectability. Syringeability refers to the handling characteristics of a suspension while drawing it into and manipulating it in a syringe. Syringeability includes characteristics such as ease of withdrawal from the container into the syringe, clogging and foaming tendencies, and accuracy of dose measurement. The term <u>injectability</u> refers to the properties of the suspension during injection; it includes such factors as pressure or force required for injection, evenness of flow, aspiration qualities, and freedom from clogging. The syringeability and injectability characteristics of a suspension are closely related to viscosity and to particle characteristics.

2. Emulsions

An emulsion is a heterogeneous dispersion of one immiscible liquid in another. This inherently unstable system is made possible through the use of an emulsifying agent, which prevents coalescence of the dispersed droplets. Parenteral emulsions are rare because it is necessary (and difficult) to achieve stable droplets of less than 1 μm to prevent emboli in the blood vessels and it is not usually necessary to achieve an emulsion for drug administration.

Parenteral emulsions have been used for several pruposes, including:

1. Water-in-oil emulsions of allergenic extracts (given subcutaneously)
2. Oil-in-water sustained-release depot preparations (given intramuscularly)
3. Oil-in-water nutrient emulsions (given intravenously)

Formulation options are severely restricted through a very limited selection of stabilizers and emulsifiers primarily due to the dual constraints of autoclave sterilization and parenteral injection. Additionally, unwanted physiological effects (e.g., pyrogenic reaction and hemolysis) have further limited the use of intravenous emulsions.

An increasingly popular class of intravenous emulsions is fat emulsions, which have been described by several researchers [50, 51]. These preparations have been available in Europe for over 20 years and in the United States since 1975. Fat is transported in the bloodstream as small droplets called chylomicra. Chylomicra are 0.5 to 1.0 μm spheres consisting of a central core of triglycerides and an outer layer of phospholipids. Intravenous fat emulsions usually contain 10% oil, although they may range up to 20% (see Table 12). These emulsions yield triglycerides which provide essential fatty acids and calories during total parenteral nutrition of patients who are unable to absorb nutrients through the gastrointestinal tract. The products commercially available in the United States range from 0.1 to 0.5 μm and have a pH of 5.5 to 8 (blood plasma has a pH of 7.4). Glycerol and glucose are added to make the product isotonic. For a more complete discussion of parenteral emulsions, other texts should be consulted [50-52].

3. Dried Forms

Sterile solids are drugs or drug products packaged in a dry form which must be reconstituted or suspended in sterile vehicles prior to administration. Many drugs, particularly the cephalosporins and penicillins, are not sufficiently stable in aqueous solutions to permit packaging them "ready to use." The pharmacist, nurse, and physician should be aware of the final form of a reconstitutable product. A dry solid may be intended to be reconstituted as a solution or as a suspension. If the final product is to be a solution, it should not be administered until all the solids are totally in solution. The key to the final product form can be distinguished from the title of the product.

Dry solids which are intended to be reconstituted by the addition of suitable solvents to yield solutions, conforming in all respects to the requirements for

Table 12 Intravenous Fat Emulsions

Component (g/100 ml)	Intralipid[a] 10%	Intralipid[a] 20%	Liposyn[b]	Infonutrol[c]	Lipofundin[d]	Lipiphysan[e]	
Soybean oil	10	20					
Safflower oil			10				
Cottonseed oil				15	10	10	15
Egg phospholipids	1.2	1.2	1.2				
Soybean phospholipids				1.2	1.2		
Soybean lecithin						1.5	2
Glycerol	2.25	2.25	2.5				
Glucose				4			
Sorbitol					5	5	5
Pluronic F-68				0.3			
DL-α-Tocopherol						0.05	0.05
Water for Injections q.s. ad	100 ml	100 ml	100 ml	100 ml	100 ml	100 ml	

[a]Cutter Laboratories, Berkeley, California, and Vitrum A.G., Stockholm, Sweden.
[b]Abbott Laboratories, North Chicago, Illinois.
[c]Astra-Hewlett, Södertäye, Sweden.
[d]Braun, Melsunger, West Germany.
[e]Egic, L'Equilibre Biologique S.A., Loiret, France.

injections (solutions for injection), will be described by a title in the form: —for Injection or Sterile—. Examples are Thiopental Sodium for Injection (USP), in which the preparation contains added substances in addition to the drug, and Sterile Nafcillin Sodium (USP), in which there are no additional ingredients only the drug. In any such labeling, the product is intended to be appropriately reconstituted as a solution. Some reconstituted products must be further diluted prior to use, an example being Methohexital Sodium for Injection (USP).

Dry products which are to be reconstituted as suspensions by the addition of a suitable vehicle to yield a product meeting all requirements for sterile suspensions will be labeled Sterile—for Suspension. An example is Sterile Ampicillin Trihydrate for Suspension. Such preparations are manufactured and packaged, therefore, as dry sterile solids by sterile filtration and freeze drying or bulk sterilization and aseptic powder filling. The sterile bulk powder in the latter process can be achieved by either aseptic crystallization or spray drying. The powder filing procedure is described in sufficient detail elsewhere [53, 54], so only a brief discussion will be included. Freeze-drying, however, will be covered in more detail.

Powder Filling. This method involves filling sterile powder into individual containers under aseptic conditions in which a measured quantity, either on a weight or volume basis, is delivered to a wide-mouth container. If the material is free-flowing, a machine method is used whereby the solid material is fed from a hopper to the container by means of an auger in the stem of the hopper or an adjustable cavity in the rim of a filling wheel.

Particle size and shape are important factors in powder filling since electrostatic charge, hygroscopicity, and flow are greatly influenced by these properties. Additionally, the dissolution rate will be influenced by particle size. The humidity of the filling room should be carefully controlled. If the room is too dry, the powder will become electrostatically charged and will not flow. If the humidity is too high, compaction will occur due to moisture in the powder.

Drugs that associate with water to produce crystalline forms are called hydrates. Water content of the hydrate forms of sodium cefazolin as a function of relative humidity is seen in Figure 17. As shown in the figure, the sesquihydrate is the most stable structure when exposed to extreme humidity conditions. This figure also reveals the importance of choosing the proper combination of hydrate and humidity conditions when designing a manufacturing process or facility.

For parenteral products the powder is generally prepared under aseptic conditions by crystallization or spray drying, which provides greater assurance of sterility within the material. In the crystallization technique the drug is dissolved in an appropriate solvent and sterilized by filtration. Then under controlled conditions, another sterile solvent in which the drug is not soluble is added to the solution to induce crystallization of the drug. The sterile crystals are removed, washed, dried, and generally tested for particle size distribution, dissolution rate, and correct crystalline form prior to filling.

In order to obtain a uniform product from lot to lot, strict adherence to the procedures developed for a particular crystallization must be followed, including control of pH, rates of addition, solvent concentrations, and purity, temperature, and mixing rates. Each crystallization procedure has to be designed to ensure sterility and minimize particulate contamination. Subtle changes, such as using absolute ethyl alcohol instead of 95% ethanol during the washing procedure in a crystallization procedure, can destroy the crystalline structure if the material being crystallized is a hydrate structure.

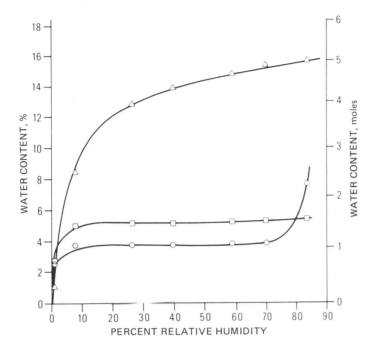

Figure 17 Relative humidity versus water content of hydrate forms of sodium cefazolin. —○—○—○—, Monohydrate; —□—□—□—, sesquihydrate; —△—△—△—, pentahydrate. (From Ref. 28.)

If the drug powder is to be prepared by spray drying, a sterile solution of the drug is prepared in a similar manner as for aseptic crystallization but instead of crystallizing the drug by adding another solvent, the sterile solution or a resultant slurry is sprayed through an atomizer with a fine orifice into a drying chamber, generally conical in shape (see Fig. 18). Upon contact with a stream of hot sterile gas, the solvent rapidly evaporates and the resulting powder is collected in a sterile chamber. The type of atomizer and method of spraying, the concentration of the solution to be sprayed, the pressure at which it is atomized, and the temperature and pressure of the gas in the chamber are factors influencing the particle size and

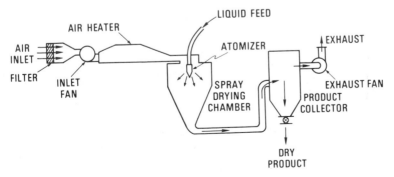

Figure 18 Schematic drawing of spray dryer.

porosity of the resultant powder. The drug powder, present as hollow spheres, is then filled into vials as a dry powder.

Freeze-Drying. From a historical standpoint the process of freeze-drying, often referred to as lyophilization, received its initial thrust during World War II when whole blood and blood plasma became lifesaving elements, and adequate supplies were jeopardized because of stability and shipping problems associated with these natural biological products. Soon after World War II, the pharmaceutical industry began considering the process for the preparation of sterile injectable dosage forms which could not be formulated into stable solutions. At the same time the food industry began employing freeze-drying to process and package foods, an application that continues to grow. Another application that has been receiving research attention is the preservation of biological substances, especially those of high worth or in short supply. Vital organs and tissues are also preserved by freeze-drying. Substances that degrade in solution become candidates for freeze-drying. This precludes storage of the product in a deep-frozen state which presents solubility problems, is costly, and there is always the risk of degradation. Often, freeze-drying offers the only means to stabilize the product or may be a convenient way to stock-pile material for defense or emergency purposes and of course shipment and storage of dry material is less expensive than that in solution form. Although there are those who would consider freeze-drying only as the last resort, there are others who view it as a panacea—a way to get into clinical trials quickly or a way to exclude contaminants and inert particles, especially in comparison with powder filling. Certainly, freeze-drying does offer the advantage over powder filling of accuracy of dosage, since the drug is filled into the final container as a solution. Microgram quantities can be filled precisely. Powder filling is used where the required dosage is represented by a large quantity of the drug or where the solubility is not adequate to freeze and as previously described with powder filling, sterilization of the powder is possible prior to filling.

The process of freeze-drying illustrated in Figure 19 involves (1) dissolving the drug and excipients in a suitable solvent, generally water; (2) sterilizing the bulk solution by passing it through a bacteria-retentive filter; (3) filling into individual sterile containers; (4) freezing the solution by placing the open containers on

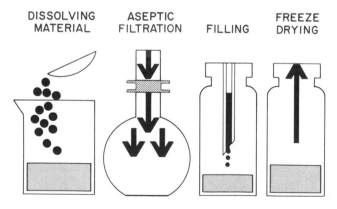

Figure 19 Freeze-drying process.

cooled shelves in a freeze-drying chamber or prefreezing in another chamber; and (5) applying a vacuum to the chamber and heating the shelves in order to sublime the water from the frozen state. The desired characteristics of a freeze-dried pharmaceutical dosage form include (1) an intact cake occupying the same shape and size as the original frozen mass; (2) sufficient strength to prevent cracking, powdering, or collapse; (3) uniform color and consistency; (4) sufficient dryness to maintain stability; and (5) sufficient porosity and surface area to permit rapid reconstitution. Of course, as with any injectable dosage form, freedom from contamination (i.e., microorganisms, pyrogens, and particulates) is an essential attribute.

The desired characteristics can be achieved by proper formulation of the product and by employing optimum freeze-drying cycles. The development of a suitable formulation and a freeze-dry cycle requires knowledge of some basic properties, such as (1) eutectic temperature; (2) temperature effect on solubility; (3) thermal properties of the frozen solution; (4) degree of supercooling; (5) heat transfer properties of the freeze-dryer shelves, metal trays, glass vials, and the frozen product; and (6) equipment design and equipment capability. Formulating the solution to be freeze-dried must be done with a view toward the characteristics required at the time of reconstitution and administration. The drug alone often does not provide the solid content or characteristics appropriate for the finished product, and inert or relatively inert substances such as lactose or mannitol must be added prior to freeze-drying to provide the necessary bulk and desired characteristics.

For a systematic approach to the development of a suitable freeze-dried product, knowledge of the various stages of the process is necessary. The main stages can be classified as freezing and drying. The initial freezing process is of critical importance since it will influence the pattern of the sublimation phase. The latter phase must occur from the solid state throughout the cycle. Appropriate cooling cycles must be determined in order to obtain an appropriate structure of the frozen mass, which is a function of the rate of freezing and the final freezing temperature. The rate of freezing also affects the size of ice crystals. The slower the rate of freezing, the larger the ice crystals that form. Freezing of the solution is most conveniently accomplished in the chamber to be employed for drying, by placing the containers of solution on a shelf that is cooled by a circulating refrigerant, such as Freon, Cellosolve, or trichlorethylene. If the frozen system exhibits metastable or amorphous-glassy structures, these structures may need to be ruptured by appropriate thermal treatments (a succession of cooling and rewarming periods), thereby inducing crystallization of the amorphous material and adequate crystal size necessary for efficient sublimation.

The most commonly employed method of drying pharmaceuticals is condensation at low temperatures whereby, through the principal mode of conduction, heat is transferred to the frozen product to effect vaporization. By further introducing a cold surface into the system at a temperature below that of the frozen product, the water vapor evolved by the drying material will be condensed as ice on the refrigerated surface. The process is illustrated in Figure 20, together with the temperature gradient during the drying cycle. Factors influencing the rate of vaporization have been discussed extensively [55, 56]. The faster heat can be applied, the faster the drying proceeds, provided that (1) the temperature of the product remains below its liquefying point, and (2) a sufficiently low pressure is maintained in the system by efficient vacuum pumps. If a sufficiently low pressure is not maintained, the temperature of the product will rise until a phase separation occurs, resulting in the partial softening or puffing of the product.

In developing a formulation for freeze-drying, the optimal formula will permit the overall cycle to be carried out in the least amount of time, while providing

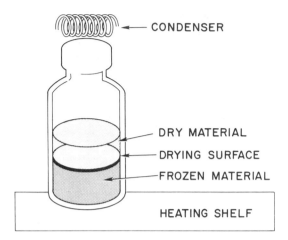

Figure 20 Drying process during freeze-drying. The temperature gradient is
shelf > dry material > drying surface > frozen material > condenser.

a stable and efficacious product which contains a low moisture content, undergoes
rapid reconstitution, and possesses the desired appearance. The potency of many
pharmaceutical agents is of such magnitude that relatively small amounts are required for the lyophilized injectable dosage form. Therefore, the need for a suitable filler of bulking agent is often indicated. The percentage of solids in the frozen plug will vary depending on the dosage and nature of the active ingredient;
generally, it whould be above 5% and not exceed 30%, with a 10 to 15% content being
optimum. Materials to choose from to add to the solution to improve the physical
characteristics of the finished cake are limited but include gelatin, mannitol, lactose, dextran, sorbitol, mono- and dibasic sodium phosphate, calcium lactobionate,
bovine serum albumin, and sodium chloride. It should be kept in mind when adding
bulking agents that drying will be accelerated if the solute concentration is kept low.
     If degradation is a risk during freezing due to concentration effects or pH
changes, stabilizers or buffers may have to be added. The problem of collapse has
been discussed earlier and if the substance is vulnerable to collapse, a rigidizer
such as glycine or mannitol may need to be added. Again it is important to point
out that dilution is also a way to avoid meltback and collapse. So compromises and
trade-offs are often necessary. If damage during freezing is a problem, a cryo-
protective agent such as bovine serum albumin may be added or to minimize damage
due to overdrying, sugars have been added. If the ingredients that are added are
found to adhere to the glass surface, such as albumin, then the containers with thin
walls, such as ampuls and tubular vials, may need to be coated with silicone to
minimize cracking. The depth of fill in a container is critical. While this depends
on the volume of the container, a rule of thumb has been 1 to 2 cm in depth but
never exceed one-half the capacity of the container.
     Most freeze-dried drug products are organic electrolytes which exhibit eutec-
tic points and supercooling tendencies. Several methods have been used for determining eutectic temperatures: (1) thermal analysis, (2) differential thermal analysis, and (3) electric resistivity. The electric resistivity method [57,58] involves
the simultaneous monitoring of resistance and temperature of a frozen sample.
Below the eutectic temperature the resistivity is very high, but when the eutectic
is reached there will be a sudden change in resistivity due to a phase change and

occurrence of liquid in the mass. An advantage of the resistance method is that
not only can eutectic temperature be determined but the degree of supercooling and
other phenomenon, such as recrystallization, can be assessed.

Examples of freezing and thawing curves are shown in Figure 21 for a 1.0
molar solution of an inorganic electrolyte, sodium chloride, together with the
warming curve for pure water. For sodium chloride, the extent of supercooling is
shown to be very significant with solidification occurring at about -30°C. In the
event that the cooling curve was used to measure eutectic temperature, inaccurate
information would be obtained as a result of the supercooling effect. The true eutectic temperature, as seen from the warming curve in the figure, occurs at
-21.6°C. The eutectic temperature is obtained from the warming curve at the point
where there is a sudden drop in resistivity or, conversely, an increase in conductivity, due to the occurrence of liquid in the cell containing the frozen mass. The
curves shown in Figure 22 for an organic pharmaceutical, methylphenidate hydrochloride, are somewhat more complex than those obtained for the inorganic electrolyte. Nevertheless, the eutectic point (-11.7°C) can be determined from the sudden
change in resistivity, indicating a phase transition.

A knowledge of the eutectic temperature of the additive is essential since the
addition of a salt such as sodium chloride to a drug with a eutectic significantly
above that of sodium chloride would only succeed in lengthening the cycle because

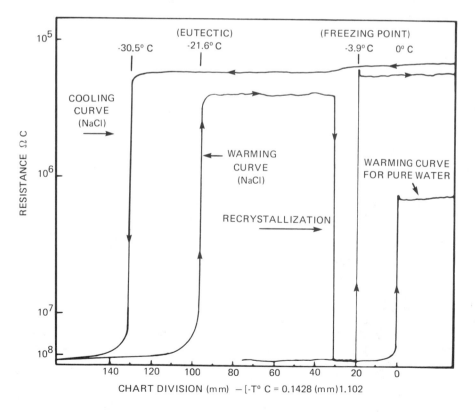

Figure 21 Resistance-temperature curves for the freezing and thawing of 1.0 M
sodium chloride solution. [From P. P. DeLuca and L. Lachman, J. Pharm. Sci.,
54:1412 (1965).]

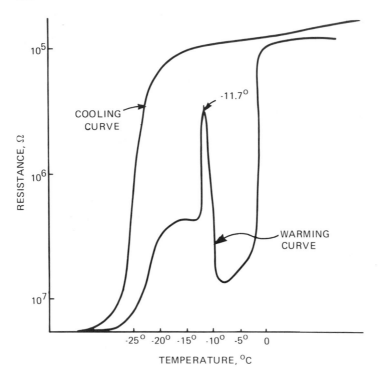

Figure 22 Cooling and warming curves for 0.3 M methylphenidate HCl solution
(From Ref. 57.)

lower temperatures would have to be maintained. In addition, some additives, such
as sodium chloride and the phosphates, tend to form crusty-appearing cakes. This
occurs during freezing and drying, probably because of the phenomenon of recrystallization. Volatile substances are generally considered to be of little value to the
finished cake but can be used if they accelerate the drying cycle. Dioxane, ethanol,
t-butanol, dimethyl sulfoxide (DMSO), and acetone are examples.

    Antimicrobial agents such as phenol, chlorobutanol, and benzyl alcohol serve
only to preserve the solution prior to freeze-drying. One must remember that if a
volatile substance is used for a temporary effect, complete removal of the substance
from the finished cake must be substantiated through adequate testing. The retention of volatile substances has been found to occur during the freeze-drying of
liquid and semiliquid foods.

    For compounds that do not form true eutectics, the variations of temperature
in a freeze-dryer often result in a finished product of varying quality. Meltback,
discoloration, and collapse are occurrences that necessitate rejections of all or
parts of the batch. Quite often a substance is not considered to be a good candidate
for freeze-drying and the process is discarded. Phase transitions that occur in the
frozen state have been shown to influence the properties of the dried product [59].
Cefazolin sodium, commercially available as a freeze-dried product, freezes as
the amorphous form and unless thermally treated to effect crystallization will remain in the less desirable amorphous state. Figure 23a is a thermogram obtained
by differential scanning calorimetry for cefazolin sodium. The first endothermic
shift occurs at -20°C (point B), an irreversible exotherm begins at -11°C (point C),
and melting of ice begins at -4°C (point F). Considering the portion of the curve

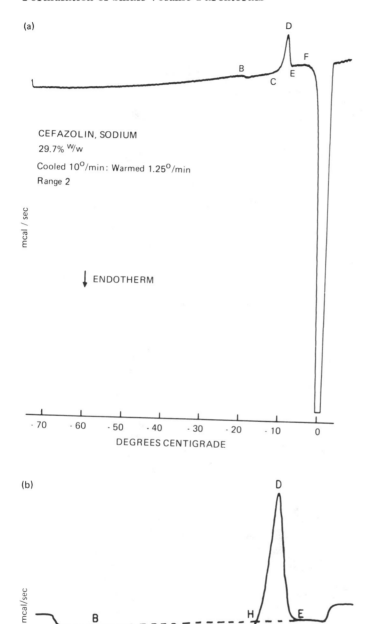

Figure 23 DSC thermogram for the warming of a frozen cefazolin sodium solution.
(a) Temperature range between 0 and –70°C. (b) Endothermic and exothermic
areas of the thermogram of cefazolin sodium. Solid curve corresponds to warming
following freezing to –30°C; dashed line corresponds to the warming curve of the
previous solution which was recooled after warming to –6°C. (From Ref. 59.)

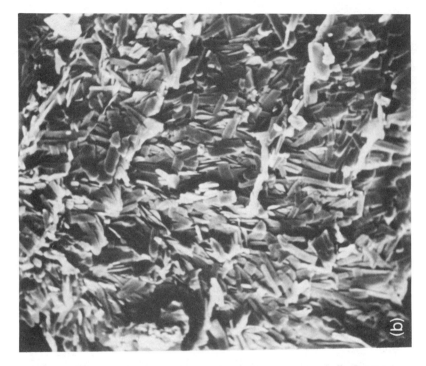

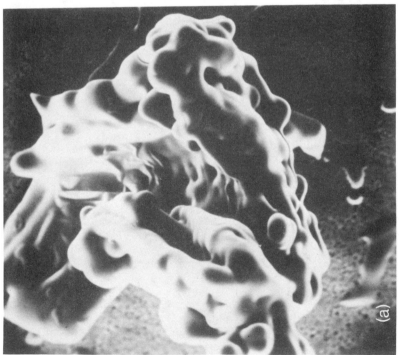

Figure 24 Scanning electron micrographs of freeze-dried cefazolin sodium. (a) Dried without thermal treatment. (b) Frozen mass warmed to −10°C and held 15 min before cooling and drying. Original magnification: 1200 X 10 kV. (From Ref. 59.)

Beginning just below the initial endotherm and to just above the irreversible exotherm, if warming were to proceed to just beyond the exotherm, say -6° C, and the system recooled to -25° C, upon rewarming, the dashed curve shown in Figure 23b, would result. This indicates that the frozen material has undergone transition. If, however, cefazolin was frozen and dried below -22° C (presumably the glass transition temperature), with no thermal treatment, the resulting product would be amorphous. This was confirmed using optical microscopy, scanning electron microscopy, and x-ray diffraction on freeze-dried material that was dried with and without thermal treatment. Material treated at -10° C exhibit birefrigence under crossed polars, defined shape by scanning electron microscopy (Fig. 24) and an x-ray diffraction pattern consisting of peaks of various intensity. All of these are indications of crystalline structure. Kinetic studies show that the crystallization can occur above -20°C (point B in Fig. 23b) and is very rapid above -11°C (point C).

Freeze-dried products are generally packaged in ampuls or vials. Ampuls would only be used for single-dose administration, and provide even drying because the tubing is thin and bottoms are reasonably flat. However, they must be sealed after removal from the chamber and reconstitution is sometimes cumbersome if shaking is required. Additionally, the generation of glass particles is a problem. Vials are used for both single- and multiple-dose application. If molded glass is used, there is greater incidence of variation of thickness and uneven bottoms. The containers must be sealed with a closure that can be accomplished inside the chamber, lessening the risk of contamination and providing an opportunity to seal under an inert gas or under vacuum. Reconstitution is much easier, but there is the risk of introducing rubber particles. Butyl rubber is preferred over neoprene due to low moisture vapor transmission.

Temperature and pressure curves for a typical cycle are illustrated in Figure 25. With the circulating temperature set at 60° C, all the probed samples passed through 0° C within 6.5 hr. The heat was lowered gradually to 40° C and allowed to remain at this temperature until the run was terminated. From the temperature and pressure curves, it can be seen that maximum drying took place between 1 and 6 hr. The maximum vapor pressure difference between chamber and condensor occurred between 2 and 5 hr, with the chamber pressure reaching a minumum value of 15 μm after 10 hr. The leveling off of the product temperature several degrees below the eutectic point (-11° C) during the primary drying phase was an indication that the heat applied was not excessive.

The application of freeze-drying to processing biological and diagnostic products has been growing. With this increased application, new problems are beginning to surface, such as the awareness that freeze-dried products can undergo structural and/or chemical modifications which might affect their physical properties, therapeutic effectiveness, and even their safety in clinical uses.

II. CONTAINER EFFECTS ON FORMULATION

Containers for parenteral products serve several purposes; facilitate manufacturing; maintain product protection, including sterility and freedom from pyrogens; allow inspection of the contents; permit shipping and storage; and provide convenient clinical use. The container components illustrated in Figures 26 and 27 must be considered as integral parts of the product because they can dramatically affect product stability, potency, toxicity, and safety, and therefore must be evaluated carefully with a variety of tests.

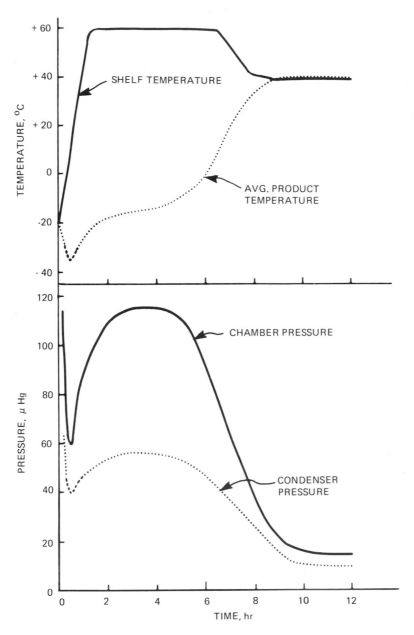

Figure 25 Temperature-time and pressure-time curves characteristic of the drying cycle for methylphenidate hydrochloride. [From P. P. DeLuca, J. Pharm. Sci., 60:778 (1971).]

A. Glass

The three types of glass recognized by the USP for parenteral use are listed in Table 13. Type I is borosilicate and is the least reactive as measured by a standardized alkalinity test run on powdered (ground) samples. Types II and III glass are

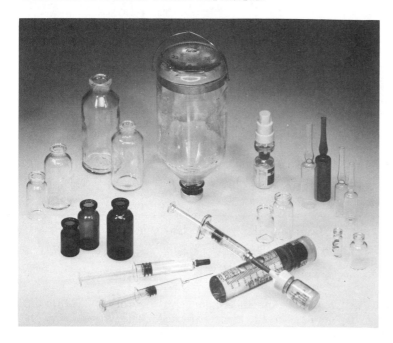

Figure 26 Representative parenteral containers.

soda lime, with type II being surface treated with sulfate, sulfite, or sulfide to make it less reactive. Type I glass is, theoretically, the best all-purpose glass for injectables and should be the only glass that is used with alkaline products. However, it is significantly more expensive than types II and III. Type II glass is

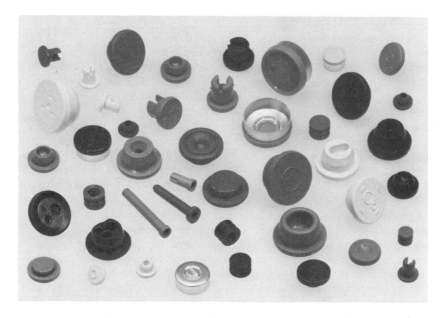

Figure 27 Representative parenteral closures.

Table 13 Parenteral Glass Types and USP XX Test Limits

| | | | Limits | |
Type	General description[a]	Type of test	Size[b] (ml)	Milliliters 0.020 N acid
I	Highly resistant, borosilicate glass	Powdered glass	All	1.0
II	Treated soda-lime glass	Water attack	100 or less	0.7
			Over 100	0.2
III	Soda-lime glass	Powdered glass	All	8.5

[a]The description applies to containers of this type of glass usually available.
[b]Size indicates the overflow capacity of the container.
Source: USP XX, p. 949.

often used for solutions that remain below pH 7.0 during their shelf life, while type III glass can be used for dry powders that are reconstituted. The particular glass container intended for use must be an integral part of the product stability program to be described later.

Unfortunately, specifying the type of glass is not sufficient to ensure the consistency needed. Manufacturers have different recipes that bear designations, such as N-514A, CA-2, KG-33, and KG-35. Table 14 lists the compositions of various glasses. The glasses vary in additives—such as oxides of boron, sodium, potassium, calcium, iron, and magnesium—which alter physical and chemical properties of the glass. For example, when formulating sulfate salts (e.g., drug substances or antioxidant), the glass container should have minimal amounts of calcium and barium to prevent the formation of insoluble inorganic sulfates [30]. To meet this requirement KG-33 type I should be specified.

Amber glass containers are often used where the product is suspected of being light sensitive. The amber color is imparted by the addition of iron and manganese oxides, the cations of which are known to catalyze oxidative reactions. Studies have shown that these ions are extracted from glass [60] and that the decomposition rate of several drugs, thiomerosal [61], amitriptylene [62], and L-ascorbic acid [63] is enhanced in amber glass containers.

The Parenteral Drug Association has published guidelines on the processing and selection of glass containers [64]. Various surface treatments are used to improve chemical resistance and decrease alkalinity. For example, exposing hot containers to sulfur dioxide reduces sodium content at the surface and a brief treatment with ammonium bifluoride effectively cleans the surface by dissolving a portion of it.

Containers should be washed in a clean area in which particulate and microbiological contamination is low. Containers are frequently shrink-wrapped with plastic to maintain low particle levels after they are manufactured and to reduce the amount of cardboard introduced into the parenteral manufacturing area. The washing of the glass must effectively clean the surface and remove particulates. The procedure consists of a rinse of deionized water, followed by a detergent wash and finally a thorough rinse with Water for Injection. If pyrogen-free water is not used, the glass should be sterilized and depyrogenated by dry heat immediately after washing.

Table 14 Representative Compositions[a] of Pharmaceutical Glass Containers

Chemical composi- tions	USP classification/manufacturer's designations USP type I glass containers						
	Kimble KG-33	Kimble KG-35	Kimble N51A	Wheaton NS-33	Wheaton NS-51	Wheaton NSV	Wheaton type I flint
SiO_2	80	69	71	81	73	73	70
B_2O_3	13	13	11	13	10	10	10
Al_2O_3	3	6	7	2	6	6	6
Fe_2O_3	0[b]	0	0	0	0	0	0
ZnO	0	0	0	0	0	0	0.5
TiO_2	0	0	0	0	0	0	0
MnO	0	0	0	0	0	0	0
BaO	0	2	2	0	2	2	2
CaO	0	1	1	0	1	0.5	1
MgO	0	0	0	0	0	0	0.5
Na_2O	4	8	6	4	6	7	9
K_2O	0	1	2	0	1	1	1

Chemical composi- tions	USP classification/manufacturer's designations						
	USP type I glass container			Type II and III glass containers			
	Wheaton type I amber	Kimble amber RN-3	Kimble amber 203	Kimble amber CA-2	Kimble R-6	Wheaton type III flint	Wheaton type III amber
SiO_2	66	67	69	73	68	72	73
B_2O_3	9	9	10	0	2	0.5	0.5
Al_2O_3	7	6	6	3	3	2	2
Fe_2O_3	1	1	1	0	0	0	0.2
ZnO	0.5	0	0	0	0	0	0
TiO_2	0	0	3	0	0	0	0
MnO	6	6	0	0	0	0	0
BaO	1	1	2	0	2	0	0
CaO	0.5	2	1	10	5	8	9
MgO	0	0	0	0	4	3	1

Table 14 (Continued)

Chemical composi-tions	USP type I glass container			Type II and III glass containers			
	Wheaton type I amber	Kimble amber RN-3	Kimble amber 203	Kimble amber CA-2	Kimble R-6	Wheaton type III flint	Wheaton type III amber
Na_2O	8	7	16	13	15	14	14
K_2O	1	1	2	1	1	0	0

The table header above the two container groups reads: USP classification/manufacturer's designations

[a]Approximate percentage compositons.
[b]A value of zero indicates that the material is not a component of the formulation; it may be present at trace levels. Type II and III containers differ only in surface treatment; their bulk composition is identical.
Source: Parenteral Drug Association, Glass Containers for Small Volume Parenteral Products: Factors for Selection and Test Methods for Identification, Tech. Methods Bull. No. 3 (1982).

B. Rubber Closures

The following classification lists most of the polymers utilized as parenteral closures:

1. Unsaturated elastomers

    a. Polybutadiene
    b. Polychloroprene
    c. Polyisoprene—natural or synthetic
    d. Nitrile butadiene rubber
    e. Styrene butadiene rubber

2. Saturated elastomers

    a. Copolymer of polyisobutylene and polyisoprene (butyl)
    b. Ethylene propylene rubber
    c. Ethylene propylene diene rubber
    d. Silicone rubber

Rubber closures are formulated from many ingredients. The resultant products are exceedingly complex and difficult to characterize fully chemically. Ingredients used in addition to the basic polymer might include:

Accelerators: Amines, thiol and thiuram compounds, sulfamides, ureas
Activators: Stearic acid, zinc oxide, zinc stearate
Antioxidants: Amines, diethiocarbamates, paraffin waxes
Vulcanizing agents: Sulfur, organic peroxides, phenolic resins
Pigments: Carbon black, chromium oxide, iron oxide

Plasticizers and lubricants: (processing acids): Paraffin, mineral oils, fatty oils,
    organic phosphates, phthalates
Reinforcing agents (fillers): Aluminum and calcium silicates, titanium dioxide,
    carbon black, silica, barium sulfate

The elastomer and additives are combined by kneading them into a homogeneous mass, which is then vulcanized into the desired closure shape. During vul-
canization heat is applied to the mixture. This causes a chemical curing of the formula into its permanent shape and properties. Production variations that may
occur during the manufacture of stoppers can affect the quality and the properties
of the stopper. To maintain batch-to-batch uniformity of a particular formulation,
strict control of the manufacturing process is necessary. Ethylene propylene elastomers require very few additives compared to many of the others; thus they usually have less extractables.

The quantitative or qualitative formula of an elastomeric closure is rarely
available to the drug product formulator. Rubber manufacturers do submit a master file to the Food and Drug Administration (FDA), including the quantitative composition of their closures. However, this information is regarded as confidential
and therefore is not available from the FDA. This position is perhaps somewhat
understandable for competitive reasons within the rubber industry, but this secrecy
severely hampers the pharmaceutical chemist in evaluating formulas and conducting
compatibility and stability studies. With better methods of analysis, the selection
and control of elastomeric closures are beginning to be based on something more
than empirical evaluation.

1. Physical Properties

Guidelines for the selection and processing of elastomeric closures have been
proposed by the Parenteral Drug Association [65, 66]. A number of physical properties have been identified as being important in the selection and control and should
be understood by the formulator.

1. Compression set: Some rubbers deform permanently when held under pressure,
   thereby reducing the sealing characteristics of the closure with the glass vial.
2. Coring: Coring occurs when a small plug or fragment of rubber is cut and dis-
   lodged from the stopper as the needle is inserted. The elastomer type, formulation, and closure design (including thickness of target area) and the needle-
   point design all influence the coring rate.
3. Durometer: This is a measure of the hardness of rubber. In general, a value
   of 30 to 35 is soft, 35 to 45 average, and above 45 is hard. High durometer
   values usually mean increased resistance to puncturing. A high durometer
   value is needed for syringe plungerheads.
4. Moisture vapor transmission (MVT): MVT is an important consideration when
   selecting a closure for hygroscopic powders, lyophilized products, and for
   products in which an inert gas is overlayed. MVT is inversely proportional to
   the thickness of the barrier. Generally, increasing the filler will decrease
   MVT. Butyl elastomers provide good MVT protection, whereas natural rubber
   is poor.
5. Puncture resistance: The pressure required to insert the needle through the
   closure is an important physical characteristic. Injections which are normally
   administered with small-diameter needles (23 to 25 gauge) must have lower puncture resistance than those administered with needles having a comparatively
   larger diameter.

6. Resealability: Resealability will vary with rubber stocks. Since stoppers must reseal to prevent contamination and leakage, resealability is an important char- to evaluate.
7. Tackiness: For ease of handling, stoppers should not stick together or clump during processing. This usually occurs when stoppers are heated during sterilization.

2. Product Compatibility

Normally, if enough tests are run, a closure that is compatible with the parenteral product can be obtained by this empirical approach. The most common compatibility problem which occurs with stoppers is the leaching of ingredients from the stopper and the reaction of these ingredients with the product. Another problem is the sorption by the closure of preservatives, as described earlier, or other ingredients in solution resulting in subpotency or inadequate preservation. Due to the large variety of ingredients in most elastomeric formulations and chemical reactions they undergo, specific ingredients that might leach into the product, and possibly cause discoloration, turbidity, or precipitation, are often difficult to identify. Qualitative and quantitative determinations of ingredients from extracts of various stopper formulations, obtained under accelerated storage conditions, using various solvents, pH conditions, and so on, often provide the formulator with additional insight in selecting the proper elastomeric formulation for a product.

The USP XX–NF XV has a section on the biological and physical–chemical testing of plastic and rubber closures. The biological tests include acute systemic toxicity and intracutaneous reactivity tests. Other tests outlined include measurement of turbidity, reducing agents, heavy metals, total extractables, and pH.

Stoppers are normally prepared by washing them in household or commercial washers using detergents such as tetrasodium pyrophosphate or trisodium phosphate. In some cases a preextraction in an autoclave or with hot water may be required prior to detergent treatment to remove paraffin or surface wax. Gentle agitation with minimum tumbling should be used to avoid generation of particulate matter. Generally, an overflow process is employed to minimize agitation. Stoppers should be sterilized and dried immediately after washing. The sterilization cycle (autoclave) should be terminated with a vacuum cycle.

Special treatments of stoppers may include treatment with dilute acid or base solutions, solvent extractions, or extraction in a chelating agent to remove surface metals from the stoppers [67]. An oxiglaze (oxidation) treatment is sometimes employed to create a slightly harder and slicker surface. This is normally done to facilitate automatic handling during packaging. The oxiglaze process is carried out by treating the stoppers with 5% sodium hypochlorite in diluted hydrochloric acid. Stoppers are generally coated with a thin film of silicone to facilitate handling or insertion into the vials. This is usually applied while tumbling the closures in a closed container in the presence of a carefully measured quantity of silicone.

III. STABILITY EVALUATION

A. Compendial and Regulatory Requirements

Since 1976, the official compendia have required all official products to bear an expiration date. In the period between manufacturing and the expiration date, all products listed in the compendia must meet the requirements of the applicable monograph, provided that these products have been stored at the prescribed storage conditions.

Current Good Manufacturing Practice regulations require that all drug dosage forms marketed under an approved New Drug Application (NDA) or Abbreviated New Drug Application (ANDA) bear an expiration date that is supported by adequate data obtained with a stability indicating analytical method. FDA regulations also require adequate stability information prior to approval of a new NDA or ANDA.

B. Solutions

The stability of the majority of injectable products (i.e., solutions) should be evaluated by several parameters. These parameters include potency, pH, color, clarity, odor, stopper appearance, particulate matter, toxicity, container/closure integrity, and preservative effectiveness. As with other dosage forms, a variety of time, temperature, and humidity conditions should be used when predicting the stability of injectable drug products. A brief discussion of the significance of each attribute follows.

Most injectable products are permitted, by either the compendia or government regulations, to contain not less than 90% of the label claim of active ingredient at the expiration date. A stability-indicating assay is critical to determining compliance with this requirement. In recent years, high-performance liquid chromatography (HPLC) methods have been widely used for this purpose. In addition to determining accurately the amount of active ingredient in this product, HPLC assays, when combined with isolation and identification techniques, can be used to identify and quantitate known breakdown products. Knowledge of the breakdown products is very important when evaluating toxicology and chemical degradation data. Actually, the majority of stability failures or limitations with injectable products is due to factors other than low potency.

A change in the pH of a drug solution during stability testing can be indicative of either degradation of the active ingredient or interaction of one or more of the constituents of the solution with either the container (plastic or glass) or the rubber closure. For example, a significant increase in the pH of a neutral or acidic solution could indicate that alkaline materials are leaching from the glass container into the solution. This would be particularly true if type III glass (soda-lime) is used instead of type I glass (borosilicate). Another example would be a lowering of pH of a highly alkaline sodium barbiturate derivative, resulting in precipitation of the free acid of the drug. If a change in pH becomes important to control, a buffer system (previously discussed) may be required.

Color changes frequently occur with solutions of injectable drugs stored at high temperatures (40°C or higher). This is usually due to accelerated decomposition of the drug (especially if it degrades by oxidation) or interaction of metals from the rubber closure with one or more of the ingredients in the solution. A color change can usually be prevented by replacing the air (oxygen) in the vial or ampul headspace with an inert gas, such as nitrogen or carbon dioxide, or by the addition of a chelating agent, such as of ethylenediaminetetracetic acid, to the solution.

Turbidity in a solution can be seen utilizing the Tyndall effect. Suspended particles adsorb or scatter (diffract, refract, and reflect) light. Turbidity is the reduction in light transmission through the solution as a result of suspended particles. Generally, solutions of injectable drugs should maintain a light transmission of 70% or more during the shelf life of the product. Most solutions undergo a decrease in transmission with time, as measured in a nephelometer. Ideally, a solution immediately after manufacturing will have light transmission of 92 to 97% and will not decrease to less than 70% over a 3 to 5 year period. Factors that can cause an increase in turbidity include generation of particulate matter (usually from a solution/container interaction), precipitation of a constituent of the solution because of drug/preservative, drug/closure, preservative/closure or similar reaction, or growth of microorganisms, generally due to preservative loss.

Periodically, a container should be opened and examined for change in odor. Sometimes decomposition can be detected, particularly in solutions with sulfur-containing drugs or antioxidants. Rubber closures should be removed periodically and examined visually and microscopically for changes in color and texture. Many drug solutions, particularly those of high or low pH or oil-based, interact with rubber closures. This interaction can be accelerated by storing vials inverted under various conditions of temperature. Detectable changes in the appearance of stoppers should be investigated to determine if there are changes in properties of the product.

Several batches placed on stability should be characterized for the level of particulate matter 10 μm and larger. Periodically, these batches should be reexamined under "normal" storage conditions (i.e., 5°C and 25°C) utilizing similar methodology, for any change in particulate levels. Particulate methodology is difficult to reproduce, even under carefully controlled conditions, and care must be excersied when evaluating the results obtained. Numbers may increase (most likely) or decrease (least likely) depending on solution/container interaction, ingredient instability brought on by pH or other changes or solubilization of drug with time.

LD_{50} or LD_0 (safety test) data should be gathered initially and at intervals during the storage period to assure that no toxic breakdown or interaction products are forming. If the LD_{50} value changes significantly, the formulator should confer with chemists and toxicologists who are knowledgeable about the drug to explain this change in the safety test data.

Products in multiple-dose vials are preserved primarily to prevent the growth of microorganisms inadvertently introduced during the use of the product in the hospital, clinic, or physician's office. Therefore, a microbial challenge test must be conducted initially and at yearly intervals on samples stored at ambient (25°C) conditions. Procedures to be used are found in USP XX. Antimicrobial agents can decompose, be rendered ineffective due to pH changes or chelation with metals leached from rubber closures, or be absorbed into rubber closures. Early in the development of a product, the minimum effective concentration (MEC) or minimum inhibitory concentration (MIC) of antimicrobial agent needed in the formula must be determined. A stability indicating assay should be developed for the antimicrobial agent and samples stored at normal storage conditions (5°C and 25°C) should be assayed at regular intervals to monitor the level of antimicrobial agent. Normally, this level will gradually decrease during storage. Of course, the level should not be permitted to fall below the MIC during its shelf life.

C. Sterile Solids

Reconstituted sterile injectable solids should be inspected for most of the attributes that pertain to liquids: potency, pH, color, clarity, odor, stopper appearance, particulate matter, and toxicity. In addition, the dry sterile powder must be evaluated for color uniformity, moisture content, and reconstitution rate. Most of these parameters were discussed in the preceding section under solutions but two that deserve additional discussion are moisture content and reconstitution rate.

Most dry solids, whether dry fill, spray dried, or freeze-dried, have an optimal moisture range for stability. With rare exceptions, vials of dry sterile solids utilize butyl rubber closures with low MVT. Not only can the presence of excess moisture accelerate chemical degradation, but often determines the polymorphic or hydrate form of the drug. The crystalline form of the drug is often vital to the chemical stability of the drug, examples being the cepholasporin antibiotics. Injectible drugs that require reconstitution should dissolve rapidly, generally in 1 min or less. Chemical changes, such as formation of less soluble degradation products or a different crystalline form, can cause a slowing of the reconstitution rate.

D. Suspensions

Parenteral suspensions exhibit instability in ways not applicable to solutions and dry solids. Physical properties such as viscosity, rheological behavior, suspendibility, syringability, and particle size distribution need to be monitored as a part of a stability program. Figure 28 shows typical graphs of these properties for prednisolone acetate suspension.

The viscosity of a suspension is a measure of the resistance to flow upon shear. Through the use of a recording viscometer, the rheological behavior as well as viscosity can be determined. As shown in Figure 28a, the flow behavior for prednisolone acetate suspension is nearly Newtonian with a slight hysteresis loop. The linear and consistent sedimentation rate, as shown in Figure 28b, indicates stability of particle size and particle size distribution and, further, that particle aggregation is minimal or nonexistent. Figure 28c shows a force-displacement profile of the

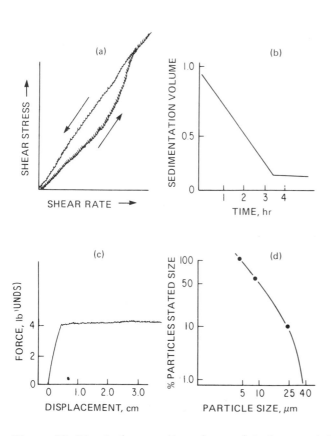

Figure 28 Physical properties of a prednisolone acetate suspension.

ejection of the suspension from a syringe. From this the force required to eject the suspension can be determined. A consistent force and shape of the curve is indicative of physical stability. Particle size distribution is shown in Figure 28d.

E. Stability Protocol

A complete stability evaluation on the final formulation in the proposed final package includes storing representative samples at at least three elevated temperatures and room temperature and in the light. The accelerated schedule (i.e., samples at elevated temperatures and in the light) generally lasts for 12 weeks. A typical schedule is shown in Table 15.
　　From the data collected over 12 weeks the decision to continue the product can be made. Most degradations being hydrolytic in nature follow first-order or pseudo-first-order kinetics. The chemical stability of the drug substance can be predicted by first plotting the temperature data as shown in Figure 29 and determining the rate constants from the slopes of the lines. The example shown is for a first-order reaction in which the substance degrades to products at a rate that is directly proportional to the concentration of the reacting substance.

$$\text{Rate} = -\frac{dC}{dt} = kC \tag{31}$$

where

　　　C = concentration of reacting substance

　　　k = reaction rate

　　　t = time

Converting Equation (31) to

$$\frac{dC}{C} = -k \, dt \tag{32}$$

Table 15 Typical Accelerated Stability Schedule for a Parenteral Solution[a, b]

Time (weeks)	Room temp.	Temperature (°C)			Light
		40	50	60	
0	X				
1			X	X	X
3	X	X	X	X	
6	X	X	X	X	X
12	X	X			X

[a] X, perform all determinations.
[b] Continue study at room temperature for 6, 12, 18, 24, 30, and 36 months.

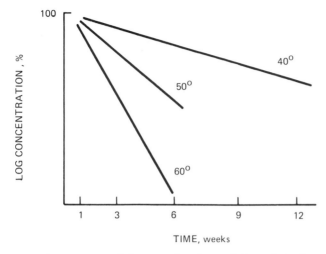

Figure 29 Typical first-order degradation plot of concentration versus time at three temperatures.

gives

$$\log C = \frac{k}{2.303} t + \text{constant} \qquad (33)$$

By plotting the concentration versus time on semilog graph paper, the reaction rate can be determined from the slope of the line.

The influence of temperature on reaction rate has been shown by Arrhenius.

$$\log k = -\frac{\Delta H_a}{2.303R} \frac{1}{T} + \log S \qquad (34)$$

where

R = gas constant (1.987 cal deg^{-1} mol^{-1})

T = absolute temperature

S = frequency factor

ΔH_a = heat of activation

By plotting the rate constants obtained at accelerated temperatures versus the reciprocal of absolute temperature (Fig. 30), the heat of activation can be calculated from the slope. The value represents the energy the molecules must reach to undergo reaction. By extrapolating the line as shown to room temperature, the rate constant at ambient conditions can be determined. From this, the time for 10% degradation can be calculated using the following expression:

$$t_{10\%} = \frac{2.303}{k_{25°C}} \log \frac{100}{90} \qquad (35)$$

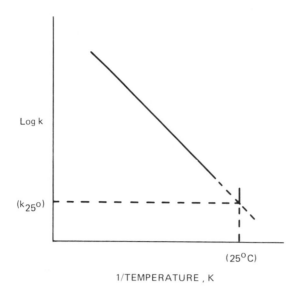

Figure 30 Arrhenius-type plot of log rate constant versus the reciprocal of absolute temperature.

In addition to the drug, the loss of antimicrobial agents and antioxidants that can be absorbed or consumed should be tested in the same manner. Such accelerated treatment allows decisions to be made on further plans for the product. For example, if the company is confident of the 12 week data, plans to submit as NDA or ANDA can proceed. Most likely by the time the FDA could act on the submission, 6 month or 1 year room-temperature data would be available. Generally, the FDA accepts accelerated data contingent upon receiving sufficient room temperature information. The expiration date will determine the amount of information required. With less than 1 year's data, an expiration date of no more than one year will be allowed. As sufficient data are accumulated, a longer expiration date can be included. For more comprehensive treatment on stability evaluation, readers are encouraged to consult other texts [68].

IV. PROCESS EFFECTS

The processing of parenteral products has been covered elsewhere in this textbook, but some specific cautions associated with the effects on formulation will be highlighted. Parenterals are processed by either nonaseptic methods and terminal sterilization or aseptically using filtration sterilization. Although parenteral solutions filled into ampuls or vials for terminal sterilization do not require aseptic processing, the final product must be sterile and free of pyrogens and particulate matter. Consequently, containers and closures are generally subjected to final rinsing with water for injection. Steam sterilization, which offers the greatest assurance of sterility, can be expected to cause some changes in the product, however subtle. Drugs are reactive substances and autoclave temperature (121°C) for 15 to 30 min could give rise to degradation processes and interactions with the container. Additionally, materials could leach from the rubber closure. In addition to loss of drug, antimicrobial agents and antioxidants can be absorbed or consumed during sterilization.

There comes a point in the development process of a product to characterize the production process and assess its effect on the formulation. This requires scale-up procedures to identify the process and equipment variables and with knowledge of the formulation and package variables assess how product quality and manufacturing productivity will be affected. In the manufacture of a sterile product, the assurance that the finished product possesses the desired quality control characteristics depends on a number of independent but interrelated events commencing with the initial design of the dosage form and carrying forth through the process design and validation and culminating with the establishment of standard procedures for manufacturing.

To provide for the assurance that all quality attributes will be achieved on a repetitive basis, the following are essential: (1) the dosage from is designed with knowledge of the desired functional and quality control characteristics of the finished product; (2) the qualification procedures are adequate to ensure reliability of the equipment, effectiveness of the process, and the integrity of the processing environment; (3) personnel are trained in contamination control techniques; and (4) there is adequate documentation of all procedures and tests. Such a development sequence combined with validation requirements suggests a formalized program culminating in a product that can be reliably processed. The process characterization is a principal step in assuring that the process can be translated to manufacturing on a routine production basis. Although this chapter is not intended to cover processing in the broad sense, those responsible for developing formulations should have an understanding of:

1. Scale-up procedures
2. Preliminary technical documentation
3. Design of processing and validation protocols
4. Qualification/validation runs
5. Final technical documentation and authorizations

The overall approach must be organized, scientific, and thorough.

REFERENCES

1. DeLuca, P. P., and Rapp, R. P., in Pharmaceutics and Pharmacy Practice, J. B. Lippincott, Philadelphia, 1982, p. 238.
2. The United States Pharmacopeia XX, National Formulary XV, The United States Pharmacopeial Convention, Inc., Rockville, Md. 1980, p. 861.
3. Hildebrand, J. H., and Scott, R. L., The Solubility of Nonelectrolytes, Dover, New York, 1964.
4. Carstensen, J. T., Theory of Pharmaceutical Systems, Vol. 1, Academic Press, New York, 1972, p. 123.
5. Connors, K. A., A Textbook of Pharmaceutical Analysis, Wiley, New York, 1967, p. 255.
6. Mader, W. J., Organic Analysis, Vol. 2, Interscience, New York, 1954.
7. Dielectric Constants, in Handbook of Chemistry and Physics, 63rd ed., CRC Press, Boca Raton, Fla., 1982-1983, pp. E-50 to E-54.
8. Margott, A. A., and Smith E. R., Table of Dielectric Constants of Pure Liquids, Natl. Bur. Stand. Circ. 514, U.S. Government Printing Office, Washington, D.C., 1951.
9. Sorby, D., Bitter, R., and Welb, J., J. Pharm. Sci., 52:1149 (1963).
10. Moore, W. E., J. Am. Pharm. Assoc. Sci. Ed., 47:855 (1958).

11. Paruta, A. N., and Irani, S. A., J. Pharm. Sci., 54:1334 (1965).
12. Paruta, A. N., and Sheth, B. B., J. Pharm. Sci., 55:1208 (1966).
13. Mauger, J. W., and Paruta, A. N., J. Pharm. Sci., 58:574 (1969).
14. Breon, T. L., and Paruta, A. N., J. Pharm. Sci., 59:1309 (1970).
15. Gorman, W., and Hall, G., J. Pharm. Sci., 53:1017 (1964).
16. Spiegel, A. J., and Noseworthy, M. M., J. Pharm. Sci., 52:917 (1963).
17. Hem, S. L., Green, R. H., Manni, P. E., Bourgeois, M. F., Lipper, P. A., and Blaha, J. M., Drug Dev. Commun., 1:471 (1974).
18. Newton, D. W., and Kluza, R. B., Am. J. Hosp. Pharm., 37:1647 (1980).
19. Newton, D. W., and Kluza, R. B., Drug Intell. Clin. Pharm., 12:546-554 (1978).
20. Schroeder, H. G., and DeLuca, P. P., Bull. Parenter. Drug Assoc., 28:1 (1974).
21. Schwartz, P. A., Rhodes, C. T., and Cooper, J. W., Jr., J. Pharm. Sci., 66:994 (1977).
22. Kostenbauder, H. B., and Higuchi, T., J. Am. Pharm. Assoc. Sci. Ed., 45:518 (1956).
23. Haleblian, J. K., J. Pharm. Sci. 64:1269 (1975).
24. Carless, J. E., Moustafa, M. A., and Rapson, H. D. C., J. Pharm. Pharmacol., 18:190S (1966).
25. Hamlin, W. E., Nelson, E., Ballard, B. E., and Wagner, J. G., J. Pharm. Sci., 51:432 (1962).
26. Ballard, B. E., and Nelson, E., J. Pharmacol. Exp. Ther., 135:120 (1972).
27. Lawrence, A. S. C., Trans Faraday Soc., 33:815 (1937).
28. Boylan, J. C., and Fites, A. L., Modern Pharmaceutics, Marcel Dekker, New York, 1979, pp. 458-459.
29. Freypuss, J., Shaw, J. M., and Ross, J. J., J. Pharm. Sci., 65:1310 (1976).
30. Boddapati, S., Butler, D. L., Im, S., and DeLuca, P. P., J. Pharm. Sci., 69:608 (1980).
31. Flynn, G. L., J. Parenter. Drug Assoc., 34:139 (1980).
32. Yeh, S., and Lach, J. L., J. Pharm. Sci., 50:35 (1961).
33. Akers, M. J., J. Parenter. Sci. Technol., 36:222 (1982).
34. Schroeter, L. C., J. Pharm. Sci., 50:891 (1961).
35. Schroeter, L. C., J. Pharm. Sci., 52:559 (1963).
36. Riegelman, S., and Fischer, E. Z., J. Pharm. Sci., 51:206 (1962).
37. Coates, D., Mfg. Chem. Aerosol News, 44:41 (1973).
38. Yousef, R. T., El-Nakeeb, M. A., and Salama, S., Can. J. Pharm. Sci., 8:54 (1973).
39. Lachman, L., Sheth, P. B., and Urbanyi, T., J. Pharm. Sci., 53:211 (1964).
40. Kostenbauder, H. B., in Disinfection, Sterilization and Preservation, 2nd ed. (S. S. Block, ed.), Lea & Febiger, Philadelphia, 1977, pp. 912-932.
41. Lachman, L., Weinstein, S., Hopkins, G., Slack, S., Eisman, P., and Cooper, J., J. Pharm. Sci., 51:224 (1962).
42. The United States Pharmacopeia XX, National Formulary XV, The United States Pharmacopeial Convention, Inc., Rockville, Md., 1980, p. 873.
43. British Pharmacopoeia, Vol. II, Cambridge University Press, Cambridge, 1980, p. 578.
44. Martin, A. N., Swarbrick, J., and Cammarata, A., Physical Pharmacy, 2nd ed., Lea & Febiger, Philadelphia, 1969.
45. Gatlin, L., Kulkarni, P., Hussain, A., and DeLuca, P. P., Am. J. Hosp. Pharm., 36:1357 (1979).

46. Ober, S. S., Vincent, H. S., Simon, D. E., and Frederick, K., J. Am. Pharm. Assoc. Sci. Ed., 47:667 (1958).

47. Boylan, J. C., Bull. Parenter. Drug Assoc., 19:98 (1965).

48. Boylan, J. C., and Robison, R. L., J. Pharm. Sci., 57:1796 (1968).

49. Nash, R. A., Drug Cosmet. Ind., 98:39 (1965-1966).

50. Groves, M. J., Parenteral Products, William Heinemann, London, 1973, pp. 30-40.

51. Pelham, L. D., Am. J. Hosp. Pharm., 38:198-208 (1981).

52. Turco, S., and King, R. E., Sterile Dosage Forms, 2nd ed., Lea & Febiger, Philadelphia, 1979, pp. 169-171.

53. Lachman, L., Lieberman, H. A., and Kanig, J. L., eds., The Theory and Practice of Industrial Pharmacy, 2nd ed., Lea & Febiger, Philadelphia, 1976.

54. DeLuca, P. P., Dev. Biol. Stand., 36:41 (1977).

55. DeLuca, P. P., J. Vac. Sci. Technol., 14:620 (1977).

56. Greaves, R. I. N., J. Pharmacol., 14:621 (1962).

57. DeLuca, P. P., and Lachman, L., J. Pharm. Sci., 54:621 (1965).

58. Rey, L., Ann. N.Y. Acad. Sci., 85:510 (1960).

59. Gatlin, L., and DeLuca, P. P., J. Parenter. Drug Assoc., 34:398 (1980).

60. Moretti, C., Boll. Chim. Farm., 103:69 (1964).

61. Lipper, R. A., and Nevola, M. M., "Influence of Amber Glass on the Decomposition of Thiomerosol in Aqueous Solution." In press.

62. Enever, R. P., LiWanPo, A., and Shotton, E., J. Pharm. Sci., 66:1087 (1977).

63. Kassem, M. A., Kassem, A. A., and Ammar, H. O., Pharm. Acta Helv., 44:611 (1969).

64. Anschel, J., Bull. Parenter. Drug Assoc., 31:47 (1977).

65. Parenteral Drug Association, Elastomeric Closures: Evaluation of Significant Performance and Identity Characteristics, Tech. Methods Bull. 2 (1981).

66. Anschel, J., Bull. Parenter. Drug Assoc., 31:302 (1977).

67. Motola, S., and Clawans, C., Bull. Parenter. Drug Assoc., 26:163 (1972).

68. Lachman, L., and DeLuca, P., in The Theory and Practice of Industrial Pharmacy, 2nd ed., (L. Lachman, H. A. Lieberman, and J. L. Kanig, eds.), Lea & Febiger, Philadelphia, 1976, pp. 32-78.

6

The Processing of Small Volume Parenterals and Related Sterile Products

JOEL BENTON PORTNOFF, RICHARD J. HARWOOD, *
and EDWARD WILLIAM SUNBERY

Merck, Sharp and Dohme Research Laboratories
West Point, Pennsylvania

Small volume parenterals (SVPs) are sterile, pyrogen-free injectable products which are packaged in volumes up to 100 ml [1]. Generally, SVPs range in size from less than 1 up to 50 ml. This is a major distinguishing feature of SVPs as contrasted to large volume parenterals (LVPs), which are normally packaged in volumes up to 1000 ml. There are limits to the volume of liquid that the extravascular tissues can tolerate at any one time. For this reason, LVPs are administered by intra- or extravascular routes, depending on composition. Products that are administered directly into the bloodstream, with rare exception, are administered as aqueous solutions. Sterile suspensions and nonaqueous solutions cannot be administered intravenously because of possible untoward effects that may occur in the cardiovascular system when an insoluble substance is administered. Some SVP aqueous solutions can be administered only by the intravenous route because of local irritation. Topically applied ophthalmic and otic formulations, although not injected, are prepared in much the same manner as small volume parenteral products. These formulations can be considered as small volume sterile products.

Small volume parenteral products can be formulated and packaged in several ways and include a wide variety of products. Small volume sterile products can be classified into one or more of the following categories:

1. Pharmaceutical products consist of organic or inorganic chemical entities in solution, as a suspension, in emulsions, as a freeze-dried product for reconstitution, or as a powder for constitution.
2. Biological products are prepared from biological sources and include vaccines, toxoids, tissue extracts, or biological extracts.
3. Diagnostic agents are used to diagnose clinical conditions. This category of products includes a wide variety of formulations such as x-ray contrast media, dyes to test organ function, material to assess blood volume and hemopoietic function, and biologicals to ascertain disease state or susceptibility to disease.

---

*Present affiliation: William H. Rohrer, Inc., Fort Washington, Pennsylvania

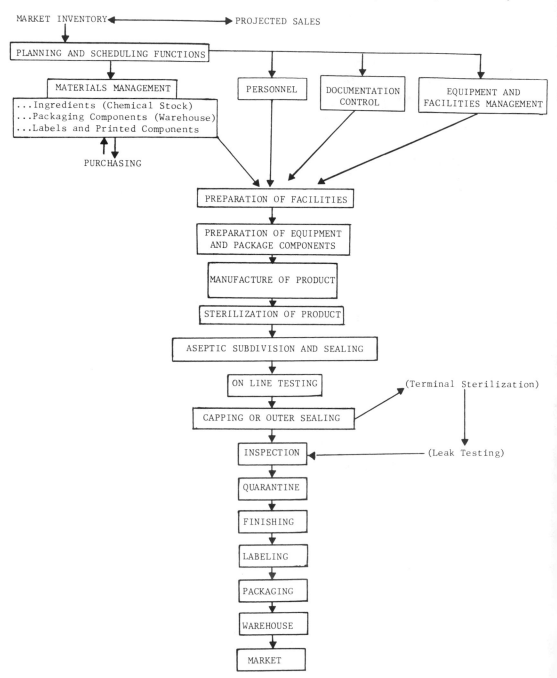

Figure 1 Overview of the manufacturing of small volume parenteral products.

4. <u>Allergenic extracts</u> are extracts of potentially allergenic substances specially
    prepared and sterilized for detection (or treatment) of patient sensitivity.
5. <u>Radiopharmaceutical products</u> are administered parenterally for the detection,
    diagnosis, and/or treatment of disease.

6. Dental products, such as local anesthetics, are used for injection into the oral tissues.

Basically, the same principles apply to the preparation or processing of all small volume sterile products. The responsibility of the production department is to provide a product that is of the desired potency, sterile, pyrogen-free, clean, physically acceptable, aesthetically packaged, and properly labeled. The manufacturing procedures, which are discussed in this chapter, are differentiated by product type (i.e., solution, suspension, freeze-dried powder, or dry-filled powder). Packaging components and/or configuration (i.e., vial, ampul, syringe, bottle, or syringe cartridge) are discussed as well.

An overview of the processes and auxiliary support functions required to manufacture small volume parenterals and related sterile products is presented in a simplified fashion in Figure 1 and can be used as the basis for discussion throughout this chapter.

Market Inventory and Projected Sales. A combination of product inventory and projected sales determine, in large measure, "when" and "how much" product is to be made by a production department. The scope of this chapter is to cover the technological aspects concerned with the preparation of SVP products. Suffice it to say that many nonproduction-related factors determine "when" and "how much" of a product is manufactured.

I. PRELIMINARY STAGES IN THE PROCESSING OF SMALL VOLUME PARENTERALS

The preparation of a sterile pharmaceutical product is the culmination of a series of actions by a diversity of personnel who support the various functions outlined in Figure 1.

A. Planning and Scheduling

Planning and scheduling activities are the key to the successful production of small volume parenterals. Once the decision is made to manufacture a given product, four groups of personnel (materials management, personnel management, equipment and facilities maintenance, and documentation control) set the manufacturing process in motion and provide the necessary goods, equipment, personnel, and facilities for the production department.

B. Materials Management

This group of personnel is responsible for providing the materials necessary to manufacture the product. Materials management personnel coordinate the activities of chemical stock, package component warehouse, printing, and purchasing so that there are sufficient supplies of chemicals, package components, and printed components to keep up with the needs of production, and makes certain that these supplies are available in a timely manner.

C. Personnel Management

The key factor in the large-scale manufacturing of high-quality products is a properly motivated production staff. The personnel must be attentive to the minute details and have a special commitment to perform a good job. The production staff
must enjoy doing the work and should be motivated by a sense of responsibility and
accomplishment. Personnel should sense real pride in helping to process a sterile
and safe product that will be administered via injection to another human being.
The production personnel are the "priceless ingredients" in a sterile operation and
they must be carefully selected for the job. This aspect is covered in greater detail in Chapter 10.

D. Documentation Control

Documentation is the control and verification of the critical activities in a pharmaceutical process production and control cycle. From a manufacturing standpoint,
documentation is necessary to keep an accurate record of the entire history of the
manufacturing process and, if done properly, enhances the ability to produce high-
quality products batch after batch. Documentation has both a current and historical
aspect. The elements of good documentation include the following:

1. Master file
2. Batch records
3. Process logs
4. Material logs
5. Distribution records
6. Complaint files
7. Retained sample storage area records
8. Returned goods records

    The master file is a perpetual record of the production and control cycles on
all batches of a particular product. The master file is a composite of the remaining
seven portions listed above. The batch record is the complete record of the manufacture, control, and distribution of a single batch of a product and includes the
following:

1. Formulation identification number
2. Formulation name and concentration of active ingredients
3. Identity and quantity of each component
4. Stock and/or control numbers for each component together with quality control
    approval and hazardous material labeling for appropriate chemicals
5. Starting and completion time for each operation
6. Chemical weight check and quality assurance counter check
7. Identification of all processing equipment
8. Process details such as mixing times and stirring rates, and sterilization times
    and temperatures
9. Labeling requirements for processing equipment and semifinished and finished
    products
10. In-process sampling procedures and test requirements, such as chemical
    purity, sterility, fill volume, pyrogen, and safety testing
11. Material accountability

<u>Process logs</u> are written verification by a responsible person that the facilities and equipment used during a pharmaceutical process have been cleaned, maintained, calibrated, and/or operated in an acceptable manner. The process logs consist of the following documents:

1. The <u>formulation manufacturing record</u> is a description of the formulation and the steps required to produce a bulk product from raw materials and includes material accountability.
2. The <u>component processing record</u> is a history of the use of packaging and processing equipment and packaging supplies. It also includes the washing and sterilization processing and validation records.
3. The <u>filling ticket</u> is a description of the subdivision procedures, such as type of package, fill volume, storage requirements, and accountability.
4. A <u>label control report</u> is a description of the label required on the final package. The package shipment requirements and product and label accountability are also included in this document. The formulation manufacturing record, the component processing record, the filling ticket, and the label control report are prepared by the production scheduling department in conjunction with the marketing department's projected needs.
5. <u>Product release sheets</u> are prepared by the quality assurance department. This document records the physical and chemical properties of the finished product for comparison against previous batches. Audit and reconciliation of the entire batch folder is required before release of product to the marketplace.

<u>Material logs</u> are a verification that the raw materials used in a pharmaceutical process are acceptable. An integral part of these logs are the <u>raw material release sheets</u>, which are prepared by the quality assurance department. These logs record the history of chemicals or packaging components which are used in the process of manufacturing the sterile product. Information such as suppliers and desired and/or undesired physical or chemical properties of the raw materials are recorded for comparison against previously used materials. Only materials meeting predetermined specifications are used in the final process.

The elements of documentation described above are ongoing and are continually updated as the production process proceeds. Once a document is completed, it is then considered part of the historical record (master file) of the batch and should be maintained. Each document should be easily accessible for inspection at any time. The following set of records should be maintained as well.

<u>Distribution records</u> are maintained so that the manufacturer can determine the location of all manufactured products at all times. In addition, a <u>complaint file</u> is maintained as a backup to in-house monitoring of product performance. Complaint files include inquiries or complaints on product and/or package defects or adverse product reactions. In addition to the complaint file, a <u>retained sample storage area</u> is maintained as a comparative reference source to assist in the reply to product inquiries and complaints.

The <u>returned goods record</u> is a record of products returned to the manufacturer as a result of complaints or products exceeding their shelf life before being consumed. In any case, returned goods are an important indicator of product market demand and acceptance of a product.

E. Equipment and Facilities Management

The proper type and size of equipment must be made available for each particular processing step. There are several types of equipment that are used in the overall processing of small volume parenteral products. A large variety of machinery and devices are used to accomplish a myriad of tasks. Examples of equipment to perform these tasks are: (1) washing equipment for glass, plastic, and rubber components; (2) mixing equipment to manufacture the bulk product; (3) filtering equipment to clarify and/or sterilize the product; (4) storage tanks to hold the bulk product prior to subdivision; (5) filling or subdividing equipment; (6) stoppering and/or sealing equipment; and (7) terminal sterilizing equipment. This equipment will be discussed in detail later in the chapter.

The condition of the facility in which the product will be manufactured is a very important factor in the efficient manufacture of a product in a reproducible manner. The facility must be largely self-contained and have sufficient room within which to carry out all of the manufacturing and packaging steps. The facility must be dedicated to the manufacture of parenteral products.

Control of personnel movement in the production area is vital to producing a clean, sterile product of high quality and, for this reason, the layout and design of the facility are important. Generally, the traffic of goods and personnel goes in one direction—from the "dirtiest" area to the "cleanest" area with no return or crossover. Figure 2 shows one concept of a floor plan of a facility for preparing small volume parenteral products. If one follows this floor plan, it will be noted that there are main areas which are categorized by the air quality:

1. General air conditioning: warehouse, general laboratory, and finishing areas
2. Controlled air: components preparation area, formulation preparation area, airlock entry into component preparation room
3. Sterile area: airlock into sterile areas and sterile cubicle
4. Humidity-controlled sterile areas: liquid filling and lyophilization rooms

A properly designed floor plan of a facility will not provide a good environment for preparing small volume parenteral products unless special construction design and special materials of construction are used [2]. The facility must have walls, ceilings, and floors that are smooth, nonshedding, and easily sanitizable. The facility must be designed to have minimum cracks or crevices and ledges where particles can collect. Fixed horizontal surfaces should be minimized or eliminated so that dust and/or bacteria cannot accumulate. The walls, floors, ceilings, fixtures, and partitions are clean, cleanable, smooth, impervious to cleaning/sanitizing solutions, and must resist chipping, flaking, or deterioration, for example, stainless steel or an epoxy covering.

F. Preparation of Facilities

Before the raw materials are assembled and before the equipment and the package components are prepared for the manufacture of a small volume parenteral product, the facility must be cleaned. This cleaning operation must be planned in advance. To eliminate or reduce the potential of cross-contamination, the service area is usually cleaned first, the clean room next, and the sterile area is cleaned last. As a general rule, the cleaning sequence proceeds from the ceiling to the floor.

The following are suggested procedures to be followed for starting up a new or previously dormant facility for the preparation of small volume parenteral products.

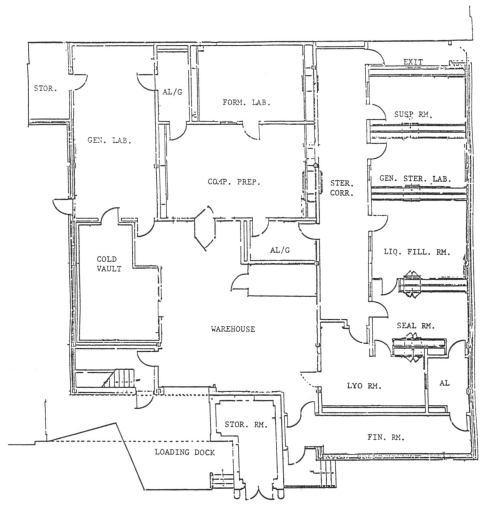

Figure 2 Floor plan of a pilot plant facility which can be used to manufacture small volume parenteral products. (Courtesy of Merck, Sharp and Dohme Research Laboratories, West Point, Pennsylvania.)

1. Cleaning of Service Areas

For purposes of definition, a "service area" includes offices, rest rooms, storage rooms, mechanical support rooms, lockers, and labeling/cartoning rooms. The ceilings are wiped down with a disinfectant detergent and water using a non-shedding sponge. The sprinkler heads are dusted with a soft-bristled brush and light diffusers are cleaned using synthetic detergent and water. A vacuum cleaner equipped with a brush tool is used to dust drapes, if present. The air supply and return vents are washed with a degreasing germicide detergent and water using a nonshedding cloth or sponge. A disinfectant detergent and water are used to wipe down the walls, doors, and partitions. A nonshedding cloth or sponge is always used in such operations to reduce particulation. The windows are washed with a suitable window cleaner. Accessible areas of office furniture and other miscellaneous equipment are damp-wiped using a disinfectant detergent and water with a nonshedding cloth.

Rest room areas are especially hard to clean and great care must be exercised in cleaning such areas. Sink bowls and related plumbing hardware are washed with a germicidal detergent and water using a nonshedding cloth. The interior surfaces of all bowls are cleaned with a hydrochloric acid solution. The exterior surfaces of all bowls are washed with a germicide detergent.

In mechanical support rooms, lockers and storage rooms, accessible floor areas, and cove bases are vacuumed and then machine-scrubbed. When appropriate, a detergent stripping solution is used to remove old floor finish. After floors are rinsed with clean water, the old floor finish and stripper solutions are removed from accessible floor areas using a floor mop or tank-type wet-pickup vacuum cleaner. This procedure is repeated until all of the old floor finish and stripper solutions are removed. A fresh floor finish is applied to accessible floor areas using a nonshedding synthetic-strand mop. The floor drains and drinking fountain drains are flushed with a germicidal detergent and water.

As noted earlier, these procedures are usually followed when starting up a new facility. After startup, routine maintenance of the service area is absolutely essential. Tables 1 through 5 summarize the typical maintenance procedures and their frequency (i.e., daily weekday, monthly, etc.) to be used for the service areas of a SVP manufacturing facility.

2. Preparation of Clean Room Areas

Clean room areas are those places in which packaging components and processing equipment are cleaned and/or prepared for sterilization and in which chemicals are blended into clean bulk formulations.

The ceiling, lighting fixtures (inside and outside), sprinkler heads, and air supply vents are thoroughly washed with a germicidal detergent using a nonshedding cloth. Burned-out light bulbs are replaced with new ones that have been washed with a germicidal detergent. Similarly, the walls, including baseboards, doors, door frames, and air return vents, are thoroughly washed and then all of the horizontal surfaces, fixtures, equipment, and furniture are washed with a germicidal detergent using a nonshedding cloth.

Accessible floor areas and cove bases are vacuumed and old floor finishes are removed and refinished as outlined in the preparation of the floors in the service area. Then, all of the drains in the area are flushed with a germicidal detergent and water.

The floors are washed down with a germicidal detergent and water using a nonshedding cloth. After startup, routine maintenance as outlined in Table 6 should be followed.

3. Preparation of the Sterile Room

The sterile rooms in which the bulk formulations are sterilized and subdivided are cleaned using the procedures outlined under the preparation of the clean room. One significant difference between a clean room and a sterile room is that the sterile room does not have any drains. Drains are a potential source of microbial contamination for a sterile room area. Liquid spills in sterile rooms are removed with a wet/dry vacuum equipped with a high-efficiency particulate air (HEPA)-type filter. This is followed by a damp germicidal detergent wipe-down.

Table 1 Daily Maintenance Procedures for Service Areas in a Facility for Manufacturing Small Volume Parenteral Products

---

Office Areas

Dry-mop acessible floor area using a treated dry mop. Pick up sweepings from floor.

Empty waste containers and reline with plastic bags when necessary.

Empty ashtrays and wipe clean with a damp cloth with synthetic detergent and water.

Rest Rooms and Lockers

Sweep accessible floor area using a synthetic-fiber push broom. Pick up sweepings from floor.

Damp-mop accessible floor area using a cotton/synthetic-strand mop and disinfectant synthetic detergent in water.

Wash sink and hardware using creme cleanser and a damp sponge; rinse clean and wipe dry.

Wash mirror using a suitable window cleaner solution and wipe dry with a clean cloth.

Restock towel dispenser and spot-clean dispenser using a synthetic detergent with a sponge or cloth.

Restock toilet tissue dispenser.

Clean interior surfaces of commode bowl using a hydrochloric acid formulated bowl cleaner with a bowl mop. Wash exterior surfaces of bowl, seat, and hardware using a synthetic detergent and water; wipe dry.

Empty large waste receptacles and replace plastic liners as required.

Spot-clean walls using a synthetic germicide detergent and water with a cellulose sponge.

The maintenance procedures outlined in Table 1 should be followed on a routined basis as required.

G. Preparation of Equipment

Preparation, like planning, is a vital part of the manufacturing process. Preparation of equipment entails the cleaning, sanitizing, assembling, and in many cases, sterilizing and/or depyrogenation of equipment. The equipment includes such diverse items as tanks (portable or stationary), filtration assemblies, mixers, transfer lines, homogenizers, filling assemblies, vial trays, stopper containers, component preparation equipment, and the work area in general. The proper cleaning of all equipment that comes in contact with the product is particularly critical for parenteral products. Concern must be demonstrated for general cleanliness as well as for the equipment and area, so that one must be sure that the area and equipment

Table 2 Weekly Maintenance Procedures for Service Areas in a Facility for Manufacturing Small Volume Parenteral Products

---

Office Areas

   Dust ledges using a treated synthetic cloth.

   Dust accessible partition areas using a treated synthetic cloth or small treated dry mop.

   Dust picture, bulletin board, or wall ornament using a treated synthetic cloth.

   Damp-wipe stainless steel push plates and kick plates using a synthetic detergent and water with a cloth or sponge, then polish with an industrial-grade stainless steel polish and cloth.

   Dust accessible areas of office furniture using a treated dust cloth.

   Dust accessible areas of other equipment using a treated dust cloth.

Rest Rooms and Lockers

   Damp-wipe stall partitions using germicidal synthetic detergent and water with a sponge or cloth.

Storage Rooms and Mechanical Support Rooms

   Vacuum floors and backs of equipment.

   Empty trash.

   Remove empty pallets.

Aisles

   Sweep accessible floor area using a synthetic-fiber push broom. Pick up sweepings from floor.

   Wet-mop accessible floor area using a cotton/synthetic-strand mop and disinfectant synthetic detergent in water.

---

are free from cross-contamination from products processed just previously or those being processed nearby. The bioclean aspects of the operation are of utmost importance as well. The goal of manufacturing a sterile, pyrogen-free product requires maintenance of a minimum microbial load throughout the process in order to increase the probability of success. Furthermore, the presence of bacteria in or on the equipment will lead to pyrogen contamination even after successful "kill" of live organisms. As discussed in the chapter on "Industrial Sterilization" in Volume 2, pyrogens are essentially metabolic by-products of vegetative microorganisms. One way to assure that the equipment and general area have received proper treatment prior to use is to monitor the area and equipment periodically for the type of living organisms present, and to determine their relative levels. The microbiological flora of each manufacturing facility are likely to differ between each other, and decontamination plans should be tailored accordingly. This approach is better than attempting to try to decontaminate the area(s) for all organisms ("shotgun" decontamination). Additionally, many organisms grow resistant to a particular bacteriacide or a fungicide. Alternating the type of "cidal" agent on a random basis eliminates this protential problem.

The first step in maintaining clean equipment is the practice of ordinary good housekeeping principles. Orderliness and cleanliness are prerequisites for a proper sterile operation. Equipment should never be put away dirty. Cleaning up as

Table 3 Monthly Maintenance Procedures for Service Areas in a Facility for Manufacturing Small Volume Parenteral Products

Office Areas

Buff accessible floor area using a buffing solution and a rotary floor buffing machine.

Spot-clean walls using a synthetic detergent and water with a cellulose sponge.

Dust doors, louvers, and frames using a treated synthetic cloth or vacuum with a brush tool.

Damp-wipe accessible parts of a telephone using a synthetic detergent and water with a cloth or sponge.

Damp-mop floors.

Vacuum shelves.

Rest Rooms and Lockers

Dust air return vents using a dry pickup vacuum equipped with a brush tip or a treated dust cloth or other suitable brush.

Damp-wipe stainless steel push plates and kick plates using a synthetic detergent and water with a cloth or sponge, then polish with an industrial-grade stainless steel polish and cloth.

Dust accessible areas of walls and woodwork using a treated synthetic cloth or small treated dry mop.

Dust doors, louvers, and frames using a treated synthetic cloth or vacuum with a brush tool.

Flush floor drains and drinking fountains using a synthetic germicidal detergent and water.

Aisles

Machine-scrub accessible floor area using a stripper solution to remove old floor finish.

Scrub cove base using a stripper solution and a suitable tool to remove floor finish. Rinse clean.

Apply acrylic water-base floor sealer to accessible concrete or terrazzo floor using a cotton/synthetic-strand mop.

Wash walls and ceiling using a germicidal solution. Vacuum heating element.

Table 4 Biannual Maintenance Procedures for Service Areas in a Facility for Manufacturing Small Volume Parenteral Products

---

Offices Areas

Wash accessible areas of walls using a synthetic detergent and water with a cellulose sponge.

Wash air supply and air return vents using a degreasing detergent and water.

Scrub cove base using a stripper solution and a suitable tool to remove floor finish. Rinse clean and remove old floor finish and stripper solution from accessible floor area using a floor mop or tank-type wet pickup vacuum. Apply floor finish to accessible floor area using a cotton/synthetic-strand mop.

Damp-wipe with a cloth or sponge accessible partition areas using a synthetic detergent and water.

Dust drapes using a tank-type vacuum equipped with a brush tool.

Dust air return vents using a dry pickup vacuum equipped with a brush tip or a treated dust cloth or other suitable brush.

Dust accessible areas of upholstered chairs using a tank vacuum equipped with a brush tool.

Damp-wipe with a sponge or cloth vinyl-covered areas of chairs using a synthetic detergent and water.

Wash walls and ceiling, including sprinkler heads, with phenolic detergent. Clean light fixtures.

Machine-scrub accessible floor area using an ammoniated detergent stripper solution to remove old floor finish.

---

soon as possible after an operation has been completed is a good practice. Dirty equipment can provide a growth medium for microorganisms. This can contaminate other portions of the facility with microorganisms and pyrogens. Nothing takes the place of good, nonabrasive scrubbing with detergent and water. Of course, fiber and particle shedding cloth or brushing utensils should be avoided. Copious amounts of water must be employed following detergent scrub to ensure no soap residue.

Because some equipment is very complex, particularly stationary tanks and pipes, chemical tests are employed to detect residual detergent in the rinse water. Rinsing is continued until the level of residue is below maximum acceptable limits. The final rinse should be made with clean 180°F pyrogen-free water for injection. Finally, equipment should be dried thoroughly with shed-free cloth materials or allowed to air-dry in a laminar flow area. Glassware should be dried and depyrogenated simultaneously in a hot air oven at sterilizing temperatures of 250°C and above. All clean equipment should be covered with shed-free materials and stored in a clean, dry area until used.

Facilities such as walls, ceiling, tabletops, work surfaces, and equipment should be periodically monitored for surface contamination by living organisms. This consists of swabbing objects and incubating the swabs on sterile nutrient plates or employing plates which are placed in direct contact with the surfaces and then incubated. Should bacterial contamination be noted, disinfection steps must be instituted, particularly where resistant spores are suspected or isolated.

Spaulding [3] has tabulated the antimicrobial efficacy of selected classes of compounds as measured by their relative level of activity as disinfectants, antiseptics, or germicides, as may be seen in Table 8. Because of the rapidity of action and effectiveness, glutaraldehyde is becoming more popular over the widely used phenolic compounds. Stonehill, Krop, and Boric [4] have demonstrated the comparative sporicidal action of activated glutaraldehyde against Bacillus megaterium as a test organism. The data are presented in Table 9.

Equipment treated with disinfectants or germicides must be copiously rinsed with pyrogen-free water to ensure absence of residual compound before thoroughly drying and storage. Rinsing the equipment with hot pyrogen-free water is recommended just prior to use with the product.

Any equipment that is intended for use in the sterile part of the manufacturing operation should be treated to render it sterile. Depending on the characteristics of the materials of construction of the equipment, there are various options available in the method of rendering the item sterile. Dry heat sterilization in a drywall oven

Table 5 Annual Maintenance Procedures for Service Areas in a Facility for Manufacturing Small Volume Parenteral Products

---

Office Areas

Clean light diffusers using synthetic detergent and water.

Dust sprinkler heads using a soft-bristled brush.

Wash air supply and air return vents using a degreasing detergent and water.

Damp-wipe with a cloth or sponge accessible areas of office furniture using a synthetic detergent and water.

Damp-wipe with a cloth or sponge accessible areas of miscellaneous equipment using a synthetic detergent and water.

Clean and treat accessible areas of wooden desks using a suitable wood polish with a cloth.

Rest Rooms and Lockers

Clean light diffusers using synthetic detergent and water.

Wash painted ceiling using a synthetic detergent and water with a cellulose sponge.

Dust sprinkler heads using a soft-bristled brush.

Note: On an as-needed-basis, perform the following maintenance procedures:

Aisles

Clean light diffusers using synthetic germicidal detergent and water.

Replace lamp outages.

Replenish soap in dispenser and damp wipe exterior with a sponge or cloth using synthetic detergent and water.

Remove graffiti using an industrial-grade graffiti and ink remover.

Table 6 Routine Maintenance Procedures for the Clean Room Area in a Facility for Manufacturing Small Volume Parenteral Products

Frequency	Description
Weekly	Vacuum accessible floor area using a vacuum cleaner with a HEPA-filtered vent.
Weekly	Damp-mop accessible floor area using a cotton/synthetic-strand mop and disinfectant synthetic detergent in water.
Weekly	Spot-clean walls and doors using a disinfectant synthetic detergent and water with a nonshedding sponge.
Weekly	Wash mirrors using a suitable window cleaner and wipe dry with nonshedding material.
Weekly	Wash sink and hardware using creme cleanser and a damp sponge; rinse clean and wipe dry.
Weekly (or as required)	Damp-wipe all horizontal surfaces with a disinfectant synthetic detergent and water with nonshedding material. Vacuum ventilator grills.
Weekly	Wash window glass using a suitable window cleaner and squeegee or wipe dry.
Weekly	Dust ledges using a treated synthetic cloth.
Weekly	Dust doors, louvers, and frames using a treated synthetic cloth or vacuum with brush tool.
Weekly	Dust accessible areas of office furniture using a treated dust cloth.
Weekly	Dust accessible areas of other equipment using a treated dust cloth.
Monthly	Buff accessible floor area using a buffing solution and a rotary floor buffing machine.
Monthly	Dust accessible parts of safety shower ceilings using a treated dust cloth.
Monthly	Clean stainless steel surfaces using a synthetic detergent and water with a sponge or cloth followed by application of stainless steel polish on a cloth.
Monthly	Damp-wipe accessible parts of a telephone with a cloth or sponge using a synthetic detergent and water.
Monthly (or as required)	Wash walls (including baseboards, doors, doors frames), ceilings, light fixtures (inside and outside), and sprinkler heads and air return vents using a disinfectant synthetic detergent and nonshedding material.
Twice/year (or as required)	Machine-scrub accessible floor area and cove base using stripper solution with a floor mop or tank vacuum. Rinse floor area with clean water. Repeat rinse procedure as necessary.

Table 6 (continued)

Frequency	Description
Twice/year	Apply finish to floor using a synthetic-strand mop. Repeat procedure as necessary.
Twice/year	Scrub cove base using a stripper solution and a suitable tool to remove floor finish. Rinse clean. Remove old floor finish and stripper solution from accessible floor area using a floor mop or tank wet-pickup vacuum cleaner. Rinse scrubbed accessible floor area to remove remains of old floor finish and stripper solution. Repeat procedure as necessary. Apply floor finish to accessible floor area using a cotton/synthetic-strand mop.
Twice/year	Dust air return vents using a dry pickup vacuum equipped with a brush tip or a treated dust cloth or other suitable brush.
Twice/year	Damp-wipe with a cloth or sponge accessible areas of lab bench fronts using synthetic detergent and water.
Twice/year	Damp-wipe with a cloth or sponge accessible areas of the face of lab hoods using a synthetic detergent and water.
Twice/year	Damp-wipe with a cloth or sponge accessible areas of office furniture using a synthetic detergent and water.
Twice/year	Damp-wipe with a cloth or sponge accessible areas of other or miscellaneous equipment using a synthetic germicide detergent and water.
Twice/year	Damp-wipe with a sponge or cloth vinyl-covered areas of chairs using a synthetic germicide detergent and water.
Twice/year	Wash waste baskets using a synthetic germicide detergent and water using a cloth or sponge and wipe dry.
Annually	Wash accessible areas of walls with a cellulose sponge using a synthetic detergent and water.
Annually	Clean light diffusers using a synthetic detergent and water.
Annually	Dust sprinkler heads using a soft-bristled brush.
Annually	Wash air supply vents using a degreasing detergent and water.
Annually	Wash air return vents using a degreasing detergent and water.
As needed	Replace lamp outages on a need basis.

at temperatures of 170°C or above for 1 to 3 hr at temperature is the preferred method [5]. This method is particularly useful for glass or nonsoldered metal objects. Although lower temperatures may be used with a longer exposure time, the process must be shown to be as effective as the parameters stated. Unfortunately,

Table 7 Routine Maintenance Procedures for Sterile Areas in a Facility for Manufacturing Small Volume Parenteral Products

Frequency	Description
Weekly (when in use)	Vacuum accessible floor area using a vacuum cleaner with a HEPA-filtered vent.
	Empty waste containers; wash and reline with plastic bags when necessary. Spot-clean walls and doors with a non-shedding material using a synthetic germicidal detergent and water.
	Wash drinking fountains and sinks using creme cleanser or a disinfectant synthetic detergent in water with a sponge; rinse clean and wipe dry.
Weekly	Wash window glass and ledges using a suitable window cleaner; squeegee or wipe dry.
	Damp-wipe all horizontal surfaces using a disinfectant synthetic detergent and water with a nonshedding material. Vacuum air supply and air return vents.
	Damp-mop accessible floor area using a synthetic-strand mop and disinfectant synthetic detergent in water.
Monthly	Wash walls (including baseboards, doors, door frames), ceilings, light fixtures (inside and outside), sprinkler heads, air return vents, and intercom using a disinfectant synthetic detergent and nonshedding material. Replace lamp outages as needed.
	Damp-wipe using a disinfectant synthetic detergent and water with a nonshedding material the inside of shoe cabinets and gown locker compartments.
Twice/year	Machine-scrub accessible floor areas and cove bases using a stripper solution to remove old floor finish. Remove old finish and stripper solution with floor mop or tank vacuum cleaner. Rinse floor area with clean water. Repeat rinse procedure as necessary.
	Apply floor finish to floor area using a synthetic-strand mop. Repeat the procedure as necessary.

most other materials cannot withstand the high temperatures necessary for drywall sterilization. Although not the preferred method for sterilizing equipment, steam sterilization in an autoclave at 121°C and 15 to 18 psig for a sufficient time period to render the object sterile (usually 20 min or more) has been routinely used [6]. This second method is quite effective in sterilizing but not efficient in depyrogenating objects. Items to be autoclaved should be prerinsed with 180° F pyrogen-free water to try to eliminate pyrogenic substances.

Table 8   Relative Antimicrobial Efficacy of Selected Compounds

Product	Concentrations	Relative activity level[a] as:		
		Disinfectant	Antiseptic	Germicide
Glutaraldehyde solution	2%	+3	0	High
Formaldehyde + alcohol	8% + 70%	+3	0	High
Formaldehyde solution	3–8%	+1 to +2	0	High to intermediate
Iodine + alcohol	0.05% + 70%	0	+4	intermediate
Alcohols	70%–90%	+2	+3	intermediate
Chlorine compounds	500–5000 ppm (as available chlorine)	+1	±	intermediate
Phenolic compounds	1–3%	+3	±	intermediate
Iodine solution	1%	0	+2	intermediate
Iodophors	75–150 ppm (as available iodine)	+1	+3	intermediate to low
Quaternary compounds	1:750 to 1:500	+1	+2	low
Hexachlorophene	1%	0	+2	low
Mercurial compounds	1:1000 to 1:500	0	+1	low

[a]+4 indicates maximum usefulness, 0 indicates little or no usefulness.
Source: Ref. 3.

Should the equipment be sensitive to heat or pressure generated in a sterilizing procedure in an autoclave, gas sterilization by ethylene oxide is a third option.
Caution must be exercised in eliminating any residuals of ethylene oxide or its
breakdown products on the equipment.   A final option is the use of ionizing radiation,
for sterilization.   Many disposable items, such as rubber gloves, plastic items, and
even sterilizing filters, are sterilized via ionizing radiation by the manufacturers
of such items.   Radiation is not a practical method for the parenteral manufacturer
unless the manufacturer has access to a convenient source of gamma or high-energy
electron beam radiation on the plant site.

Table 9   Relative Sporicidal Action of Several Antimicrobial Agents Against
B. Megaterium

Test agent	Approximate Number of Surviving Organisms X 100 as a Function of Contact Time (min)					
	Initial	0	30	60	120	240
2% Glutaraldehyde	4000	1700	300	4 4	0 0	0
1% Saponated cresol	3700	3000	3600	2400	2300	2220
2% Saponated cresol	3700	2900	3100	3000	2700	1300
2% Formaldehyde	4000	3200	2300	1900	20	10
Water	4100	4000	4000	4100	4000	3900

Source: Ref. 4.

Items such as filtration apparatus and associated sterilizing membranes, tanks, bottles, mixing equipment, filling machinery, vent filters, utensils, stoppering equipment, and other items brought into the sterile area, such as tools, must be sterilized just prior to use in the sterile operation. The sterilization processes for equipment sterilization must be validated and documented in exactly the same way as the sterilization procedure for components or products. The concept of validation and documentation (e.g., load description, load sizes, load patterns, mapping of same, heat distribution, and heat penetration) are discussed in greater detail in the chapter on Industrial Sterilization in Volume 2. The reader should keep in mind that equipment sterilization is just as complex as product or package sterilization and it is vital to the total sterile operation. To produce a sterile product, equipment handling deserves a great deal of attention and shortcuts must not be tolerated.

H. Preparation of Packaging Components

A sterile package consists of primary and secondary packaging components. Secondary packaging components are not in direct contact with a sterile product. The function of the secondary component is to aid in the shipment, identification, or market appeal of a product. A box or a shrink wrap are examples of secondary containers. The primary packaging components are in direct contact with the sterile product and are designed to protect the product from loss of sterility and provides an environment that minimizes physical and chemical decomposition. Examples of primary packaging components are ampuls, vials, syringes, syringe cartridges, squeeze bottles, and rubber or plastic stoppers. It is the intent of this section to discuss how to prepare primary packaging components for use in packaging a sterile product.

The preparation and sterilization of primary packaging components for parenteral or other sterile products are very important steps in the overall manufacturing scheme. The primary components must be clean and sterile. There are numerous methods for cleaning primary packaging components. However, only the general methods for cleaning and sterilizing rubber, glass, and plastic components as practiced by many pharmaceutical companies will be discussed in this section. The type of processing available for primary packaging components are limited by the chemical nature of the component (e.g., rubber components are heat labile and therefore cannot be sterilized by dry heat without charring the rubber).

1. Rubber Components

Rubber components such as vial stoppers, syringe parts, and ophthalmic dropper bulbs should be stored until used in cool, clean areas. Since rubber degrades with time when exposed to air and elevated temperatures, staging and tight first in/first out inventory control for these packaging components are critical. The actual processing of rubber components involves the following operations: (1) washing, (2) sterilization, and if necessary, (3) siliconization.

Washing. The primary goal of washing is to remove particulate matter (such as dirt and/or surface contaminants) from the rubber. The washing process may be carried out with or without the assistance of a detergent. The use of detergents should be considered carefully because, potentially, residual amounts of detergents can be difficult to remove from the rubber. Ordinary clothes washers have been used to wash rubber components. There are two problems associated with ordinary clothes washers: (1) the tumbling action of the washer produces rubber abrasion, resulting in excess particle formation, and (2) the gravity drain at the bottom of the washer forces the dirty effluent liquid to be drained through the clean stoppers at the end of the wash cycle. These problems have been reduced because washing equipment has been tailored for the specific problems associated with stopper washing. The Huber Company (Fig. 3) has eliminated most of the gravity drain problem by adding an overflow rinse cycle to "float" dirt and debris away from the stoppers toward the top of the liquid surface and out to a separate drain system. This prevents drainage of wash water back through the clean bed of closures. In addition, the Huber washer is equipped with a punch card-type cycle controller. A wash cycle may be embossed onto the surface of the card by punching holes at the appropriate locations. The card is then fed into a reader (A in Fig. 3) that controls the wash cycle, thus making it easy to duplicate a wash cycle. One disadvantage of the Huber is that it is still a rotary drum washer similar to ordinary clothes washers. The tumbling action of the inner basket (B in Fig. 3) may cause the stoppers to

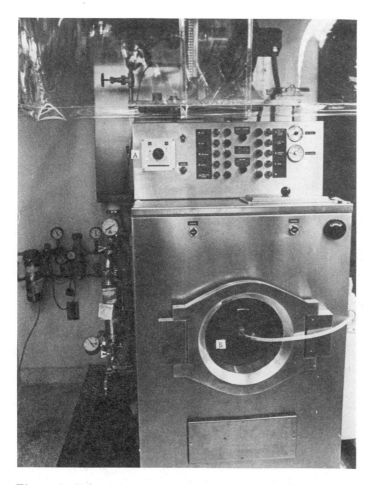

Figure 3 Huber stopper washer under laminar flow. (Courtesy of Merck, Sharp and Dohme Research Laboratories, West Point, Pennsylvania.)

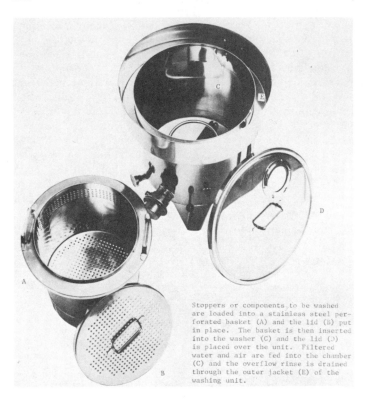

Stoppers or components to be washed
are loaded into a stainless steel perforated basket (A) and the lid (B) put
in place. The basket is then inserted
into the washer (C) and the lid (D)
is placed over the unit. Filtered
water and air are fed into the chamber
(C) and the overflow rinse is drained
through the outer jacket (E) of the
washing unit.

Figure 4 Capsolut washing machine. (Courtesy of Production Equipment, Inc.,
Division of the Burnet Co., Rochelle Park, New Jersey.)

abrade against each other or against the drum. The Capsolut washer (Fig. 4) has
eliminated both the drain and abrasion problems associated with clothes washers.
The Capsolut washer gently agitates the stoppers via filtered air, which is directed
toward a basket containing the stoppers. The "dirt" or debris floats to the surface
while the tank is being flushed with clean water from below. The debris is removed
by overflow through a drain system at the top of the tank. This prevents contamination of the clean stoppers by dirty drain water and also limits stopper abrasion as
seen in the rotary drum-type washers. The Capsolut does not have a card controller like the Huber. However, recent models have been modified to provide reproducible cycles.

The washing time and temperature of the rinse water will depend on specifications developed for the type, size, and quality of rubber components being washed
per load. Both water and air entering the washer unit must be filtered before use.
Frequently, a 0.22 μm cartridge-type filter is used and the filter is checked periodically for integrity and/or clogging. This is usually accomplished by keeping a
regular record of the pressure drop across the filter unit. The filter cartridges
are changed when there is a noticeable pressure change or when the pressure drop
exceeds the maximum allowable limit for water passage. The frequency of changing
the filters depends on the extent of usage and the quality of water and air.

Finally, Nishimura et al. [7] have described a new system in which each stopper (both lower and upper surfaces) is washed individually. Table 10 summarizes

Table 10 Average Particle Size of Particulate Left on Rubber Closures Postwashing by Different Types of Washing Systems

Particle size (μm)	Unwashed	Average particle count per 5 X 20 mm closures after washing in			
		Individual washer	Domestic clothes washer	Rotary cage washer (Capsolut type)	Rotary drum washer (Huber type)
25-50	TNTC[a]	10	63	94	93
50	25-115	1	23	63	24

[a]Too numerous to count.
Source: Ref. 7.

the average particle count obtained for three sets of stoppers which were washed by each of the types of stopper washers and compares the results to that obtained with a conventional washer.

The degree of cleanliness of the rubber components being washed is usually measured in relation to previous batches. The insurance or validation that a reproducible and acceptable washing process has been achieved can be viewed from two positions. One approach is based on achieving reproducibility through the use of various controllers, like the Huber, to produce a consistent cleanliness for each cycle. The second approach is to monitor each wash cycle by evaluating the incoming wash water and the outgoing rinse water for particulates, clarity, and in some cases pH. Washing in this instance is continued until the cleanliness parameters of previous batches have been met. Microscopic counting, visual inspection, or electronic counting using light blockage (HIAC), light scattering (Climet), or laser beam techniques (Spectrex) are being used to evaluate particulate matter. In essence, the washing cycle is continually being validated in this manner. After washing, the rubber components are packed in clean glass, polypropylene, non-shedding synthetic bags, or stainless steel containers with sealable tops. The washed components are then transferred for lubrication or sterilization.

Sterilization. The washed, packed (and often siliconized) rubber components are generally sterilized by autoclaving (moist heat). Moist heat is the process of choice with rubber because of the rapid heat penetration. The slow heat penetration of dry heat may dry and crack the rubber while a sterilant gas such as ethylene oxide may be difficult to release from the rubber matrix within a practical time period. Moist-heat exposure time for rubber components is established for microbial kill rates based on batch size and loading patterns. Exposure times are critical. Underheating may not produce an adequate microbial kill, while overheating may cause problems such as tackiness or decomposition (cracking) or the rubber. After autoclaving, the rubber components must be dried. This is done either by applying vacuum right in the autoclave or by drying them at low temperatures in vacuum or forced-air ovens. The parameters for these processes must be established for each rubber compound. A typical cycle would be 1 to 2 hr at 100°F in an autoclave.

The sterilized, dried stoppers are then stored in a cool, humidity controlled, clean area, preferably under laminar airflow. There is usually a time period beyond which the stopper should not be used if there is a delay in processing the product. The time factor is largely dependent on the characteristics of the rubber compound and the individual production/quality control policy on storing of sterilized components prior to use. This period of time is usually based on the assessed risk factor for contamination of the stored sterile rubber components.

Siliconization. Siliconization of rubber components is usually necessary to facilitate insertion of the rubber components into container openings via high-speed automatic filling and sealing equipment. Without siliconization, shingling, or jam-up of the rubber components (stoppers) in feed chutes is common because of the high friction of untreated rubber. Additionally, during high-speed stoppering operations, the lubricity imparted by siliconization is required to compensate for slight misalignment between the vial and stopper position and allows for easy insertion under mechanical stress. The situation is akin to putting a dry rubber hose over a dry glass or stainless tube. A small amount of water for lubricity makes the job much easier. At one time, stoppers were stored in sterile water after washing and sterilizing. These were then aseptically removed and inserted into the vials by hand. The availability of silicone lubricants has largely enabled this technique to be eliminated. Wet closures increase the risk of mold contamination and chemical attack (swelling) in the presence of water. Furthermore, dry products such as lyophilized or powder fill products could not tolerate the moisture levels.

Either a plain silicone oil or an aqueous emulsion of a silicone oil is used to siliconize SVP rubber components. The aqueous emulsion makes it easier to ensure a more uniform application of silicone oil. It may be applied by boiling rubber components in the emulsion or by simply rinsing the rubber in the emulsion. However, the use of plain silicone oils, such as Dow-Corning DC-360 Medical Fluid, is becoming more commonly used than the commercial emulsions in water. Many companies have found it prudent to use the neat silicone fluid because emulsions tend to become contaminated by mold. This contamination increases the risk of pyrogen contamination of the product. One method for applying silicone oil to rubber is to rotate the components (very slowly to avoid rubber abrasion) in a tablet coating pan or a rotary washer like the Huber and slowly add small amounts of silicone oil (e.g., 1 ml per 1000 to 10,000 components, depending on rubber component size, design, and desired lubricity). Some manufacturers prefer to apply the silicone to the dry rubber components, whereas others prefer applying the silicone to wet rubber. There does not appear to be any difference in the resultant lubricity using either method.

In general, rubber components should not be reprocessed because the conditions of washing, sterilization, siliconization, and drying provide a great deal of physical and chemical stress on the rubber. If one desires to reprocess rubber components, extensive testing may be necessary to prove that there are no adverse effects upon the rubber after reprocessing.

2. Glass Components

Glass components such as vials, ampuls, bottles, syringe cartridges, and syringes are more chemically stable than rubber components and therefore may be stored at a higher temperature and at high humidities for a longer period of time. Glass components such as rubber have to be washed and sterilized and, if necessary, may have to be siliconized.

Washing. The washing of glass components for sterile products is a unique challenge. Glass is not as inert as often supposed. Sanga [8] has described the mechanism and nature of the chemical attack on glass surfaces, particularly by water. The inorganic chemical components of glass vary considerably [9], not only among types of glass (USP types I, II, and III), but between tubing glass and molded glass (see the chapter on Glass Containers for Parenterals in Volume II for a discussion of glass components). Furthermore, the composition of glass can vary from manufacturer to manufacturer. Typical compositional variation in type I and II molded and type I tubing glass was demonstrated by Sanga [8]. Inorganic ions can react with the product or water itself and can be extracted into the parenteral solutions. Imperfections in the glass surface will allow escape of these ions into the liquid medium bathing the glass surface. In addition, minute imperfections on the surface of the glass may flake off as glass "chips." The glass manufacturers have been taking steps to maintain a clean surface on the inner walls of the glass containers as supplied to manufacturers of parenteral products.

There are several methods of treatment to increase the durability of the surface of glass. These methods of treatment include:

1. Heating: To remove sodium by volatization via fire polishing.
2. Clay contact: To remove Na^+ and O^{--}.
3. Sulfur treated: To remove alkali by heating to 1000 to 1200°F and then exposure to sulfur trioxide or sulfur dioxide gas in the presence of moisture.
4. Acid treated: To remove alkali by forming a sodium salt that can be washed from the surface of the glass, using hydrochloric acid, sulfuric acid, ammonium sulfate, ammonium chloride, or sulfur at 1200°F.
5. Fluoride treated: Fluoride ions replace the pendent oxygen or hydroxyl groups on the glass, thus improving the surface durability of the glass. The fluoride ions also react with sodium to form the insoluble fluoride salt. The glass is essentially etched and the surface layer removed.

Some companies have experimented with fluoride rinsing of the glass containers [10] and found that the reduction of particulates is not sufficient to warrant its use. The use of fluoride presents increased financial cost and safety risks in handling because residual fluoride compounds must be removed from the glass.

Aside from chemical interactions and physical breakdown of the glass surface, there is a major problem of dust, cardboard and paper particles, glass chips, and other debris that find their way into the container some time between manufacture and use by the pharmaceutical company. The glass industry has made great strides in reducing the potential particulate contaminants by introducing the use of shrink wrap around glass containers. The containers are wrapped in a plastic film immediately after they are manufactured. The film is stretched over the container, making a tight seal over the mouth and body of the entire packet of containers (e.g., 1000 vials in one shrink-wrapped unit). The packets are then packed into conventional cardboard boxes. Previously, vials and bottles were packaged directly into cardboard boxes with cardboard separators between each container. This led to cardboard slivers and dirt associated with shipping and handling. These cardboard particles, which are quite difficult to remove from the containers, found their way into the containers. During container washing, the heavier cardboard particles often cling to the walls of the vial or bottle when wetted and are not rinsed out of the container by the washing machine. Furthermore, the shipped containers often were shocked and jarred during shipment and handling, leading to glass chips in the vial or bottle. In addition, dust, insects, and debris which had found its way into the cardboard boxes were easily able to enter the open, exposed container. Shrink wrapping tightly seals the opening of the container and holds each vial or bottle in a rigid, fixed position, thus reducing the incidence of glass chip formation when the cartons are jarred during handling. Despite the advantage of shrink wrap, containers are still prone to particulate contamination, and physical washing treatments are still necessary for producing clean containers for parenteral products.

There are a number of commercially available washing machines for cleaning vials, bottles, ampuls, plastic containers, syringe barrels, and syringe cartridges. Basically, a series of water washes under pressure and air jet treatments in a variety of pressure and time sequences are employed to cleanse the containers. Some units employ steam as part of the liquid wash cycle. One of the most popular methods of washing ampuls, vials, and similar containers is the use of a stationary rig of stainless steel nozzles (washing needles) in a fixed position plate through which alternate cycles of air, steam, or water are forced under pressure into inverted containers resting on a holder that maintains them at a fixed distance from the end of the washing needles.

The Metromatic washer (Fig. 5) is an example of a typical semiautomatic washer used to clean a variety of containers and a number of container sizes. The air and water entering the washing machine should be filtered to reduce particulate contact with the containers during washing. A 0.22 μm cartridge is the most common porosity, although 1 to 5 μm sizes are being used to give a higher flow rate. The once common use of city water or deionized water is diminishing and is almost nonexistent. Manufacturers are using hot, pyrogen-free distilled water as the washing and rinsing fluid.

A typical wash cycle, allowing 1 min for each step, would be:

Inside wash: Hot filtered pyrogen-free water
Outside wash: Hot filtered pyrogen-free water

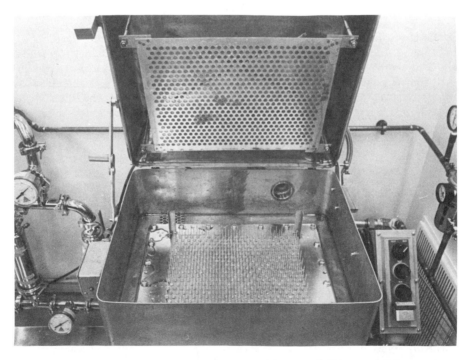

Figure 5 Metromatic washer for cleaning glass containers. (Courtesy of Merck, Sharp and Dohme Research Laboratories, West Point, Pennsylvania.)

Inside: Filtered air
Inside wash: Hot filtered pyrogen-free water
Outside wash: Hot filtered pyrogen-free water
Inside: Filtered air
Inside wash: Hot filtered pyrogen-free water
Inside: Filtered air
Inside: Filtered air

The vials or ampuls are then removed in trays for sterilization.

Although the stationary washer approach is sufficiently rapid for most production systems, there are continuous washing systems (such as the Cozzoli or Strunck) that can be incorporated into a unit operation tunnel. That is, vials/ampuls are washed, sterilized, filled, and sealed in one continuous operation. Figure 6 shows a washer for such a system.

   Sterilization. After washing, glass components are sterilized by dry heat. Dry heat is the process of choice for sterilizing glass components. Advantage may be taken of the fact that the glassware is dry at the end of the cycle [11]. Dry containers can be kept sterile during storage more easily than wet equipment. Glass containers generally have the largest surface area of any of the primary packaging components. As such, the glass container is the most probable source of pyrogen contamination (see the chapter on Industrial Sterilization in Volume 2). Dry heat is the only method of sterilization that will consistently destroy pyrogens [12]. Dry heat destroys pyrogens by cleaving the large organic molecules that make up a pyrogen into basic elements such as carbon, nitrogen, phosphorus, and so on. These basic elements will not trigger the pyrogen heat response like the larger organic molecules. Like moist heat, exposure time for dry heat is established for microbial kill rates and depyrogenation and is based on batch size and loading patterns. Exposure times for dry heat are longer than moist heat. Dry heat has a slower penetration rate. A typical cycle would be 4 hr at 250°C in a drywall oven. Figure 7 shows a typical hot air sterilizer.

   The sterile, depyrogenated glass containers are stored in covered stainless steel trays in a cool, humidity-controlled, clean area, preferably under laminar airflow.

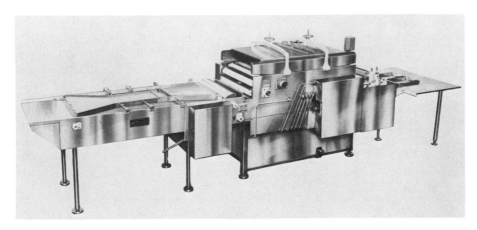

Figure 6 Cozzoli Model AW9 continuous washing system. (Courtesy of Cozzoli Machine Company, Plainfield, New Jersey.)

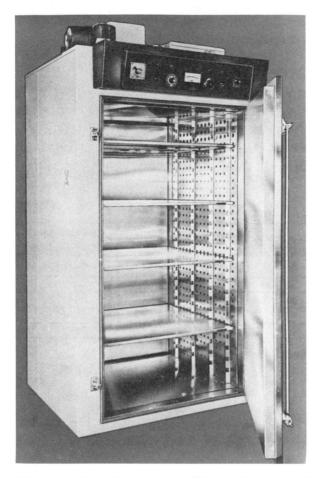

Figure 7 Hotpack hot air sterilizer. (Courtesy of Hotpack Corporation, Philadelphia, Pennsylvania.)

Siliconization. Siliconization of glass containers is usually necessary to facilitate the draining of solid products (suspensions and dry powder) from the walls of the containers. This drainage factor may help improve the appearance of the product as well as help the dose uniformity by inhibiting drying of the solid portion of a suspension on a vial wall, resulting in a reduction of the solids delivered per volume of suspension.

Siliconization is carried out with a freshly prepared aqueous emulsion (the composition of which varies with each user's requirements) which is sprayed into the vial via a standard vial washing machine as described previously in this section. After the silicone emulsion has been applied, the siliconized vials are baked in a dry wall oven at 250°C for 5 hr. This baking procedure bakes the silicone onto the surface of the glass component. This procedure is done last in the processing step, so that it serves as a depyrogenating step as well. The sterile, siliconized, depyrogenated glass containers are stored in covered stainless steel trays in a cool, humidity-controlled, clean area, preferably under laminar airflow.

3. Plastic Containers

Plastic Ophthalmic Dispensers Plastic containers, such as ophthalmic dispensers, are usually washed in much the same manner as glass but are sterilized by means requiring low temperature because of the low melting point of the plastic used. Polypropylene or high-density polyethylene parts, such as caps, can be steam sterilized. However, low-density polyethylene plastics that are usually employed for flexible-walled ophthalmic packaging cannot be steam-sterilized, due to the distortion encountered during the normal autoclaving cycle. Therefore, plastic ophthalmic dispensers usually are sterilized with ethylene oxide. The washed plastic components are placed in polyethylene or parchment bags which allow adequate penetration of the gas for sterilization and proper venting after sterilization to remove the sterilant. The sterilizing cycle (time, temperature, gas concentration, and relative humidity conditions) has to be determined for each material and for each load pattern used.

Spore strips and/or color change strips should be strategically placed according to the type of load and its configuration, size, and location in the sterilizer chamber. Once the cycle has been completed, the articles are removed and deaerated rapidly in a forced-draft hot air oven (low temperature, range 60 to 100°C) or laminar flow hood for several hours to allow for the discharge of excess gas into a well-ventilated area so that less than 1 ppm of ethylene oxide can be detected on suitable monitoring equipment. The color-change strips are examined to see if they were adequately exposed to ethylene oxide gas and the spore strips are placed in culture medium and incubated. All sterilization charts are maintained and identified. Samples of material being sterilized are submitted for sterility testing and determination of residual gas. While awaiting release test results, the sterilized components are stored in a clean, isolated area. Samples are also tested for sterility and subjected to NF and USP plastic toxicity tests, as appropriate.

Exposure to cobalt-60 gamma rays or to the high-energy electron beam source is another method employed to sterilize plastic components and is usually done on a contract basis. Electron beam and cobalt-60 sterilization are being used with increasing frequency.

Plastic Syringes Plastic syringes are rarely used to package unit dose injections. The pharmaceutical industry in the United States has not marketed prefilled plastic syringes. This is mainly due to potential plastic extractives, weight loss by virtue of water vapor loss, plastic-product interaction, and regulatory acceptance barriers. Such devices would be sterilized by a gas sterilant or by exposure to radiation.

II. MANUFACTURE OF THE PRODUCT

Except for the added restraints of maintaining an exceptionally clean area with low bioburden, of keeping equipment ultraclean, and keeping raw materials at the lowest bioburden, the manufacture of small volume sterile products in bulk for later subdivision into packages is carried out like any pharmaceutical process. A high level of cleanliness must be imposed to minimize the risk of product contamination by extraneous debris, viable organisms, or pyrogenic substances.

Beyond these restraints, the majority of formulations fall into three pharmaceutical product categories: (1) solutions, (2) suspensions/dispersions, and (3) solids for constitution.

The formula and suggested method of manufacture, sterilization, and subdivision will be explained on a step-by-step basis. The formulas and procedures that have been selected for discussion in this chapter are typical of those used in the pharmaceutical industry.

A. Preparation of a Small Volume Parenteral Solution

A sterile solution is the most common small volume parenteral dosage form. The composition of a typical solution formula is presented in Table 11. The preparation of a solution involves the dissolution of all the ingredients into an appropriate solvent system. The most common solvent is water. However, cosolvent systems, such as aqueous/glycol mixtures, have been used when water alone lacks sufficient solvent power to dissolve the active drug. Occasionally, nonaqueous systems such as vegetable oils are used when aqueous and cosolvent systems are found to be inadequate to dissolve the active drug. Solutions are the parenteral dosage form of choice because they offer convenience in their diversity of end use (intravenous, intramuscular, or subcutaneous) and content uniformity is easily obtained during manufacture and administration.

The composition of a sterile solution is often uncomplicated in nature. In addition to the soluble drug, a sterile solution may contain one or more of the following agents:

1. Osmotic pressure adjusters such as sodium chloride or mannitol are used.
2. Bacteriostatic agents are required for multiple-dose containers. Benzyl alcohol is commonly used for injectables and benzalkonium chloride is commonly used for ophthalmic solutions.
3. Buffering agents such as phosphates, acetates, and citrate salts have been used. The choice of which system to use is determined by the desired pH and the compatibility of the active ingredient with the buffer system.
4. pH adjusters such as sodium hydroxide or hydrochloric acid are used in combination with suitable buffering agents. Occasionally, the pH can be adjusted without the aid of additional buffering agents.
5. Antioxidants such as bisulfite, ascorbate, and citrate compounds are used to preserve oxygen-labile drugs.
6. Chelating agents such as disodium edetate (EDTA) are used to sequester heavy metals which can catalyze degradation reactions.

The preparation of a sterile solution might appear to be a simple matter. However, clean room conditions must be maintained and special preparation techniques must be used to minimize particulate and microbial contamination. Therefore, preparation of a sterile solution product can be quite difficult. This will become obvious when one considers the difficulties in using the procedures that are presented in the example below if they were to be used to prepare a formula consisting mainly of Sterile Water for Injection, USP.

Figure 8 depicts the process flow diagram for one way to produce a sterile solution such as that presented in Table 11. In this example it should be assumed that the soluble drug is heat labile and, as such, cannot be terminally sterilized via autoclaving. The method of processing is discussed in detail below.

Figure 8: Operation 1—Nonsterile Formulation

1. Place water for injection into a clean, vented, glass-lined or stainless steel pressure tank. A starting volume in excess of 10% of the final volume is

Table 11 Formulation for a Multiple-Dose Sterile Ophthalmic or Injectable Solution[a]

Dosage

10 mg	Soluble drug	Active drug
8.30 mg	Sodium phosphate monobasic (monohydrate)	Buffering agent
11.29 mg	Sodium phosphate dibasic (anhydrous)	Buffering agent
0.1 mg	Benzalkonium chloride	Ophthalmic preservative
	or	
9.0 mg	Benzyl alcohol	Parenteral preservative
q.s. pH 6.8 to 7.0	Sodium hydroxide	pH adjustment
q.s. ad 1 ml	Water for Injection, USP	Solvent

[a]Product: soluble drug solution (10 mg ml^{-1}).

recommended to cover losses due to evaporation during heating. Seal the pressure tank.

2. Heat the water for injection to 121°C and maintain for 20 min while gradually releasing tank pressure. Then cool to 60°C.

3. Remove and place in a separate vented stainless steel or glass container of suitable capacity a quantity of water for injection equal to about 30% of the final formula volume, and save for final volume adjustment.

4. To the remaining water for injection (at 60°C), from step 2, add and dissolve with stirring the sodium phosphate monobasic (monohydrate) and sodium phosphate dibasic (anhydrous). Care must be taken that the phosphate salts are all dissolved; hydrates are formed in solution which increase the time for complete dissolution rate. Addition of phosphates at higher temperatures (60°C) and high mixing shear will be helpful.

5. Allow the solution from step 4 to cool to room temperature (25 to 30°C). Then, add and dissolve with stirring the water-soluble drug and the preservative. Check the pH of the solution. If required, adjust the pH to 6.8 to 7.0 with approximately 1 N sodium hydroxide (NaOH) solution.

6. Bring the bulk to final volume with water for injection and mix well.

Note: The water for injection for volume adjustment is obtained from a portion of the material saved in step 3.

Figure 8: Operation II—Sterilization

1. Sterilize the bulk solution from operation I, step 6, by filtration through a sterile sterilizing membrane, with an appropriate nonshedding preclarification filter.

2. Collect the sterile filtrate directly from the sterilizing membrane via sterile tubing and siphon into a sterile, clean, closed, vented stainless steel tank or glass vessel.

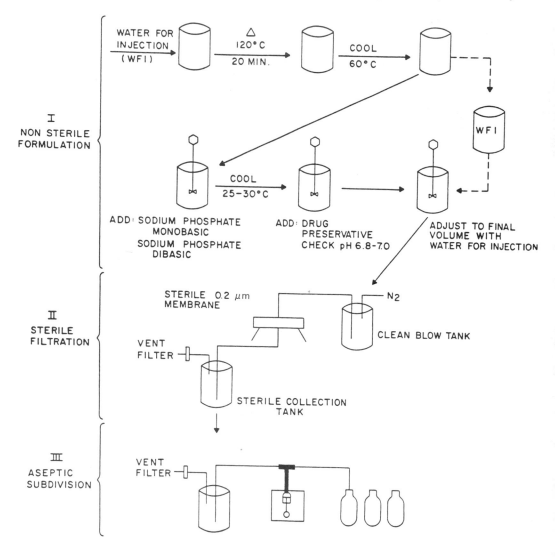

Figure 8   Production of a sterile solution.

Figure 8: Operation III—Sterile Subdivision

1. Aseptically subdivide the sterile bulk solution into an appropriate sterile
   container.
2. Aseptically apply sterilized closure systems to the container and seal.
3. Sample across the filling operation at intervals determined by quality control
   standards for sterility tests and volume fill checks.
4. Visually inspect all units for defects and particulates against a well–lighted
   black–and–white background.
5. Submit samples to the quality control laboratory for release assays.

In certain countries (e.g., Scandinavia) "cold" sterilization (e.g., filtration) is not
recognized as the primary method of final product sterilization. The preferred

method of sterilization in these countries is terminal heat or radiation sterilization in the package. However, many organic medicinals lack sufficient stability in solution during irradiation or heating such as is found in high-pressure steam autoclaves. An alternative method has been to steam or dry heat sterilize those portions of the formula that are not heat labile and incorporate sterile chemical components or chemical components of known low bioburdens (low microorganism counts).

An alternative sterilization process for the Scandinavian countries for the production of the formulation discussed in Figure 8 is presented in Figure 9. A detailed discussion of the alternative sterilization process is presented below.

Figure 9: Operation I—Nonsterile Formulation of the Vehicle

1. Place water for injection into a clean, vented, glass-lined or stainless steel pressure tank. A starting volume in excess of 10% of the final volume is recommended to cover losses due to evaporation during heating. Seal the pressure tank.
2. Heat the water for injection to 121°C and maintain for 20 min while gradually releasing tank pressure. Then cool to 60°C.
3. Remove and place in a separate vented stainless steel or glass container of suitable capacity a quantity of the water for injection equal to about 30% of the final formula volume. Seal the vessel and save for final volume adjustment.
4. To the remaining water for injection (at 60°C), from step 2, add and dissolve with stirring the sodium phosphate monobasic (monohydrate) and sodium phosphate dibasic (anhydrous).
5. Seal the pressure tank for autoclaving.

Figure 9: Operation II—Thermal Sterilization of the Vehicle

1. Autoclave both of the vessels from operation I, steps 3 and 4, for 30 min at 121°C, timed at product temperature.

Figure 9: Operation III—Aseptic Formulation of the Active and Preservative

1. Cool the sterile vessels from operation II, step 1, to room temperature (25 to 30°C), then aseptically add and dissolve with stirring the water-soluble drug and the preservative.
2. Aseptically check and adjust the pH to 6.8 to 7.0 if required with approximately 1 N NaOH solution.
3. Aseptically bring the bulk to final volume with water for injection.

Note: The water for injection for volume adjustment is obtained from a portion of the material saved in operation I, step 3, and autoclaved in operation II, step 1.

Figure 9: Operation IV—Filtration

1. Filter the bulk solution from operation III, step 3, through a sterile membrane, with an appropriate nonshedding preclarification filter pad.
2. Collect the sterile filtrate directly from the membrane via sterile tubing and siphon into a sterile, clean, closed, vented stainless steel tank or glass vessel.

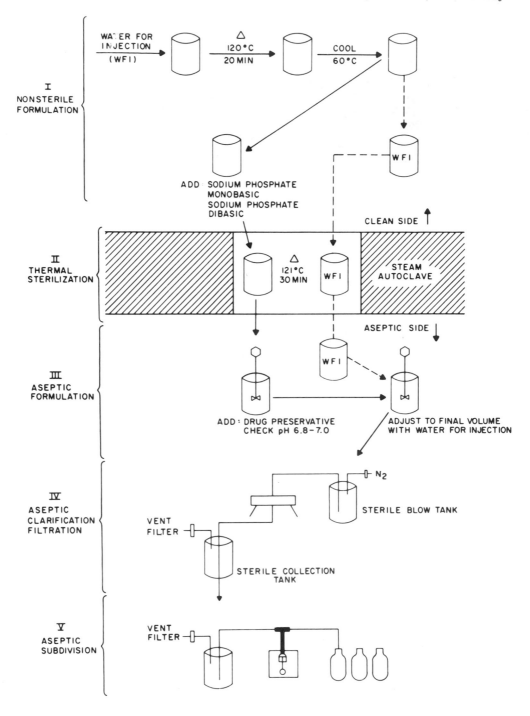

Figure 9 Production of a sterile solution by an alternative sterilization process.

Figure 9: Operation V—Sterile Subdivision

1. Aseptically subdivide the sterile bulk solution into an appropriate sterile container.

Some multinational pharmaceutical companies export concentrated solutions of final product to subsidiary foreign companies. This procedure not only satisfies some regulatory requirements that prohibit importation of finished packaged goods but also provides an economical advantage for shipping bulk rather than packaged solution. The offshore company then makes arrangements for dilution and subdivision. This third method of manufacture is shown in Figure 10 and is discussed below.

Figure 10: Operation I—Nonsterile Formulation of a 5X Concentrate

1. Place water for injection into a clean, vented, glass-lined or stainless steel pressure tank. A starting volume in excess of 10% of the final volume of the concentrate is recommended to cover losses due to evaporation during heating. Seal the pressure tank.
2. Heat the water for injection to 121°C and maintain for 20 min while gradually releasing tank pressure. Then cool to 60°C.
3. Remove and place in a separate vented stainless steel or glass container of suitable capacity a quantity of water for injection equal to about 30% of the final formula volume. Seal the vessel and save for final volume adjustment.
4. To the remaining water for injection (at 60°C), from step 2, add and dissolve with stirring sodium phosphate monobasic (monohydrate) and sodium phosphate dibasic (anhydrous).
5. Allow the solution from step 4 to cool to room temperature (25 to 30°C) and then add and dissolve with stirring the soluble drug and a preservative. Check the pH of the solution. Adjust the pH to 6.8 to 7.0 if required with approximately 1 N NaOH solution.
6. Bring the bulk to final volume of the concentrate with water for injection and mix well.

Note: The water for injection for volume adjustment is obtained from a portion of the material saved from step 3.

Figure 10: Operations II, III, and IV—Sterilization, Subdivision, and Shipment of 5X Concentrate

1. Sterilize the bulk solution from operation 1, step 6, by filtration through a sterile sterilizing membrane, with an appropriate nonshedding, preclarification filter pad.
2. Collect the sterile filtrate in a clean, sterile, tared, tightly sealable stainless steel vessel for shipping; and also collect samples for assay and sterility testing.
3. Record the empty tare weight and the gross weight of the filled shipping vessels, on the vessel, prior to shipping.
4. Ship the concentrate.

Figure 10: Operation V—Dilution of 5X Concentrate to Provide a Bulk Solution

1. Place water for injection into a clean, vented, glass-lined or stainless steel pressure tank. A starting volume in excess of 10% of the final volume, less the

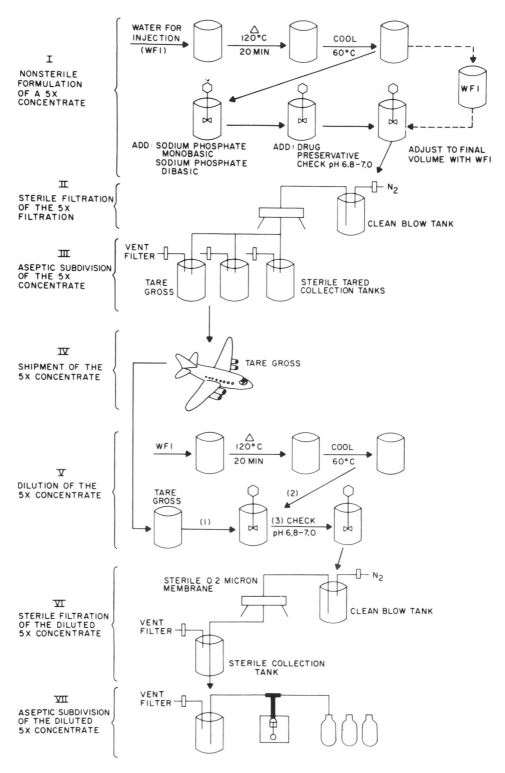

Figure 10   Production of a sterile solution via a 5X concentrate.

concentrate volume, is recommended to cover losses due to evaporation during heating. Seal the pressure tank.

2. Heat the water for injection to 121°C and maintain for 20 min while gradually releasing tank pressure. Then cool to 60°C.

3. Remove and place in a separate vented stainless steel or glass container of suitable capacity about 15% of the water for injection. Seal the vessel and save for final volume adjustment.

4. Cool the remaining 85% of Water for Injection from step 2 to room temperature (25 to 30°C); add and dilute 5X concentrate with stirring.

5. Check the pH of the solution. Adjust the pH to 6.8 to 7.0 if required with approximately 1 N NaOH solution.

6. Bring the bulk to final volume with water for injection and mix well.

Note: The water for injection for volume adjustment is obtained from a portion of the material saved from step 3.

Figure 10: Operation VI—Sterile Filtration of the Diluted 5X Concentrate

1. Sterilize the bulk solution from operation III, step 6, by filtration through a sterile sterilizing membrane, with an appropriate nonshedding preclarification filter pad.

2. Collect the sterile filtrate directly from the sterilizing membrane via sterile tubing and siphon into a clean, sterile, vented stainless steel tank or glass vessel.

Figure 10: Operation VII—Aseptic Subdivision of the Diluted 5X Concentrate

1. Aseptically subdivide the sterile bulk solution into an appropriate sterile container.

2. Aseptically apply sterilized closure systems and seal.

3. Sample across the filling operation at intervals determined by the local quality control director for sterility tests and volume fill checks.

4. Visually inspect all units for defects and particulates against a well-lighted black-and-white background.

5. Submit samples to the quality control laboratory for release assays.

Typical small volume parenteral sterile solution formulations which may be processed in the manner described above are presented in Table 12 for comparative purposes.

B. Preparation of a Typical Suspension Formula

Table 13 shows a typical suspension formula. It is for either a sterile ophthalmic dosage form or it can be used as an injectable product. The primary difference is related to the preservation system. Benzyl alcohol is commonly used in injectable products, while benzalkonium chloride is not normally injected by the intravenous route and therefore is restricted to ophthalmic use.

Sterile suspensions for injection or for ophthalmic administration are more complicated in composition than are sterile solutions. Consequently, they are more difficult to process and sterilize than solutions. Usually, portions of the suspension composition are prepared and sterilized separately. Later, these portions are combined aseptically to yield a final sterile bulk product for aseptic subdivision.

Table 12 Typical Small Volume Parenteral Solutions

R_X	Dosage	Ingredient category
Hydrocortisone sodium phosphate	50 mg	Active drug
Benzyl alcohol	9 mg	Preservative
Sodium citrate	10 mg	Buffering agent
Sodium bisulfite	3 mg	Antioxidant
Sodium hydroxide	1 mg	pH adjustment
Water for Injection qs. ad	1.0 ml	Solvent
Cyanocobalamin	100 μg	Active drug
Sodium chloride	8.3 mg	Tonicity additive
Methylparaben	1.5 mg	Preservative
Propylparaben	0.2 mg	Preservative
Water for Injection qs. ad	1.0 ml	Solvent
Thiamine hydrochloride	20 mg	Active drug
Riboflavin	2 mg	Active drug
Pyridoxine hydrochloride	1.9 mg	Active drug
Nicotinamide	100 mg	Active drug
D-Panthenol	10 mg	Active drug
Ascorbic acid	100 mg	Active drug
Cyanocobalamin	50 mg	Active drug
Mannitol	50 mg	Tonicity additive
Phenol	5 mg	Preservative
Water for Injection qs. ad	1.0 ml	Solvent
Phenytoin sodium	50 mg	Active drug
Propylene glycol	0.4 ml	Cosolvent
Alcohol	0.1 ml	Cosolvent
Sodium hydroxide qs.	pH 12	pH adjustment
Water for Injection qs. ad	1.0 ml	Solvent
Prochlorperazine (as edisylate)	5 mg	Active drug
Sodium biphosphate	5 mg	Buffering agent
Sodium tartrate	12 mg	Buffering agent
Sodium saccharin	0.9 mg	Antioxidant
Benzyl alcohol	7.5 mg	Preservative
Water for Injection qs. ad	1.0 ml	Solvent

The very nature of the particulate solid in suspension precludes the use of a filtration step to sterilize the total composition. Obviously, the suspended product, which has an average particle size of 5 to 10 μm and which may even have larger aggregates, will be filtered out by a 0.2 or 0.45 μm filter. The solid active ingredient may be sterilized prior to compounding into a suspension in a number of ways, such as dry heat, autoclaving, ethylene oxide, radiation, sterile precipitation, and/or crystallization.

Organic chemicals, because of their relatively low melting points and heat sensitivity, are not usually stable to dry heat sterilizing temperatures in the range 250°C and up. Sterilizing a suspension product using autoclaving with steam under pressure is not a very common practice since aqueous solubility is increased with temperature and there is the chance that the solid will dissolve and subsequently

Table 13 Formulation for a Sterile Ophthalmic or Injectable Suspension[a]

Dosage	Ingredient	Ingredient category
800 mg	Insoluble drug	Active drug
0.20 mg	Polysorbate 80, USP	Surface-active agent
6.67 mg	Sodium chloride, USP	Tonicity additive
5.00 mg	Sodium carboxymethyl-cellulose	Viscosity building agent
9.00 mg	Benzyl alcohol	Parenteral preservative
	or	
0.12 mg	Benzalkonium chloride	Ophthalmic preservative
qs. ad 1.0 ml	Water for Injection	Solvent

[a]Product: insoluble drug suspension (8 mg ml^{-1}).

decompose or recrystallize in an uncontrolled fashion when the material is cooled. Saturated solutions of a solid which crystallize on cooling can result in different crystal forms, habits (shapes), or sizes. The physical form of the recrystallized solid may not be suitable in the final formulation. It has been shown, however, that some compounds can be prepared as a concentrated slurry in saturated sodium chloride and autoclaved without untoward effects [13].

Ethylene oxide treatment is another way to sterilize a powder for incorporation into a sterile suspension system. However, residuals of this toxic gas and/or its by-products may remain on the powder. Additionally, the very reactive ethylene oxide moiety can chemically interact with the active solid to form a new chemical entity or can decompose the product. Radiation is being investigated as a means of sterilizing powders. However, since radiation energy can break chemical bonds and/or form new ones [14], a large number of organic molecules cannot withstand the rigor of exposure to sterilizing doses of radiation.

Because of the limitations of other methods for sterilizing chemical compounds, sterile crystallization or precipitation is the most practical method of preparing a sterile solid for suspension. This key step is not usually a part of the pharmaceutical processing. It is more likely to be a step handled during or after synthesis of the compound by a chemical engineering group. Even though it is beyond the scope of this chapter to discuss this methodology in detail, a brief description of how sterile crystallization can be accomplished is in order. The active ingredient is dissolved in a solvent, usually an organic solvent or cosolvent. These solutions are sterilized by filtration through a sterilizing membrane disk or cartridge of suitable porosity (0.2 μm or less) and collected in a sterile vessel containing a sterile liquid in which the drug is insoluble. As the nonaqueous drug solution mixes with the nonsolvent, the drug precipitates as a crystalline solid or as an amorphous mass. The final precipitate is then aseptically collected using suitable filtration equipment and is washed with a sterile nonsolvent. The washed precipitate is then either maintained as a wet cake for incorporation into a suspension, or dried either by air in a laminar flow enclosure or in a conventional sterile hot air or vacuum oven. By controlling the rate of precipitation and by choosing the proper conditions, including the choice of cosolvent system, a uniform controlled particle size can be produced. Some sterile solids may have to be aseptically milled to reduce particle size and/or break up hard aggregates of solid if the crystallizing or precipitation procedure does not produce a uniform particle size.

Ball milling or glass bead milling of solids has been used quite extensively. A sterile slurry of the powder, either by itself or in a portion of the vehicle, is rolled on a roller mill with ceramic or glass beads contained in a sealed sterile bottle. The ball milling is continued until proper particle size is obtained. With the modern concern for particulate contamination and its sources, this technique has largely been discontinued. Conventional powder handling mills such as the Fitzpatrick mill are commonly used under stringent clean, sterile conditions, to reduce the particle size of a sterile solid. Air attrition mills such as the Jetomizer, Micronizer, and Jet Pulverizer are being employed more commonly. Since air force is the principle of these milling devices, the air must be sterile (by filtering) and the equipment must be sterilized. It is advisable to conduct all milling in a laminar flow area or clean room. Once the sterile solid of proper particle size is available, the manufacture of a sterile suspension can commence. The milled solid is collected in clean, sterile containers, and cleanly sampled for particle size determination, crystal form, cleanliness, and assay.

A method of manufacture of a suspension described by O'Neill [13] for the in-process sterilization of the active drugs is depicted in the process flow chart (Fig. 11) and is discussed below.

Figure 11: Operation I—Preparation of Saturated Sodium Chloride and Drug Paste

1. Place into a tared, clean, Pyrex glass wide-mouth bottle, which has been calibrated to a desired volume, all of the sodium chloride required for adjustment of the toxicity of the formula and water in a quantity that is insufficient to dissolve all the sodium chloride.
2. Mix well, either by magnetic bar or standard electrical mixer.
3. Slowly sift in the required amount of insoluble drug.
4. Wet the solid, by mixing, as well as possible. Note: All the solid may not be completely wetted.
5. Seal the bottle by wiring a stopper containing a stainless steel (type 316) tube sealed on the end; the sealed portion of the tube should extend into the center of the paste. The stopper should also contain a suitable nonshedding air vent.
6. For safety purposes place the bottle in a metal can and hold the sealed container for autoclaving.

Figure 11: Operation II—Sodium Carboxymethylcellulose (Sodium CMC) Solution

1. Place into a suitable vessel a predetermined quantity of water for injection suitable to dissolve the sodium CMC (180°F).
2. Start agitation with a mixer such as Lightnin' mixer to create a vortex.
3. Slowly, sift into the vortex the desired quantity of sodium CMC.
4. Mix vigorously until no visible powder or gelatinous lumps are visible and, while still hot, clarify through a coarse clarification filter.
5. Bring the sodium CMC solution to the desired volume by rinsing the clarification filter using water for injection (180°F).
6. Collect the clarified sodium CMC solution in a suitable clean, Pyrex bottle. Place in a metal can for safety purposes in the event the bottle ruptures during transport or autoclaving. Partially insert a stopper, cover the bottle neck, and stopper with parchment or kraft paper. Tie securely to the neck of the bottle.
7. Place the bottle in a metal can for safety purposes in the event the bottle ruptures during transport or autoclaving. Hold the wrapped container for autoclaving.

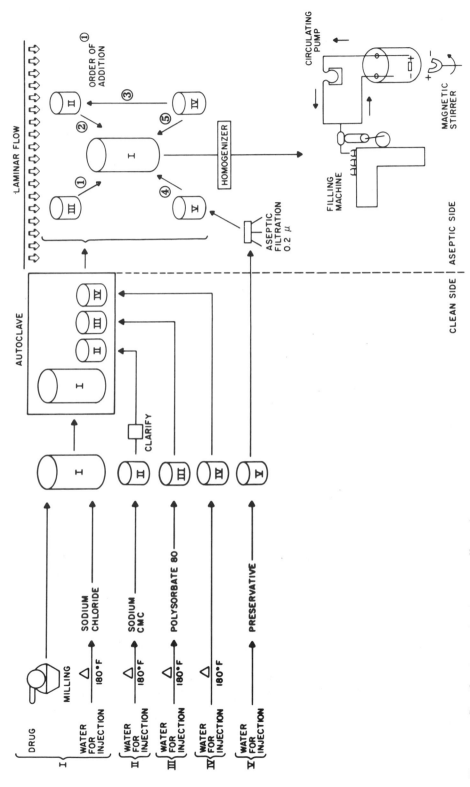

Figure 11 Sterile suspension process flow chart.

Figure 11: Operation III—Polysorbate 80 Solution

1. Place into a suitable container the desired amount of polysorbate 80.
2. Add sufficient water for injection (180° F) to make the solution up to the desired volume.
3. Place the polysorbate 80 solution into a suitable clean, Pyrex glass bottle and partially insert a stopper covered with parchment or kraft paper. Tie securely to the neck of the bottle.
4. Place the bottle in a metal can for safety purposes in the event the bottle ruptures during transport or autoclaving. Hold the wrapped container for autoclaving.

Figure 11: Operation IV—Sterile Water for Injection

1. Place into a suitable Pyrex glass bottle an excess of water for injection (180°F) for final volume adjustment of the bulk suspension.
2. Partially insert a stopper covered with parchment or kraft paper. Tie securely to the neck of the bottle.
3. Place the bottle in a metal can for safety purposes in the event the bottle ruptures during transport or autoclaving. Hold the wrapped container for autoclaving.

Figure 11: Operation V—Preservative Solution

1. Dissolve the preservative in a sufficient quantity of water for injection in a suitable container.
2. Mix well and transfer to a stainless steel pressure vessel.

Figure 11: Autoclave Step

1. Containers of the following components are placed in a steam autoclave.
   I. Insoluble drug slurry in saturated sodium chloride
   II. Sodium carboxymethylcellulose solution (sodium CMC solution)
   III. Polysorbate 80 solution
   IV. Water for injection
2. Approximately 3 ml of a medical-grade silicone oil are placed into the stainless tube in the stopper on the drug paste container. A thermocouple that has been precalibrated at 0°C and 121°C is placed into the tube. The tip of the thermocouple and several inches of wire should be covered with silicone oil to facilitate uniform heat distribution around the thermocouple. Placement of the stainless tube is inspected to ensure that the thermocouple in the stainless tube is located in the middle of the drug paste. Refer to Figure 12 for a diagram of the apparatus.
3. The autoclave is closed. The autoclave is then charged with steam at a sufficient pressure to yield 121°C.
4. The sterilization cycle is complete when the temperature recorded by the thermocouple in the drug paste reaches 121°C for a sufficient time period to produce an F_0 of 22 with F_0 calculations beginning at 100°C or maintaining the temperature at 121°C for a specific time period consistent with previously determined D values necessary to destroy inoculum in the product.
   F values define the time at temperature required to kill a microorganism. D values are the rate at which death of a microorganism occurs with respect to

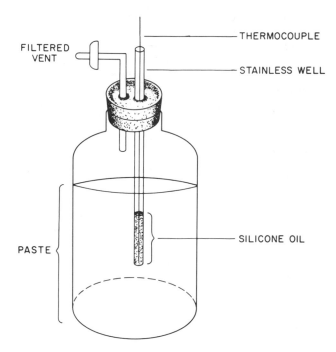

Figure 12 Apparatus for controlling the sterilization of a suspension paste. The sterilization cycle is controlled by the temperature measured at the thermocouple in the center of the paste.

time. D values are expressed as the time required to reduce a microbial population by one decimal or by one $\log_{10}$ unit. F_0 is related to both F and D values and is more fully discussed in the chapter on Industrial Sterilization in Volume 2.

5. The steam in the autoclave is exhausted on the slow cycle used for liquids. The containers are removed from the autoclave when sufficiently cool to handle after the completion of the cycle.
6. The following preparations are placed in a sterile room and allowed to cool to room temperature.
    I. Sterile drug/saline paste.
    II. Sterile sodium CMC solution.
    III. It should be noted that the sterile polysorbate 80 solution is gently agitated before cooling to room temperature in order to prevent solidification.
    IV. Sterile water for injection.
7. When the four solutions have cooled to room temperature, the stoppers are aseptically inserted into the neck of each bottle.

Figure 11: Aseptic Formulation in the Laminar Flow Area

1. Aseptically, under laminar flow, transfer with mixing (sterile magnetic bar or sterile mixer) part III (sterile polysorbate 80 solution) to part I (sterile insoluble drug/saline paste). Mix until a smooth paste is obtained.
2. Aseptically under laminar flow, transfer with mixing part II (sterile sodium CMC) to part I/III (sterile polysorbate 80/insoluble drug/saline paste) above.

3. The vessel from part II may be rinsed with sterile water for injection to effect complete transfer. Mix well until uniform.
4. Aseptically filter through a 0.22 μm sterilizing membrane with a suitable non-shedding prefilter, part V (preservative solution) into the mixture of part I, II, and III (insoluble drug/saline paste, polysorbate 80, sodium CMC).
5. Aseptically bring the volume of the suspension to final volume by rinsing the pressure tank previously containing preservative solution with water for injection (part IV) through the sterilizing membrane. Mix well until uniform.

Figure 11: Aseptic Homogenization

1. Aseptically homogenize the sterile suspension using a suitable sterilized homogenizer such as a Manton Gaulin.
2. Recirculate the suspension through the homogenizer for 5 to 10 min with no pressure.
3. Apply pressure to 1500 to 2000 psig and continue to recirculate the suspension for 10 to 15 min (depending on batch size).
4. While the suspension is still being pumped through the homogenizer under 1500 to 2000 psig, aseptically divert the flow of suspension from the homogenizer to a clean, sterile Pyrex glass bottle equipped with a sterile Teflon stirring bar or sealable mixer. This may be performed by transferring the outlet portion of the homogenizer or by using the closed transfer system depicted in Figure 13.
5. Agitate the suspension continuously until subdivision or intermittently for 3 to 4 hr periods daily if there is a delay in filling.

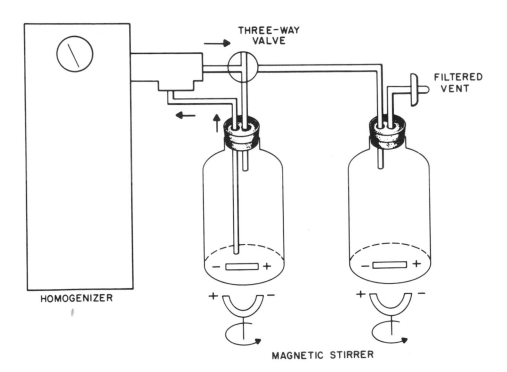

Figure 13 Homogenization apparatus: aseptic setup.

Figure 11: Aseptic Subdivision

1. Aseptically transfer the sterile bulk suspension to a suitable filling apparatus as discussed in Section III.B.
2. With constant stirring, aseptically subdivide the suspension into suitable packages.
3. Aseptically insert a stopper with an appropriate apparatus.
4. Sample periodically for sterility testing, fill volume, and uniformity of suspension.
5. Segregate the suspensions by number or time until uniformity has been established.
6. Inspect each package visually for defects, obvious fill variation or obvious extraneous particulate matter.

Typical small volume parenteral suspension formulations that may be processed in the manner described above or via analogous processes are presented in Table 14 for comparative purposes.

C. Preparation of a Typical Freeze-Dried Powder Formula

Freeze-drying (lyophilization) is a drying process applicable to the manufacture of pharmaceuticals, biologicals, serums, and hormones which are thermolabile or otherwise unstable in aqueous solution for prolonged storage periods, but which are stable in the dry state [15]. By removing the solvent by the physical process of sublimation, heat-sensitive drugs or biologicals can be dried with a minimum of degradation of the product. Degradation is minimized by (1) reduction of heat input during drying, and (2) avoidance of prolonged solution of the drug in liquid solvent during the solvent removal phase. By comparison, an evaporative process requires heat to remove the solvent. The evaporative process continuously makes a more concentrated solution. These two factors can accelerate the degradation kinetics.

A product to be freeze-dried is prepared, sterilized, and subdivided as a sterile solution or sterile suspension. After the desired amount of material is filled into a container, the container is subjected to freezing by any one of the following processes.

1. Freezing in standard freezer chests at -18 to -50°C for a prolonged period of time
2. Freezing on refrigerated shelves of a lyophilization chamber at -50°C or below
3. Freezing in a liquid nitrogen tunnel at a predetermined rate of movement via a moving belt through the tunnel

The frozen mass, once in the lyophilization chamber, is subjected to vacuum and the freeze-drying cycle is commenced. The product should be cooled to a temperature below its eutectic point [16]. The frozen solvent in the frozen product will pass from the solid to the gaseous state without becoming liquid (sublimation) after the frozen product is subjected to extremely low pressures. The freeze-drying process consists of two distinct cycles: (1) primary drying, which constitutes the bulk of the sublimation process, and removes most of the solvent and forms a "cake"; (2) secondary drying which removes vestigial solvent. The latter part of the cycle usually requires a small amount of external heat energy input and results in drying the "cake" thoroughly.

Table 14 Typical Small Volume Parenteral Suspensions

R_x	Dosage	Ingredient category
Betamethasone (as sodium phosphate)	3.0 mg	Active drug
Betamethasone acetate	3.0 mg	Active drug
Dibasic Sodium phosphate	7.1 mg	Buffering agent
Monobasic Sodium phosphate	3.4 mg	Buffering agent
Disodium edetate	0.1 mg	Stabilizer
Benzalkonium chloride	0.2 mg	Preservative
Sodium hydroxide or		
hydrochloric acid qs.	pH 6.8 to 7.2	pH adjustment
Water for Injection qs. ad	1.0 ml	Solvent
Penicillin	1.2 million units	Active drug
Penicillin G benzathine	0.9 million units	Active drug
Penicillin G procaine	0.3 million units	Active drug
Sodium citrate qs.	to pH	Buffering agent
Lecithin	0.5%	Suspending agent
Carboxymethylcellulose	0.55%	Suspending agent
Providone	0.55%	Suspending agent
Methylparaben	0.1%	Preservative
Propylparaben	0.01%	Preservative
Water for Injection qs. ad	1.0 ml	Solvent
Triamcinolone diacetate micronized	40 mg	Active
Polysorbate 80	2.0 mg	Dispersant
Polyethylene glycol 4000	3.0 mg	Cosolvent
Sodium chloride	8.5 mg	Tonicity agent
Benzyl alcohol	9.0 mg	Preservative
Sodium hydroxide or		
hydrochloric acid qs.	pH 6.0	Buffering agent
Water for Injection qs. ad	1.0 ml	Solvent

     Production-sized freeze driers are usually operated by an automatic control system. The temperature of a sample of the product is continuously monitored throughout the process. The temperature of the sample will steadily drop if no heat is introduced into the system because the vaporization of the solvent results in a removal of heat from the product. Therefore, after equilibrium has been reached, it becomes necessary to introduce heat into the system at a controlled rate. By monitoring the temperature of the sample, the rate of introduction of heat into the system is controlled in comparison with the rate experimentally found to produce a satisfactory product.

     After the drying process is completed, the vial containing the product is sealed as rapidly as possible to prevent any sorption of moisture. Some freeze driers are equipped with a mechanism to press specially slotted rubber closures firmly into the neck of the vials prior to removal from the chamber. Prior to placing the vials into the chamber, the special closures (Fig. 14) are loosely put into the neck of the vials. The slots in the closures allow solvent vapor to escape from the vials during the drying cycle.

     Table 15 gives a formula for a sterile lyophilized injectable product. The method of manufacture is discussed in detail below and is shown diagrammatically in Figure 15.

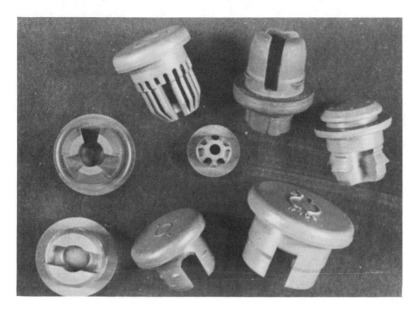

Figure 14 Slotted rubber closures.

Figure 15: Operation I—Lyophilization Chamber Preparation

Lyophilization Chamber Setup and Sterilization

1. Open the lyophilizer door and examine the inside of the chamber for a buildup of residual material. If residual material is present, rinse the chamber with hot distilled water and wipe down with a lint-free cloth.
2. Arrange the precalibrated lyophilizer thermocouples uniformly throughout the chamber and condenser. Special emphasis should be given to locate thermocouples in portions of the chamber known to be heat sinks. These cold spots are to be monitored at temperature control points during the steam sterilization of the chamber.
3. The chamber door is secured and all the external vent valves to the vacuum pumps and vacuum release lines are closed.
4. The thermocouple temperatures and chamber pressure-monitoring devices on the chamber are turned on.

Table 15 Typical Formulation for a Lyophilized Sterile Injectable Product[a]

R_x	Dosage	Ingredient category
Soluble drug	10 mg	Active drug
Mannitol qs.	qs.	Bulking agent/tonicity agent
Sodium hydroxide/ qs. hydrochloric acid	qs. pH 6.8 to 7.0	pH adjustment
Water for Injection, USP qs. ad	1.0 ml	Solvent

[a]Product: soluble drug (10 mg ml^{-1}).

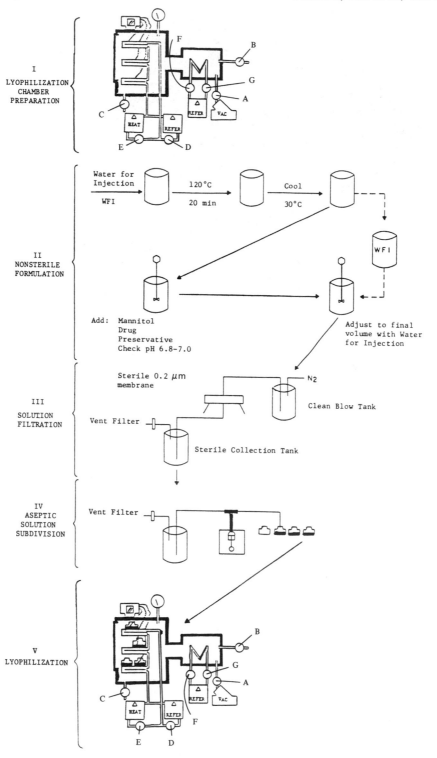

Figure 15 Process flow diagram for the production of a sterile lyophilized product.

5. The chamber vacuum pump(s) are switched on and allowed to run for 2 min. The vacuum pump valve (see A in Fig. 15) to the chamber is opened and the chamber is evacuated to approximately 28 in. of mercury.
6. Close the external vent lines to the vacuum pump(s) valve and then turn off the vacuum pump(s).
7. The clean steam line valve (see B in Fig. 15) and vent valve (see C in Fig. 15) to the lyophilization chamber and condenser is opened. Monitor the chamber and condenser thermocouple temperature and pressure with an appropriate recording device. When all the thermocouples reach 121°C, begin timing the sterilization time for the chamber and condenser. The chamber and condenser are maintained at 121°C for a period of time necessary to reach an F_0 value adequate to assure sterility of the chamber and condenser. Actual steaming times are based on validation of time at temperatures based on heat penetration and kill rates of microbial spore indicators.
8. The clean steam line valve to the lyophilization chamber and condenser and the vent valve are turned off. The temperature recording device is placed on hold. The chamber and condenser are allowed to cool down overnight.

   Chamber chill down.

9. The temperature recording devices on the lyophilization chamber are turned on.
10. The chamber shelves (open valve D in Fig. 15) and condenser plates (open valves F and G in Fig. 15) are chilled to below the freezing point of the eutectic of the product to be lyophilized.

Figure 15: Operation II—Nonsterile Solution Formulation

1. Place water for injection into a clean, vented, glass-lined or stainless steel pressure tank. A starting volume in excess of 10% of the final volume is recommended to cover losses due to evaporation during heating. Seal the pressure tank.
2. Heat the water of injection to 121°C and maintain for 20 min while gradually releasing tank pressure. Then cool to 30°C.
3. Remove and place in a separate vented stainless steel or glass container of suitable capacity, about 30% water for injection. Seal the vessel and save for final volume adjustment.
4. To the remaining 70% of the water for injection (at 30°C), from step 2, add mannitol and dissolve with stirring.
5. Add and dissolve with stirring the water soluble drug and the preservative. Check the pH of the solution. Adjust the pH to 6.8 to 7.0 if required, with approximately 1 N sodium hydroxide solution or 1 N hydrochloric acid.
6. Bring the bulk to final volume with water for injection and mix well.

Note: The water for injection for volume adjustment is obtained from a portion of the material saved from step 3.

Figure 15: Operation III—Solution Filtration

1. Sterilize the bulk solution from operation II, step 6, by filtration through a sterile sterilizing membrane, with an appropriate nonshedding preclarification filter.

2. Collect the sterile filtrate directly from the sterilizing membrane via sterile tubing and siphon into a sterile, clean, closed, vented stainless steel tank or glass vessel.

Figure 15: Operation IV—Aseptic Solution Subdivision

1. Aseptically subdivide the sterile bulk solution into an appropriate sterile container.

Figure 15: Operation V—Lyophilization

Product freezing (via the refrigerated shelf of the lyophilization chamber).

1. Open the chamber door and load the product to be lyophilized into the chamber shelves. Stoppers on vials must be only partially inserted to permit evacuation of the vial. Do not mix vial sizes on any one shelf. Any vial size may be used, provided that they are the same height on each shelf.
2. Place a thermocouple into at least one vial on each shelf. The thermocouple must be in the center of the solution to assure representative product temperature reading.
3. Close the chamber door.
4. Monitor the product temperature. When all product thermocouples reach the desired temperature to ensure crystallization, the condenser plate temperature controller is set at -60°C.

   Primary drying.

5. Monitor the condensing plate temperature on the temperature recorder. When all the condenser plate thermocouples reach approximately -50°C, the vacuum pumps are turned on and the vacuum pump valve A (see Fig. 15) to the chamber is opened.
6. Monitor the vacuum in the chamber. When a pressure of approximately 100 μm is reached, allow the product to equilibrate for at least 1 hr.
7. Heat is slowly added to the shelves by opening valve E (see Fig. 15) and closing valve D (see Fig. 15) as determined by sample temperature and a preprogrammed cycle until the product temperature reaches the shelf temperature (approximately room temperature). Maintain the product at the shelf temperature set point for the duration of the predetermined cycle.

   Secondary drying.

8. Increase the shelf temperature to 30°C or a temperature that will not degrade the product being lyophilized. Monitor the product thermocouples until the chamber shelf temperature and product temperature are the same. Maintain the chamber in this mode for a predetermined period of time that guarantees that a minimum level of solvent remains. The lyophilization cycle is complete at this point except for stoppering.

   Product stoppering.

9. The product may be stoppered within the chamber or outside the chamber. Stoppering outside the chamber is rarely done because of the risk of bacterial or particulate contamination. Internal stoppering is the most pharmaceutically

acceptable method. Within the chamber, the vials can be stoppered under vacuum, or under the pressure of an inert gas such as nitrogen or argon.

   The most common commercial method of internal stoppering entails the
hydraulic movement of the lower shelves upward. When the stoppers come in
contact with the bottom of the shelf immediately above it, the stoppers are
forced all the way into the neck of the vials. When the top shelf of vials are
fully stoppered, the operator shuts off the hydraulic cylinder and reverses the
movement of the shelves. This allows the stoppered vials to drop down on the
shelf for removal and capping.

   Typical small volume parenteral freeze-dried powders for reconstitution
formulations are presented in Table 16.

D. Preparation of a Typical Sterile Dry Fill Powder for Constitution

Freeze-drying of solutions of drugs is one way to formulate drugs which are either
thermolabile or unstable when in aqueous solution. However, freeze-drying does
not always solve formulation problems. Sometimes, freeze-dried products are not
sufficiently stable to give the desired shelf life.

   In many cases, solid-state stability over the desired shelf-life period can be
related to the extent of crystallinity. The lyophilization process does not always
produce a crystalline drug product. It has been observed that solid-state stability
is greatly affected when the lyophilization process results in either an amorphous
product or a mixture of amorphous and crystalline material [17]. When a lyophilization process is unacceptable, the alternative process consists of aseptically
placing a sterile powder into a sterile vial. This process is known as sterile dry
powder filling.

   The dry filling process is also sometimes utilized when product sales are
high. The large number of lyophilization chambers required to provide the desired
number of product units can become prohibitively expensive in space and capital
expenditure. Powder filling, on the other hand, is much more economical, particularly as the number of units produced increases. In addition, the time and energy

Table 16 Typical Small Volume Parenteral Freeze-Dried
Powders for Reconstitution

R_X	Dosage	Ingredient category
Dactinomycin	0.5 mg	Active drug
Mannitol	20.0 mg	Bulking agent
Asparaginase	10,000 IU	Active drug
Mannitol	80 mg	Bulking agent
Ethacrynate sodium equivalent to ethacrynic acid	50 mg	Active drug
Mannitol	62.5 mg	Bulking agent
Thimerosal	0.1 mg	Preservative
Doxorobicin HCl	10 mg	Active drug
Lactose	50 mg	Bulking agent

necessary to produce a freeze-dried product adds considerably to the cost and time of pharmaceutical processing.

For these reasons, the sterile dry filled powder has become a very popular sterile dosage form. Many antibiotic products are marketed as sterile dry filled powders and are prime examples of this type of product. The powders intended for formulation are sterilized and milled, if necessary, exactly as described in Section II.D.

The pharmaceutical manufacturing process is essentially a filling operation. The process is difficult because it must be able to convert a bulk material, which is clean, sterile, and pyrogen-free, into "unit doses" which are also clean, sterile, and pyrogen-free. The operation must be able to guarantee an accurate product fill which is clean, fast dissolving, and elegant in appearance. The dosage form must be clear and particulate-free upon constitution.

There are several ways to subdivide sterile powders aseptically. One such method is described below. Usually, the formula of a sterile dry filled powder consists of one active ingredient and is similar to that shown in Table 17. Sometimes excipients or additives are preblended with the active ingredient prior to subdivision.

Operation I—Subdivision

1. The sterile drug powder is aseptically transferred to the clean presterilized powder filling machine hopper. The powder is agitated in the hopper via mixer blades to insure a uniform smooth blend (see Fig. 16).
2. The powder is aseptically filled into the sterile vial using powder filling equipment such as positive piston displacement fillers or auger-type fillers (see page 254). The vials are sealed with presterilized closures and aluminum crimp seals.
3. The fill weight controller is adjusted to the proper fill. The fill weight is check-weighed. Filled vials from across the filling operation are constituted and examined for particulate matter. The closure and seal are also examined. If the fill, particulate levels, and closure seals are within specification, the filling operation may begin.
4. Containers are filled, stoppered, and sealed within a sterile area and passed through into a clean, nonsterile inspection area. Each container is wiped, washed, dried, and visually inspected to make sure that each vial has a closure and a seal.

Operation II—Subdivision Sampling

1. Filled containers are sampled at set intervals during the filling operation for checking fill, sterility, pyrogens, clarity of restored solutions, and any

Table 17 Formulation for a Small Volume Parenteral Powder for Constitution[a]

R_x	Dosage	Ingredient category
Soluble sterile drug powder	1 g	Active drug

[a]Product: soluble sterile drug powder (1 g per container).

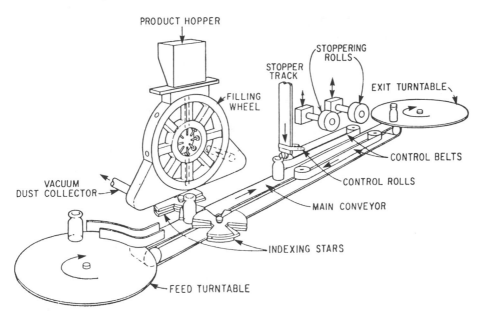

Figure 16 Schematic diagram of the Perry powder filling machine. (Courtesy of Perry Industries, Inc., Hicksville, New York.)

additional release tests (pH, color, etc.) which are required for the drug. The time to conduct these tests is slower than the filling operation. Therefore, filled containers are segregated by filling time and stored in numbered totes or boxes so that test samples can be identified. Additional quality control testing can be done at a later date by resampling the appropriately numbered isolated trays.

Typical formulations for small volume sterile powders for constitution are given in Table 18.

Table 18 Typical Small Volume Parenteral Powders for Constitution

R_x	Dosage	Ingredient category
N, N', N''-Triethylenethiophosphoramide	15.0 mg	Active drug
Sodium chloride	80.0 mg	Tonicity agent
Sodium bicarbonate	50.0 mg	Buffering agent
Cephalothin sodium	1 g	Active drug
Sodium bicarbonate	qs. pH 6–8.5 on constitution	Buffering agent
Mechlorethamine HCl	10.0 mg	Active drug
Sodium chloride	qs.	Tonicity agent
Methylprednisolone sodium succinate (equivalent to methylprednisolone)	40 mg	Active drug
Sodium biphosphate anhydrous	1.6 mg	Buffering agent
Sodium phosphate dried	17.4 mg	Buffering agent
Lactose (hydrous)	25 mg	Bulking agent

III. PACKAGING AND SEALING

A. Inert Gas Treatment

Very often, oxygen-sensitive parenterals require that they be packaged in inert atmospheric conditions. This condition can be achieved in a number of ways. The easiest product to package under inert atmosphere is one prepared by lyophilization. One can aseptically seal the product under vacuum as one way of removing oxygen or one can proceed to purge the chamber with a filtered-sterilized inert gas at a pressure of 2 to 3 psig just before stopper insertion. Nitrogen is commonly used, but many manufacturers have found that argon, although more expensive than nitrogen, is more efficient. This efficiency is due to the fact that argon is heavier than air and will enter the vial, as compared to nitrogen, which will tend to rise out of the vial because it is lighter than air.

Dry filled powders are more difficult to purge. However, by proper design of purge needles, careful control of gas flow, gas pressures, purge needle size, and proximity and positioning of the purge needle with respect to the vial opening, as well as how close the last purge station is to the stoppering step, efficient gas purging can be achieved. The speed of the vials going down the line is also an important factor. The pressure of gas must be kept constant. This can be accomplished by a dual pressure regulator system (one at the source of gas and another as close to the final purge stations as possible, with constant differential pressure). Also, the gas flow entering the container, just before stoppering, must be aerodynamically positioned and must be set to minimize turbulence and "blow out" of the purge gas and replacement by room air. It is often better to try to "layer" the gas into the vial rather than "blow" it in. Some companies actually set up an enclosed gas purged tunnel along the entire filling line, which encases the vials from time of filling to time of stoppering in order to guarantee efficient purging.

Liquids require a slightly different approach. With liquids, one is able to bubble (or sparge) the gas directly into the liquid, in the bulk state (particularly while cooling a liquid) and during the filling operation. Many manufacturers use a dual needle of concentric design which permits simultaneous filling of liquid and purge gas at the same time. In addition, purge needles can be positioned along the filling line, just as with powders, for final purging before the stoppering step.

In all cases involving sterile products, the inert gas must be sterilized. A convenient method is to pass all gases through a sterilized 0.45 μm filter which is placed in line. Shed-free hydrophobic Teflon-type filters are recommended for these operations as well as for venting operations during autoclaving of liquids.

B. Filling Equipment

There is a wide variety of equipment available that can be used to dispense small volume parenterals into the market container. The equipment, if properly designed, will maintain sterility, cleanness, and accuracy at delivery. As discussed in previous sections, there are several types of sterile SVP dosage formulations (e.g., solutions, suspensions, and powders). As shown in Table 19, most liquids and suspensions can be dispensed using equipment that is designed to employ the following basic mechanisms: piston, rotary chemical pump, and time/pressure. Figure 17 depicts a typical piston-type liquid filling machine. In its most simple form, the piston filler consists of a syringe or piston (A), a three-way valve (B), a cam (C), and a vernier volume adjustment (D) which allows the user to adjust the stroke travel length of the piston, thus controlling the volume delivered. The three-way valve

Table 19 Types of Filling Equipment

Mechanism of filling	Types of product filled	Types of package
Piston type (Cozzoli)	Liquid products such as solutions, suspensions, emulsions, and solutions for freeze-drying	Vials, ampuls, plastic containers, bottles, syringe cartridges, plastic minibags
Rotary chemical pump type (King Technofil)	Same as above	Same as above
Time/pressure type (Aquafil)	Same as above	Same as above
Auger (Hoflinger & Karg)	Powders	Vials, bottles, plastic minibags
Vacuum pressure displacement (Perry, Hoflinger & Karg)	Powders	Vials, bottles, plastic minibags

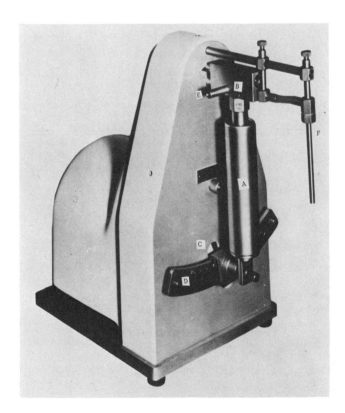

Figure 17 Tabletop piston fillers, Model F400X. (Courtesy of Cozzoli Machine Company, Plainfield, New Jersey.)

(B) is connected to the piston, the bulk product through a connection at (E), and the filling needle (F). Very often, for solutions, an in-line filter of 0.2 to 1.0 μm porosity is employed. The filter can be placed between the bulk solution and the three-way valve, or it can be placed between the three-way valve (B) and the filling needle (F). The movement of the piston (A) riding on the cam (C) at a predetermined distance governed by the setting of the lower piston on the vernier (D) actuates the three-way valve (B) so as to move a volume of liquid product from the bulk, through the valve, into the syringe barrel, and then back through the valve into the market package through the filling needle. Depending on the batch size, the equipment will vary in size and complexity. However, the principle of operation is common to the basic mechanism.

A rotary chemical pump (Fig. 18) works on the principle that a positive displacement pump is driven by a DC motor. As the gears in the housing (A) turn, the liquid is drawn into the void spaces from the bulk solution through hose B. The fluid is driven forward by the motion of the gears. The revolutions are counted and at the end of the count the motor stops. A timer circuit (C) operates and then the motor goes on again for the next filling. The liquid is ejected through hose (D) into the filling needle (E).

The time/pressure filler (fill-time controller) is quite similar in operation to the rotary chemical purge except that once the desired volume is delivered, the delivery tube is pinched shut to cut off fluid flow. The delivery of fluid is measured by the time that the delivery tube is open at a specific pressure. A schematic of one such piece of equipment is shown in Figure 19.

Basically, all liquids are filled in the same manner. Suspensions require additional attention to maintenance of uniformity through adequate mixing and/or

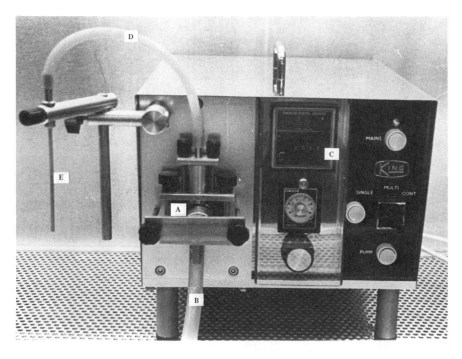

Figure 18 King rotary chemical pump filling machine. (Courtesy of Modular Packaging Systems, East Hanover, New Jersey.)

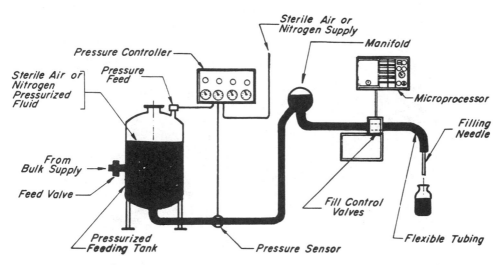

Figure 19 Time/pressure liquid filling machine. (Courtesy of Perry Industries, Inc., Hicksville, New York.)

recirculation during subdivision. Powder fillers are unique systems which work either by vacuum displacement or auger.

For powder filling, Perry Industries makes available a small "gun" piston hand filler which in principle works like a capsule filler. The inside depth of the gun barrel is set to hold a specified volume equivalent to a given weight. The guns are available in several diameters. The characteristics of the powder are important to accurate fills. These characteristics consist of particle size distribution, cohesiveness, flow properties, density, and abrasiveness. Once the powder characteristics have been established for a particular product, the depth of the gun chamber can be set to a specific length (for a specific diameter) by turning the inside piston down or up. The guns are under vacuum and the powder is drawn up and compacted in the gun. A foot pedal switches the vacuum to air pressure (sterilized via in-line filter) and the powder is ejected into the vials. The fills are check-weighed until the correct piston depth has been established.

Figure 20 shows a Perry Model LM14 powder filler which is unique for establishing the fill characteristics of a powder. The combination air pump and vacuum system are housed in casing (A). The filling gun (B) consists of a tube (C) which is the powder chamber. A piston inside the tube (C) is set to the correct depth for the desired fill volume by turning a knurled nut (D). The gun is connected to the pump/vacuum system by means of hose (E). A foot pedal (F) is used to control the cycle.

This basic principle is also employed in more sophisticated and automatic equipment. Powder is fed via a hopper to rotating filling ports which are under vacuum in order to pack the powder into the ports. Figure 21 depicts an automatic powder filler which employs the piston displacement method.

As the filling wheel (A) (Fig. 21) turns, powder from the hopper (B) is drawn through the ports (C) into the piston chambers. Powder is smoothed off of the ports by a blade (D). The cycle goes from vacuum to pressure just under the vials to dislodge the powder from the parts. The depth of the pistons can be set much like the

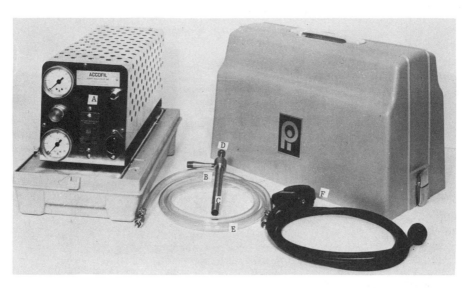

Figure 20 Powder filling machine. (Courtesy of Perry Industries, Inc., Hicksville, New York.)

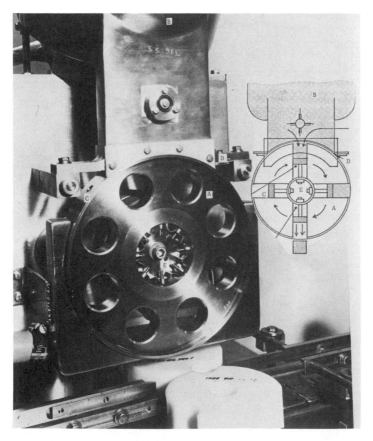

Figure 21 Automatic rotary powder filling wheel. Inset shows schematic operation. (Courtesy of Perry Industries, Inc., Hicksville, New York.)

hand gun by adjusting the threaded nuts in the center of the wheel (E). Weight
checks are made periodically for each port (8 to 12 ports usually) once the dose has
been established

Another method of powder subdivision is by auger feed. This principle is
based on volume displacement by a screw feed. Powder is fed via hopper into a
chamber that contains an auger. The auger turns and carries a fixed amount of powder to the empty vial. Size of delivery, once again, depends on such parameters as
auger size, auger rotation depth, powder density, and other powder characteristics
discussed earlier in this section. A typical auger filler such as the Hofliger and
Karg (H. & K.) is depicted in Figure 22. Note that the auger (A) turns and picks up
the powder. The depth of travel in the turn, which has been predetermined, delivers the accurate dose of powder.

C. Sealing

All containers must receive a primary sterile seal in a sterile area immediately
after filling. In addition, some containers require a secondary seal to assure the
user that the primary seal has not been opened.

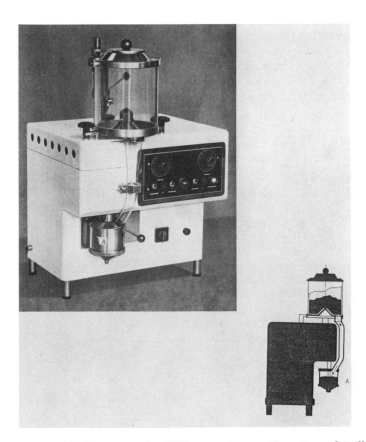

Figure 22 Auger powder filling machine. (Courtesy of Hoflinger & Karg, Robert
Bosch, GM&H, Dusseldorfer Strasse 11, D-7050 Waiblingen.)

1. Sealing Ampuls

Ampuls are unique in that the primary and secondary seal are the same. Ampuls are sealed by melting a portion of the glass in a flame. There are two types of seals:

1. The pull seal is made by heating the neck of an ampul below the tip to the molten state and then pulling the top of the neck away from the ampul body. In theory a small twisted capillary forms which is easily melt-closed by the heat of the flame.
2. The roll or tip seal is made by heating the top of the neck of a rotating ampul to form a molten bead that seals the ampul on cooling.

2. Sealing Bottles, Cartridges, and Vials

These containers have a primary seal consisting of a tight-fitting rubber or plastic closure and a secondary seal that holds the primary seal in place. Secondary seals are usually aluminum caps that are crimped on to a threadless container or aluminum or plastic screw cap which is maintained in place by a semiperforated crimp or a plastic shrink band.

3. Sealing Syringes

Syringes are unique in regard to sealing characteristics due to the need for venting the sterile package when applying a rubber seal. Some type of vacuum or sterile venting procedure is required to insert the plunger/stopper after filling the syringe. One can use the analogy of trying to fit a cork into a very full bottle; the air has to be evacuated or displaced before the cork will remain in the bottle due to the back pressure generated by compressing what little air remains. The most

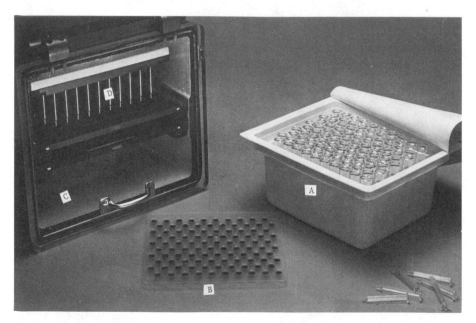

Figure 23 Hypak SCF prefilled syringe system. (Courtesy of Becton-Dickinson Pharmaceutical Systems, Rutherford, New Jersey.)

common high-speed production method involves the insertion of a fine sterile wire between the stopper and the syringe barrel during stoppering to allow air
to escape and the closure to seat properly. However, Medication Delivery Systems
(Fig. 23) has a unique system (HYPAK) which is finding increased acceptance for
pilot-size batches and for full production lots. Trays of sterile, clean syringes
[with rubber-tip cap in place or shielded needle in place (A)] are provided together
with a matching tray of clean sterile stopper/plungers (B). The sterile syringe
barrels are filled by conventional means, such as a piston displacement filler, and
placed into the specially designed pressure/vacuum chamber (C). The stopper/
plungers are placed directly above the filled barrels. When the door of the chamber
is closed, vacuum is increased. At a predetermined reading, a solonoid is tripped,
which activates a series of stainless steel plungers (D) that force the plunger-stop-
pers into the filled barrels. Pressure is then allowed into the chamber to break
the vacuum and allow for removal of the filled, assembled syringes.

IV. INSPECTION OF THE FINAL PRODUCT

One important part of the production scheme is the inspection of the units for a variety of defects, such as cracked glass, deformed glass, no stopper, no cap, poor
seal crimp, or visible particulate matter such as black specks, white specks, fibers,
rubber particles, and lack of clarity.

Most manufacturers 100% inspect all units either on the line or before labeling.
The samples are taken from segregated bulk packages or totes. Other manufacturers
inspect statistical samples of the lot. In the authors' opinion, all parenteral products should be 100% inspected on line and then a statistical sampling examined by a
separate quality assurance group.

The tried-and-true method of on-line inspection involves the use of an inspection lamp with well-lighted background and a black-and-white background to pick up
oppositely colored particles. Some companies use magnification. The accuracy of
this type of inspection is largely dependent on the training and commitment of the
inspector. Another factor affecting accuracy is that of fatigue on the part of the
inspector.

Many manufacturers are beginning to use sophisticated electronic inspection
devices which work either by light scattering, impingement or reflection, or by
video recording imagery. The problem associated with these types of detection
equipment have been many, particularly the separation of air bubbles and imperfections in the glass from real particulates. The biggest problem has been in setting
limits (i.e., "how clean is clean?"). The sensitivity of many of the electronic de-
tectors is so much greater than that of human eyes that limits could be set on the
machine that would make all units fail. The ideal is to set the machine to duplicate
the standard efficiency of the human inspectors.

V. LABELING

This chapter has covered various stages of SVP manufacture: planning, component
and equipment preparation, manufacture, sterilization, subdivision, sealing, inspection, and packaging. There remains just one more thing to be done as part of
the processing of parenterals: labeling of the filled, released units. Labeling of
packages could be the subject of a chapter in itself. Above and beyond the obvious
needs for label correctness and label control which are part of the quality assurance

program, there are problems associated with applying the label under manufacturing conditions. Speed of labeling becomes critical to keep the operation going. Such things as label composition and types of label glue are of extreme importance in proper labeling. The science of labeling involves not only the physical handling of the labels, but also includes the understanding of the physical/chemical factors necessary for bonding the label to the package. For example, siliconized glass is extremely difficult to label.

With plastics, there is sometimes a problem that the glue or printing on the label can interact with the product [18]. The proper choice of label and label glue is of extreme importance in guaranteeing a good product.

Many manufacturers use prelabeled silk screen packages rather than the conventional paper glue type. This presents other problems, such as expense, commitment to a particular batch for quantity of vials or ampuls, difficulty of washing and sterilizing prelabeled units, difficulty in properly inspecting the already labeled units, or possible damage to the label by handling after completion of the process with subsequent rejection of the entire package.

VI. CONCLUSION

This chapter has attempted to deal with the overall subject of processing of small volume parenterals. In doing so, it has overlapped with several other chapters in this book. For this, the authors offer their apologies. There are many factors that had to be discussed, if but briefly, because they are such an integral part of the processing. In general, the overall processing of parenterals and other sterile products should conform to a similar scheme outlined in Figure 1.

APPENDIX: LIST OF SUPPLIERS

Climet Instruments Company, Redlands, California
Cozzoli Machine Company, Plainfield, New Jersey
Dow-Corning Corporation, Medical Products, Midland, Michigan
W. J. Fitzpatrick Co., Chicago, Illinois
Fluid Energy Processing and Equipment Co., Hatfield, Pennsylvania
HIAC/ROYCO Instrument Division, Smithtown, New York
International Pulverizing Corporation,
Jet Pulverizer Co., Moorestown, New Jersey
Manton Gaulin Co., Inc., Everett, Massachusetts
Metromatic Products Corporation, Oyster Bay, New York
Mixing Equipment Co., Rochester, New York
Perry Industries, Inc., Hicksville, New York
Spectrex Company, Redwood City, California
H. Strunck and Co., Maschinenfabrik Lichtstrasse 30-54, Germany
Z Packaging, Inc., Nanuet, New York

REFERENCES

1. Turco, S., and King, R. E., Sterile Dosage Forms: Their Preparation and Clinical Application, Lea & Febiger, Philadelphia, 1979, p. 163.
2. Werble, W., The Gold Sheet, F-D-C Reports, Inc., Vol. 10(5), 1976, p. 2.

3. Spaulding, E. A., J. Hosp. Res., 9:5-31 (1972).
4. Stonehill, A. A., Krop, S., and Borick, P. M., Am. J. Hosp. Pharm., 20: 465-485)1963).
5. Avis, K. E., in The Theory and Practice of Industrial Pharmacy, 2nd ed. (L. Lachman, H. A. Lieberman, and J. L. Kanig, eds.), Lea & Febiger, Philadelphia, 1976, p. 563.
6. Avis, K. E., in The Theory and Practice of Industrial Pharmacy, 2nd ed. (L. Lachman, H. A. Lieberman, and J. L. Kanig, eds.), Lea & Febiger, Philadelphia, 1976, pp. 570-571.
7. Nishimura, T., Kishimoto, J., Nishida, Y., Noguchi, Y., and Imai, S., J. Parenter. Drug Assoc., 33(2):96 (1979).
8. Sanga, S. V., J. Parenter. Drug Assoc., 33(2):61 (1979).
9. The United States Pharmacopeia XX, The United States Pharmacopeial Convention, Inc., Rockville, Md., 1980, pp. 949-950.
10. Nail, S. L., J. Parenter. Drug Assoc., 33(4):177 (1979).
11. Avis, K. E., in The Theory and Practice of Industrial Pharmacy, 2nd ed. (L. Lachman, H. A. Lieberman, and J. L. Kanig, eds.), Lea & Febiger, Philadelphia, 1976, p. 570.
12. Avis, K. E., in The Theory and Practice of Industrial Pharmacy, 2nd ed. (L. Lachman, H. A. Lieberman, and J. L. Kanig, eds.), Lea & Febiger, Philadelphia, 1976, p. 588.
13. O'Neill, J. L., U.S. Pat. 3,962,430 (1976).
14. Antoni, F., Manual on Radiation Sterilization of Medical and Biological Materials, International Atomic Energy Agency, Vienna, 1973, pp. 13-35.
15. Avis, K. E., in The Theory and Practice of Industrial Pharmacy, 2nd ed. (L. Lachman, H. A. Lieberman, and J. L. Kanig, eds.), Lea & Febiger, Philadelphia, 1976, p. 681.
16. Avis, K. E., in The Theory and Practice of Industrial Pharmacy, 2nd ed. (L. Lachman, H. A. Lieberman, and J. L. Kanig, eds.), Lea & Febiger, Philadelphia, 1976, p. 619.
17. Oberholtzer, E. R., and Brenner, G. S., J. Pharm. Sci., 68(7):863-866 (1979).
18. Chrai, S., Gupta, S., and Brychta, K., Bull. Parenter. Drug Assoc., 31(4): 195-200 (1977).

7

Manufacturing of Large Volume Parenterals

NICHOLAS J. KARTINOS and MICHAEL J. GROVES*

Travenol Laboratories, Inc.
Morton Grove, Illinois

A large volume parenteral (LVP) has been variously defined, but it is presently accepted to apply to an injection intended for intravenous use and packaged in containers holding 100 ml or more, for single use, and prepared without benefit of a preservative. Preparations intended for use as irrigating solutions (pour bottles), for hemofiltration, or for peritoneal dialysis are also regarded as LVPs. These preparations may be packaged in containers designed to empty rapidly and may contain a volume of more than 1 liter.

Because these solutions are injected directly into the bloodstream (intravenous preparations), poured into open body cavities and surgical areas (irrigating solutions), have direct contact with blood (hemofiltration), or are introduced into a body cavity (peritoneal dialysis), they must be presented as sterile and nonpyrogenic preparations. Although official particulate matter standards in the United States Pharmacopeia (USP) apply only to intravenous solutions, all preparations must be substantially free of particulate matter. Thus the processing parameters presented in this chapter apply fully to these various solutions to ensure that the final products are sterile, nonpyrogenic, and substantially free of particulate matter.

LVPs are usually regarded as providing water, electrolytes, or nutrients. Certain specialty products also fall within the definition of a large volume parenteral. These are biological products and x-ray contrast agents.

The USP definitions for sterile preparations for parenteral use generally do not apply to biological products. These products are primarily albumin, purified human plasma, and related protein fractions. Because of their special nature, the Bureau of Biologics, Food and Drug Administration (FDA), governs the licensing of these materials. They are not amenable to steam sterilization but are sterilized by filtration and aseptically filled. Obviously, components of the container system must be rendered sterile and nonpyrogenic before filling. Washed and properly protected parts may be autoclaved and then dried, as required, before use. Parts such as glass containers may be washed, dried, and rendered sterile and nonpyrogenic by

---

*Present affiliation: College of Pharmacy, University of Illinois at Chicago, Chicago, Illinois

exposure to dry heat at high temperature. Temperatures in the range 160 to 170°C for a period of not less than 2 hr are employed. Higher temperatures and correspondingly shorter periods may be employed for heat-resistant articles. Lower temperatures and longer periods are employed for heat-sensitive materials. Rubber and plastic components cannot be subjected to such treatment, requiring other modes of sterilization (e.g., steam sterilization).

X-ray contrast agents make up the group of products that are LVPs and also diagnostic agents. These products are processed in a manner similar to the one described, employing either terminal steam sterilzation or sterile fill, depending on the stability of the active components.

The decade of the 1970s brought dramatic changes in the processing of LVPs in the United States and in many foreign countries. In the United States this was stimulated by the publishing of the FDA's proposed Current Good Manufacturing Practices (CGMP) regulations specifically for LVPs. At this writing, they are not official but are required reading for the fine points they detail regarding FDA compliance and inspection activities. The basic premise of these proposed CGMPs is that it is not possible or acceptable to attempt only to test for quality in the final product. Every aspect of the manufacturing process must be defined, qualified, and controlled to ensure product quality. Hopefully, the finalized CGMPs will stress the principles of control and avoid the specifics for achieving them. Thus technology will not be frozen at a point in time, and improvements may be made as the subject develops.

An LVP also may be more simply defined as water containing a drug substance and confined in a container with a secure closure system. This chapter attempts to depict the elements associated with combining water and drug substances (raw materials) into a batch of solution, filling, and sealing it into containers ready for terminal steam sterilization, and performing this in a defined and controlled manner to ensure reliably that the final product is sterile, nonpyrogenic, and substantially free of particulate matter. Specific "how-to" examples are provided for clarity, but these are not to be viewed as final or absolute.

Because these products are uniformly aqueous systems, it is appropriate to introduce the subject of processing LVPs with a brief overview of fluid dynamics—the physical and physiochemical properties of liquids as they apply to LVPs. On a commercial scale, these products are made in large batch sizes. Batch sizes as large as 20,000 liters are not uncommon. These large volumes must be pumped through pipes from tanks to filter assemblies to the filling machines, and autoclaves of commensurate size must be utilized.

I. FLUID DYNAMICS AND HEAT FLOW

The fundamental properties of fluids, such as viscosity and density, become important when considering the rates of solution flow, the power required to pump a liquid from one tank to another, or the transfer of heat during the autoclaving of a large volume parenteral. It is not difficult to imagine the difference in pressure required to filter a 70% aqueous solution of dextrose compared to a 5% dextrose or a simple 0.9% saline solution through the same system. Under some conditions, the delivery of heat from a steam line to an autoclave is critically affected by the number of bends in the pipe. Even minor obstructions or blockages in an autoclave outlet drain can reduce the total heat delivered to a product because the velocity of steam movement is reduced and heat transfer rates are slowed. If the amount of heat delivered is a critical requirement, the product could be affected because there may not be sufficient heat for sterilization or, at the other extreme, damage may result because cooling has not occurred fast enough. For these reasons, properties such as viscosity, density, and surface tension will be discussed before moving to fluid flow and heat transfer. Throughout this section the reader should not lose sight of the fact that the object of the exercise is to understand the factors that control the transfer of heat into and out of a product during a sterilization process. A balance has to be struck between having sufficient heat to sterilize on one hand, and avoiding excessive heat that might cause product degradation on the other. All the factors involved need to be considered.

A. Properties of Fluids

1. Viscosity

Intuitively, a swimmer appreciates that movement of a body through a fluid is resisted by a force. Sir Isaac Newton wrote in his Principia (1687): "Hypothesis: that the resistance which arises from the lack of slipperiness of the parts of a liquid, other things being equal, is proportional to the velocity with which the parts of the liquid are separated from one another."

This lack of slipperiness is today called the "viscosity," a term derived from the Latin word for mistletoe (Viscum album) and originally meaning stickiness. Newton also appreciated that the frictional force (F) in a fluid was a direct function of the exposed surface area (A) at right angles to the direction of movement, and that the viscosity term is the proportionality constant of this relationship.

Consider fluid moving down a pipe. The fastest movement takes place in the exact center of the pipe and the slowest at the walls (Fig. 1). This sets up a velocity gradient. The fluid movement can be considered as a series of concentric shells. Taking two of those shells, A and B, h centimeters apart, with fluid velocities of V_A and V_B, respectively, the equation for Newton's law is

$$F \propto \alpha \Delta \frac{V_A - V_B}{h}$$

$$F \propto \eta \Delta \frac{V_A - V_B}{h}$$

The coefficient of viscosity η is the ratio of the force or stress to the velocity gradient or rate of shear (also called the strain). Newton was careful to add "all other things being equal." Unfortunately, there are systems for which this simple Newtonian concept does not always apply: non-Newtonian liquids.

The unit of force is a dyne on the cgs (centimeter, gram, second) system of units, equivalent to 10^{-5} newtons (kilogram, meter, seconds) in the modern Systeme International (SI) units. The units of velocity gradient in cgs units are cm sec^{-1} cm^{-1}. The viscosity coefficient (η) is therefore defined as the frictional force in dynes exerted on 1 cm^2 of a fluid when it is in a region of unit velocity gradient. The unit of viscosity, poise, is legitimately used in either SI and cgs units.

$$1 \text{ poise (P)} = 1 \text{ g (cm s)}^{-1} - 0.1 \text{ N s m}^{-2}$$

$$= 10^{-1} \text{ Pa} \cdot \text{s}$$

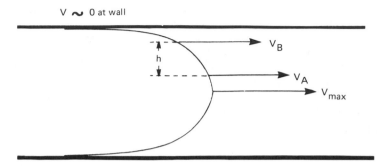

Figure 1 Cross section of flow through a pipe, illustrating the velocity gradient between V_{max} to almost zero at the walls.

where Pa = pascal = newton seconds. Because water has a viscosity of approximately one hundredth of a poise, the viscosity, more accurately the viscosity coefficient η, is often expressed as a centipoise, cP.

In industry a kinematic viscosity is often used. Kinematic viscosity is the ratio of the dynamic viscosity (in poise) to the fluid density (in g cm^{-3}), the unit being the stoke, St.

Considering the movement of gas, steam, or liquid water through a pipe, two different flow regimes may be encountered. In the first, there is slow movement through the pipe so that there are no eddies. This is usually known as streamline or laminar flow, although the term creeping flow is more evocative. In the second regime the flow is fast enough for eddy currents to be formed. This is known as turbulent flow. There is no sharp transition. The two regimes are separated by an unstable region, which is often streamline in nature but readily reverts to turbulent flow on the slightest disturbance.

Some LVP solutions such as the concentrated vegetable oil emulsions used for parenteral nutrition can demonstrate non-Newtonian behavior. This may cause problems during their manufacture such as an increase in apparent viscosity during pumping or homogenization when high shear stresses are encountered. Molding rubber compound formulations for stoppers is another example of complex flow behavior.

Many concentrated pastes or dispersions will not flow until a sufficient force has been applied to overcome internal forces or friction. This is known as the yield value and is often good initial evidence for particle-particle interactions that are manifested as non-Newtonian flow. Once these systems start moving, their flow tends to remain non-Newtonian in a number of different ways. The handling of non-Newtonian materials, especially pumping and processing, can be difficult. Unfortunately, there are few generalizations that can be applied. Each situation has to be handled on its own merits.

Because the constituent molecules become more mobile, the resistance to movement through a fluid decreases as the thermal energy of the fluid increases. The dependence of the viscosity of a Newtonian fluid upon temperature is approximated by a form of the familiar Arrhenius equation:

$$\eta \; = \; A \cdot E^{Ev/RT}$$

Here A is a constant depending on the molecular weight and molar volume of the fluid, and Ev is an activation energy term that represents an energy threshold above which molecules will flow. The gas constant (R) is present and the viscosity (η) is related to the absolute temperature (T). This equation was derived by postulating that "holes" appear in the structure of liquids formed by interactions between adjacent molecules. These holes allow loose molecules to move when the liquid flows. Analogs of rate processes familiar in chemical kinetics can then be applied. This concept has been questioned and alternative approaches made to the problem. However, interestingly enough, these lead to the same approximate relationship between viscosity and temperature, being derived as the Sheppard-Andrade equation:

$\ln \eta$ proportional to $1/T$

This equation applies to many liquids with a remarkable degree of accuracy. The major exception is liquid water, probably because water has a complex, hydrogen-bonded structure in which the ratio of bound to unbound molecules changes rapidly according to temperature and in which the presence of additives either enhance or diminish structure. Nevertheless, under a wide variety of environmental conditions, water does flow as if it were a simple Newtonian fluid.

From the previous discussion and the later section on the factors involved in heat transfer, it should be evident that the amount of heat delivered is a direct function of the viscosity of the system. The amount of heat delivered during a heat sterilization process can be quantified in terms of the F_0 value defined as

$$F_0 = \Delta t \ 10^{T-(T_0/z)}$$

where

Δt = time interval between successive product temperature measurements.

z = constant representing the temperature required for the reduction of the microbial population by 90%.

T = product temperature measured after Δt

T_0 = desired product temperature

The F_0 value is readily calculated using a thermocouple inside the autoclave and an appropriate integrator. A study by Akers, Attia, and Avis [1] provided a valuable insight into the effects produced on the F_0 values by increasing viscosity during a heat sterilization process. These authors used aqueous solutions of glycerin or sodium carboxymethyl cellulose and found that the F_0 value decreased as the viscosities increased. However, the fact that only a small change in viscosity could produce a relatively large change in the F_0 value suggests that it might be possible to use aqueous solutions of glycerol to mimic the behavior of other parenteral solutions. The behavior can be categorized in terms of the kinematic viscosity, which also takes into account the density of the solution, as well as the required F_0 value calculated in relation to that delivered for the corresponding glycerin solution. The use of aqueous glycerol solutions to assess the heat delivered is gaining ground because they are relatively stable and offer a convenient set of working standards for qualification of sterilization systems.

2. Density

The density of a substance, defined as the ratio of mass per unit volume, is a fundamental property of matter. It is a colligative property in that the density of a mixture is made up of the sum of the parts. The measurement of density can provide a great deal of information about molecules and interactions between molecules, and can be a sensitive indicator of concentration in some situations because densities due to components are additive.

$$\text{Density} \; = \; \rho \; = \; \frac{\text{mass}}{\text{volume}}$$

Units of density are g cm^{-3}, occasionally as kg m^{-3}. Because the volume of a fluid or solid can be critically affected by the temperature of measurement, the temperature is usually included as a superscript (e.g., ρ^{25}).

Density is a generic term. Other forms of density are encountered in practice. Relative density, or the obsolescent term "specific gravity" (SG), is the ratio of the density of the substance to the density of water at the same temperature.

$$\text{Relative density} \; = \; \frac{\text{density of the substance}}{\text{density of water at the same temperature}}$$

$$= \; \frac{d_s}{w_c}$$

Because relative density is the ratio of two similar functions, it is dimensionless. The specific gravity also can be used in a situation where the density of the water is defined as unity at 4°C, the temperature of maximum density. Unfortunately, later work showed that the maximum density of water occurs at 3.98°C so that ρ^4 water = 0.99997 g cm^{-3}. In most situations this difference is unimportant. However, it becomes significant if using older, tabulated data when a high degree of accuracy is required. Density ratios or relative densities can be determined for any combination of convenient materials, but obviously these materials must be specified when reporting the information.

3. Surface Tension

The rate at which heat is transferred into the contents of a container in an autoclave is affected by the properties of the surface, such as area constitution and thickness. However, the ability of the steam to "wet" the outside surface of the container is influenced by surface tension and affects the rate at which heat is transferred from the steam to the container itself. If a two-phasic system such as a dispersion or emulsion is being sterilized by heat, the interface, or the surface separating two phases in contact, becomes of interest. Heat is transferred from one phase to another through the interface. Components of the solution cross the interface during the sterilization process. Ultimately, the walls of bacterial or biological cells can be considered to be interfaces across which heat or components are being moved.

Colloidal systems, especially emulsions, characteristically have a larger surface area enclosing small volumes of material. These systems have a higher energy level than their surroundings. According to the second law of thermodynamics, there is a natural tendency for colloidal systems to lose energy. For example, emulsions consisting of a large number of small droplets tend to coalesce to one large droplet. The job of a formulator is to try to prevent that process or at least to slow it down.

Surface tension is defined as the force per unit length required to extend a surface. Because the unit of force is the dyne (cgs) or the newton, N (SI), the units are dyn cm^{-1} or N m^{-1}, respectively. Surface tension is also defined as the surface force energy change per unit area increase, sometimes called the free surface energy. In simple terms, the lower the surface tension the less work required to expand the surface area.

4. Vapor Pressure

The vapor pressure of a liquid or solid is defined as the pressure of the vapor that is in equilibrium with the substance at a given temperature. The vapor pressure of every stable compound, solid or liquid, is determined by the temperature and is a unique property of the material. The kinetic energies of molecules in a system are not uniformly distributed and some move at higher velocities than others.

The vapor pressure at a given temperature effectively represents the proportion of molecules that are fast enough (or have high enough energy) to escape from the surface of the solid or liquid and pass to the gaseous state. As the temperature is increased, a higher proportion of molecules are able to escape. If the material is placed in a container open to the atmosphere and the temperature increased, a point is reached when the vapor pressure is equal to the applied atmospheric pressure and the material boils. The boiling point of a liquid is a measurement of the forces holding the liquid together. Heat is absorbed during the process, the latent heat of vaporization, and the same quantity of heat is given out when the vapor phase condenses to the liquid state. This is one mechanism by which heat is transferred to or from a container in a steam autoclave, particularly during the initial warming-up phase, as steam condenses on the cool container and cooling-down phase as heat is extracted from the hot container by return to the liquid state.

If the substance being heated is in a closed container and is in the liquid phase, there will be a considerable increase in the pressure above the liquid surface as the vapor expands. However, the increase in pressure will itself tend to resist the vaporization of the liquid. The increase in pressure due to the conversion from a liquid to a gas phase will occur at a higher temperature. An advantage of an autoclave, especially of the counterpressure type, is that there is a high pressure applied to the outside of a container to help balance the high pressure generated inside by the contents. The heat sterilization of plastic containers would be very difficult without a means of balancing the pressure, especially because the majority of plastics used soften at sterilization temperatures. Without counterpressure (air) during the cooling phase of the cycle, the containers would swell like balloons because the vapor pressure of the heated contents is considerably higher than that of the cooler exterior.

The presence of gas in the space above a liquid decreases the rate of evaporation but does not affect the equilibrium pressure of the vapor. When a completely nonvolatile solute is dissolved in a volatile solvent, the vapor phase above the solution can come only from the volatile component. The solute may reduce the tendency of the solvent molecules to escape so that the vapor pressure of a solution is reduced proportionately to the relative number of solute molecules present. For this reason, the presence of a solute in a liquid solvent raises the boiling point of the liquid to lower the vapor pressure at a given temperature. This proposition is expressed as Raoult's law:

Vapor pressure of the solution $= P_1$

$$= P_1^{\;0} x_1$$

where

$P_1^{\;0}$ = vapor pressure of the pure solvent

x_1 = mole fraction of the solution

If the solute is air or gas, Henry's law applies in that the quantity of gas dissolved is directly proportional to its partial pressure over the solution

$$P_g = kN_g$$

where

P_g = gas partial pressure

N_g = mole fraction of gas molecules dissolved

The proportionality constant k becomes identical to the vapor pressure of the solvent in Raoult's law if the solubility of the gas is low.

The total pressure in a mixed system is the sum of the partial pressures of all of the components. However, in some cases the constituent molecules can interact with each other. In those situations, they are positive or negative deviations from Raoult's law, depending on whether or not the results of the interaction are more or less volatile than their components.

B. Flow of Fluids in an Autoclave

A fluid, either a gas or a liquid, is defined as a substance that undergoes continuous deformation when subjected to a shear stress. A surface immersed in a fluid has pressure on it. This is caused by molecules of fluid impinging upon the surface and giving up their kinetic energy in the form of a momentum change. Fluids can be classified according to the effects produced on them by a shearing stress. The volume of a liquid, for example, is little influenced by the temperature and applied pressure when flowing. This is not true for a gas, which expands significantly when heated.

When a fluid flows from one place to another, energy is usually converted from one form to another. The energy that can be attributed to the physical state of the fluid is called the internal energy. A change in the physical state, from a liquid to a vapor for example, produces a change in the internal energy. In fluid flow, the process is usually irreversible in that it is accompanied by a conversion of electrical or mechanical energy into heat or by the reduction of temperature differences between different parts of the whole system. This concept is the basis for the operation of a steam autoclave. An autoclave is in effect a closed system so that heating the contents increases the pressure inside the system.

As noted during the discussion of viscosity, the velocity of a plane at right angles to the movement of a fluid is not uniform; a velocity profile is found. The maximum velocity is found in the center of a pipe or tube and there is a minimum or zero velocity for the layer of fluid immediately adjacent to the containing wall. Two main types of flow are encountered depending on whether or not eddies can develop in the system. In streamline or creeping flow, there are no eddies to produce mixing. Movement across streamlines must occur only by molecular diffusion. In turbulent flow there are eddies or circulation currents that cause transfer of material across the streamlines and disturb the smooth transition of velocity gradient across the tube radius.

It is essential to operate an autoclave, for example, under turbulent conditions so that heat is transferred rapidly and uniformly throughout the contents. The transition from a streamline to a turbulent flow situation is mainly a function of flow velocity. In streamline flow (sometimes known as laminar flow—hence the term laminar-flow air hoods) the average velocity in the direction of flow is constant and does not fluctuate. In turbulent flow, the velocity at a point fluctuates around a mean. The transition between streamline and turbulent flow is not sharply defined. A metastable region of streamline conditions may exist where a turbulent region might otherwise be anticipated. Flow regions are usually described by the Reynold's number, Re, which is the ratio of the inertial to viscous forces in a system.

If the fluid is forced to pass over a rough surface or to make a number of sharp turns, turbulence in the major part of the flow can be induced at a much lower Reynolds number because the metastable intermediate or transition region is disturbed. However, the layer of liquid immediately adjacent to the wall (boundary layer) remains at laminar state, although as the turbulence increases, the thickness of the boundary layer decreases.

This introduction of obstacles into the system also means that the frictional resistance is increased. At the same time, however, the heat transfer and mass transfer coefficients are increased. Turbulence in steam autoclaves is desirable and is induced to increase the efficiency of both the heating and cooling stages of the sterilization process.

C. Heat Transfer

1. Concepts

Because heat is applied in some form or another in the majority of sterilization operations, the laws that describe the transfer of heat are of considerable importance. Provided that there is a difference in temperature between two parts of a system, heat flows between the parts by three processes, either singly or in combination: conduction, convection, or radiation.

Conduction Conduction is the mechanism for transferring heat by transferring vibrational energy of individual atoms or molecules without mixing. In liquids, conduction is limited to those thin layers adhering to solid surfaces when the kinetic energy is transferred from one point to another. Conduction in solids, especially metals, may occur by the movement of free electrons. Transfer of heat into a container occurs through the container wall by conduction.

Convection During convection, heat is transferred by actually mixing warm parts of the system with cooler parts. This process only occurs in fluids. In natural convection, the mixing currents are caused by local differences produced in the density of the fluid when temperature gradients appear. In forced convection, turbulent flow is induced by applying force to allow currents to carry the heat across the system.

Radiation   Radiation is the term used to describe the movement of energy
through empty space by means of electromagnetic waves. Moving through space
means that the energy cannot be diverted from its path or be transformed from one
form to another. However, if the radiant energy comes in contact with an object,
some is absorbed by the object or transmitted through it. Only the absorbed energy
is manifested as heat.

2. Thermal Resistance

Thermal resistance is easier to understand in the context of heat being conducted through a solid body. The basic law regarding heat transfer states that the
rate of transfer is directly proportional to the driving force. The driving force is
the temperature drop across the body (e.g., the rate is proportional to the driving
force, or rate = resistance × driving force).

Consider a wall of area A and thickness X (Fig. 2) and assume uniform temperatures of t_1 and t_2 are on the two faces of the wall; if a steady state exists, a
form of Fourier's law applies:

Flow of heat through area A in unit time $= \phi$

$$= \frac{kA(t_1 - t_2)}{X}$$

Because $(t_1 - t_2)$ is the driving force, the resistance to movement of heat is the term
(x/kA). The proportionality constant (k) is a property of each material of which the
wall is made and is called the thermal conductivity. Strictly speaking, k is not a
constant because it is a function of the applied temperature or temperature range

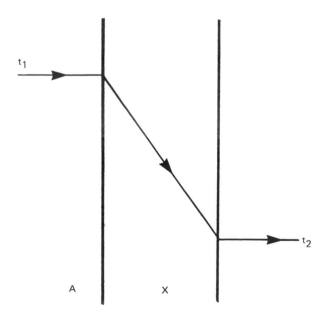

Figure 2 Thermal resistance across a wall of area A and thickness X.

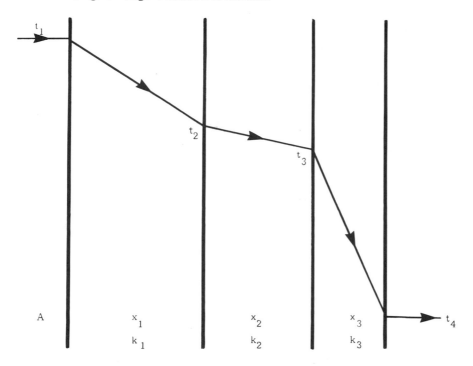

Figure 3 Heat flow across a composite wall of three layers.

over which it is measured. Generally, liquids have low thermal conductivities, and solids have high values. Assume that a container wall is actually a series of flat layers (Fig 3); each layer is composed of different thicknesses of a different material, each with its own thermal conductivity. Thus it is possible to calculate the overall thermal resistance of the wall.

Let Δt be the overall temperature drop from one side of the wall composite to the other:

$$\Delta t = \Delta t_1 + \Delta t_2 + \Delta t_3$$

This equation is rewritten as

$$\Delta t_1 = q_1 \frac{x_1}{k_1 A}$$

$$\Delta t_2 = q_2 \frac{x_2}{k_2 A}$$

$$\Delta t_3 = q_3 \frac{x_3}{k_3 A}$$

where q is the quantity of heat passing through each layer. These are summed to yield

$$\Delta t = \frac{q_1 x_1}{k_1 A} + \frac{q_2 x_2}{k_2 A} + \frac{q_3 x_3}{k_3 A}$$

Because all the heat that passes through each layer must be equal to a quantity q (i.e., $q_1 = q_2 = q_3 = q$),

$$q = \frac{\Delta t}{x_1/k_1 A + x_2/k_2 A + x_3/k_3 A} = \frac{\Delta t}{R_1 + R_2 + R_3}$$

where R_1, R_2, and R_3 are the thermal resistances of the respective layers. Thus it is not difficult to appreciate that the effective or overall thermal resistance of the total system is the sum of the individual resistances.

These considerations become important when examining the passage of heat through the wall of a container, for example, an LVP in an autoclave. The outside container has a layer of condensed steam adhering to it so that the liquid layer it-self constitutes one layer. The liquid inside the container is moving around under the influence of convection currents being set up by the heating process. Neverthe-less, there is a stationary boundary layer that constitutes the inside layer of the system. Each layer provides its own thermal resistance, which constitutes a part of the whole resistance to the penetration of heat into and out of the container. Any factor that helps to reduce this resistance is beneficial and improves the efficiency of the process. The effect of turbulent flow inside an autoclave has been mentioned because this helps to reduce the thickness of the outside boundary layer. The in-side boundary layer may be reduced by agitating the contents of the container. In static autoclaves this is not possible, but autoclaves are available in which the con-tents are rotated to provide this agitation and speed up the process of heat transfer. The agitation also reduces the cold and hot spots that are inevitably present inside an autoclave. This provides greater efficacy of the heat sterilization process.

The thickness of the boundary layer is usually not known with any certainty, although factors that contribute to its thickness can be derived empirically. Refer-ence was previously made to the effect that this boundary layer of condensed liquid on the outside of the container has on the rate at which heat can move through the walls and into the contents of the container. In point of fact it is not necessary for the thin film to be continuous. If the surface is not wettable, droplets form on the surface and fall off, continually exposing fresh surface. This is known as dropwise condensation. This condensation is actually desired for more efficient boiler oper-ation, and frequently hydrophobic materials are added to the feedwater. Most fre-quently employed are fatty acids and their derivates. If used in the boiler generat-ing steam for an autoclave, it is not difficult for entrained materials to be carried to the outside walls of the autoclave contents. Dropwise condensation on the con-tainer walls is quite likely to take place, although the usual glass and plastic sur-faces are hydrophilic. In this situation, the heat transfer rates may be higher than anticipated.

In the discussion above, the assumption has been made that the autoclave is filled only with steam. If the steam contains air, the partial pressure and the vis-cosity are lowered. The net effect is to lower the temperature of the system. Auto-claves are designed to operate with pure steam or air–steam mixtures. As stated above, the latter type is required when autoclaving LVPs in plastic containers. With either system, the sterilization process must be monitored by temperature and not by pressure.

II. WATER: THE ESSENTIAL RAW MATERIAL

A. Definition

The U.S. Pharmacopeia contains two monographs for bulk water supplies, Purified Water and Water for Injection. Purified Water is water obtained by distillation, ion-exchange treatment, reverse osmosis (RO), or other suitable process. At a minimum, the initial feedwater must comply with the Federal Environment Protection Agency (EPA) requirements for drinking water. Purified Water contains no added substances. Although Purified Water meets the bacteriological purity requirements of the regulations for drinking water, this water may be pyrogenic. It is not intended for the preparation of parenterals.

Water for Injection is water purified by distillation or by reverse osmosis and contains no added substances. Water processed by distillation or reverse osmosis, even though prepared in a properly designed, engineered, installed, and maintained system, is dependent on the design, installation, and sanitation of the downstream side of the system, particularly the piping, pumps, holding tanks, and the controls exercised over the quality of the immediate environment.

Water for Injection is used as the solvent in parenteral solutions, whether terminally sterilized in the final container or prepared under aseptic conditions and sterilized by appropriate filtration. Purified Water, deionized water, or potable water may be employed during the early phases of the manufacturing process—the preliminary cleaning of containers, parts, lines, and tanks. However, Water for Injection is more routinely employed for the final rinsing of these items and other product contact surfaces. The choice of water for these early phases depends on the locale and the chemical and microbiological quality of the specific water.

Whether one depends on municipal water supplies or on private wells, the chemical and microbiological quality of the water and the consequences of any subsequent treatments should be known. Whether Purified Water or Water for Injection is prepared by reverse osmosis or distillation, feedwater of a controlled quality must be employed to ensure maximum efficiency and minimum maintenance.

B. Pretreatment

Regardless of how Water for Injection is ultimately generated, the incoming water must be adequately pretreated to ensure its uniformity and to promote constant quality and high efficiency of subsequent treatments. No single sequence can be described that will be universally applicable, but some of the more important elements include:

1. Chlorination to suppress microbial growth throughout the system.
2. Prefiltration through depth filters (e.g., sand) to remove iron, suspended matter, and silt.
3. Flocculation for removal of suspended matter. Injecting a flocculating agent (e.g., alum) will be followed by settling of the suspended particles.
4. Water softening by ion exchange to remove the alkaline earth ions, calcium and magnesium, and thus minimize formation of scale deposits.
5. pH adjustment to the range 6.0 to 6.5 to reduce scale deposits.
6. Deionization by ion-exchange resins for the more complete removal of ions from the feedwater. Reducing the dissolved mineral content reduces scale formation and reduces corrosion.

7. Activated carbon beds for the removal of chlorine and organics. After removal
    of the chlorine other sanitizing measures (e.g., ultraviolet radiation) may have
    to be imposed to suppress microbial growth.

C. Reverse Osmosis

Reverse osmosis (RO) is defined as a process for the separation of solutes from
water by applying pressure on a more concentrated solution in contact with a semipermeable membrane to produce a less concentrated solution. The solutes may be
charged (ions) or essentially neutral (organics). Each is excluded by a different
mechanism.

Charged particles are excluded (repelled) due to interfacial tension at the
water-membrane interface. Monovalent ions are not excluded to the same degree
as the higher-valent, higher-charged ions. Organics are excluded by a sieve mechanism so that size and molecular weight are more important attributes. The higher
the molecular weight or size of a substance, the more efficiently it is excluded.
Thus bacteria, viruses, and pyrogens are removed by RO. Figure 4 depicts a typical RO system.

Both the quality and quantity of the solutes (inorganic and organic) in the feedwater can readily affect the functionality of the semipermeable membranes. Consequently, RO systems are more often a sequence of water treatment operations in
which the RO unit itself is the key component. The overall system is generally customized and depends primarily on the composition of the feedwater and the final
water quality desired. This is particularly true of large systems. In addition to
the RO unit itself, other types of water treatment equipment may include chemical
feeders of flocculating agents, chlorinators, filters, water softeners, heat exchangers, pH adjustment apparatus, pressure controls, active carbon beds, decar-
bonators, deionizers, and storage tanks.

Although potable water of suitable quality can be used directly as feedwater to
an RO unit, pH-adjusted or soft water is normally used. Of particular concern with
feedwater to RO units is the turbidity (silt concentration) and also the calcium carbonate content. These substances accelerate the plugging up of the semipermeable
membrane. Other substances often present in a water supply (e.g., iron, manganese, silica, and chlorine) can affect the efficiency and life span of the membranes
by either plugging the pores or reacting chemically. Once the RO system has been

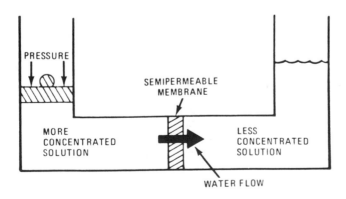

Figure 4 Reverse osmosis. (Courtesy of Osmonics, Inc., Minnetonka, Minnesota.)

designed (based on the expected feedwater quality) and installed, the task of controlling the feedwater quality will depend on the use of monitoring instruments and controls with limit settings for proper operation. The membranes in the system are subject to microbiological fouling. Therefore, the chlorine concentration in the feedwater may be deliberately kept at appropriate levels to reduce organism growth. With membranes sensitive to chlorine, other sanitizing agents (e.g., formaldehyde) are used on a scheduled basis to control the microbial level of the system. Low-molecular-weight organic substances (molecular weight 200) are not generally rejected with high efficiency by RO membranes. Certain dissolved gases such as chlorine, carbon dioxide, and ammonia may also pass through the membranes. If these organics or gases are expected to be present in the feedwater, some provision must be made for their removal. Activated carbon is generally effective in removing organics and chlorine.

Membrane integrity may be tested by use of selective molecular weight dyes, but this method is more effective in testing for large leaks. Ion exclusion tests (e.g., magnesium or sodium ions) measure membrane performance for ions. Water from reverse osmosis systems should be continuously monitored for quality by conductivity, to provide assurance of the system's level of performance.

D. Distillation

Distillation is the continuous process of heating water to its boiling (vaporizing) point in a confined environment so that the steam formed can be passed through a separator (to reduce carryover entrainment of unvaporized droplets). The steam vapor is then condensed into pure water and discharged from the apparatus. The system to accomplish this is frequently custom designed, depending on such factors as the character of the available water supply, type and quantity of energy available, and final quality and volume of product water required.

Potable water of suitable quality may be used as feedwater to distillation units. However, softened, deionized, or RO-treated water is more normally utilized to minimize mineral scale buildup, particularly calcium carbonate scale, on the heat transfer surfaces. This is one of the most common operational problems and the greatest cause of loss in efficiency. Also of concern are chloride salts and chlorine, which attack stainless steel and cause corrosion as well as cracking of the metal.

Once the feedwater pretreatment system has been designed and installed, the task of maintaining the quality of the feedwater at a consistently desirable level depends on monitoring with instruments designed to control the operation within prescribed limits. A routine program must be established for laboratory testing of periodic water samples taken at select points from the system to be evaluated for chemical and biological characteristics. Further, the feedwater pretreatment equipment must be kept sanitized by use of residual chlorine in the water, ultraviolet radiation, ozonation, heat, or periodic application of appropriate sanitizing chemicals. As stated above, some of these agents (e.g., chlorine) may have to be reduced or removed before the water enters the still.

Although there are a number of different basic designs of distillation units available on the market, the designs most prominent in LVP operations are vapor compression, multiple effect, and single-effect atmospheric stills. These stills are discussed in greater detail in the chapter on Industrial Sterilization in Volume 2.

An advantage with distillation is that the water passes through a phase change into steam at a temperature in excess of 212°F at atmospheric pressure. This aids in killing any living microorganisms and in preserving the sanitary nature of the system. Also, perfect phase change would leave behind all chemical and physical contaminants, producing very pure water vapor. After this vapor is condensed to liquid water, it is maintained at pressures greater than the water of lower purity whenever they are on opposite sides of the heat exchangers, thus guarding against possible contamination of the higher-purity fraction. One usually tests for leaks in the system by isolating specific sections and imposing hydraulic pressure to verify that each section maintains the pressure while isolated. The objective is to control the number of organisms per unit volume of the water used for final rinses of containers and equipment and the final product. Each manufacturer should establish the target limit for the product and manufacturing environment. Targets of 10 organisms per 100 ml may be representative.

When selecting either a reverse osmosis or distillation system, it is important to remember that each system has certain advantages and disadvantages. Large-capacity distillation systems normally require more energy per unit of product water produced than do RO systems, but RO systems generally require significantly more total water input per unit of product water produced. Both are largely dependent on the operating parameters involved. The water supply characteristics, the system size (capacity), and the quality of the final product water are the basic aspects governing system selection.

Both systems require that part of the feedwater be constantly "bled off" to waste because the mineral content of the feedwater captive in the system increases as pure water is separated. This constant "bleed off" is termed blow down in distillation systems and reject in RO systems. In both instances, this reduces fouling of the system with subsequent maintenance problems and reduction of the quality of the water output.

Up-to-date drawings of the respective systems should be maintained. This practice aids in achieving better maintenance of the system and simplifies future modifications, including expansion. The general operational details of the systems should be committed to writing, including procedures for descaling, passivating, and sanitizing.

Descaling: The removal of built-up mineral deposits from the surfaces of heat exchange tubes or reverse osmosis membranes. This is accomplished by the use of various acids, which dissolve the calcium carbonate and other mineral deposits.

Passivating: The treating of 300 series stainless steel with a strong oxidizing agent (e.g., nitric acid) to remove the free iron on the surface and to render the metal more chemically inactive.

Sanitizing: The use of steam and/or hot water to maintain equipment and piping at a specified minimum temperature for a defined time period to reduce the number of organisms present in the system. In the case of RO units, sanitizing is usually accomplished by exposing the water-contact surfaces to chemical sanitizing solutions (e.g., hypochlorites) for a preestablished period.

Systems producing and conveying high-purity water for LVP processing should be of a sanitary design. Material and construction should ensure that surfaces are inert, smooth, accessible, easily cleaned, and do not shed particles. Stainless steel of the 300 series with No. 4 finish (equivalent to a 150-grit polish) is recommended. Welded piping is preferred to threaded connections, but it is not always practical or necessary. Flanged connections, and an occasional threaded connection, sealed with Teflon tape have been used and found acceptable. Welds should be of a "sanitary type," that is, made by the tungsten shielded arc method using

inert gas to preclude carbide and oxide formation. The weld must have 100% penetration, so that it is smooth and free from pits, cracks, inclusions, and other defects both inside and outside.

III. RAW MATERIALS

A. Definition

Water for Injection is the universal solvent for a LVP. The range of drug substances used as solutes in the manufacture of LVPs is fairly broad. Carbohydrates
such as mono- (e.g., dextrose, fructose) and disaccharides (e.g., sucrose, maltose)
are common. Sucrose is not employed directly but is acid-hydrolyzed to a 1:1 mixture of dextrose and fructose (invert sugar). Polyols that are employed may include glycerol, mannitol, sorbitol, and xylitol. Nitrogen-containing substances
such as amino acids and protein hydrolysates are used. Lipid emulsions require
vegetable oil (e.g., soya or safflower oils) and phospholipid-type emulsifying
agents. Most of these organic materials are designed to provide nutrition. However, mannitol is not metabolized but plays a special role as an osmotic agent.
    Inorganic salts used include the alkaline (Na and K) and alkaline earth (Ca
and Mg) chlorides, and the alkaline phosphates and bicarbonates. These salts provide necessary electrolytes as well as a means to adjust tonicity. Mixed inorganic-
organic salts are frequently encountered as the alkaline metal salts (Na or K) of
organic acids (e.g., acetic, lactic, glucuronic). These function as bicarbonate
precursors and alkalizing agents. Some of the inorganic and mixed salts are prepared in situ by combining stoichiometric quantities of acid and base (sodium hy-
roxide plus lactic acid yields sodium lactate). The acids and bases, usually common ions, are also employed for pH adjustments in the manufacturer of LVPs. The
rest of the raw materials include containers and closures, and closure assemblies.
Containers may be preformed (glass or plastic) or in the form of polymer beads or
sheeting for in-plant conversion to the plastic containers.

B. Stability

The chemicals mentioned above do not constitute all the organic, inorganic, and
mixed types of materials employed as drug substances. Because of the varied
chemical nature of these materials, the storage requirements and stability characteristics of these materials differ. Heat, light, moisture, and air (CO_2 or O_2) can
adversely affect many of these materials over a period of time. The containers for
these drug substances can also be important factors in stability considerations.
The following general guidelines will aid in relating chemical types to environmental
stability factors:

1. Organic materials are generally more sensitive to heat.
2. Natural fats and oils usually contain double bonds that react with oxygen to form
    peroxides.
3. Amino acids and protein hydrolysates can be adversely affected by heat, light,
    air, and moisture.
4. Anhydrous materials can pick up moisture from the environment.
5. Hydrated substances may deliquesce or effloresce.
6. Basic materials (e.g., NaOH) may absorb CO_2 from the air.

In view of these guidelines, appropriate stability profiles specifying the manufacturing storage conditions should be developed. The research and development function, in cooperation with the quality control group, should develop appropriate programs to assess stability during storage. Packaging, containers, and the environmental factors that must be controlled should be specified. Suppliers are very often valuable sources of good information.

Inventories of materials used frequently and in large amounts are turned over rapidly. Because they are stored for relatively short periods, they usually do not present a problem. However, the situation is different for materials used infrequently and in small amounts. These materials may be stored for longer periods of time and the containers are subjected to repeated entries. Each entry and withdrawal exposes the material to moisture, air, and light, thus altering the state of the headspace. Stability considerations for raw materials can be minimized by following sound inventory practices.

An automatic reassay schedule is indicated. No fixed schedule can be prescribed that applies to all materials in all plant environments. Data from stability studies and historical reassay values can be integrated to arrive at an appropriate and current program. Although there is much less concern for storage and stability controls for containers and container components, their stability must be considered in any program.

C. Receiving

A specific, isolated area is usually dedicated as a delivery point for the receipt of raw materials. All raw materials must be inspected, identified, documented, and sampled in accordance with written procedures. Stock numbers are usually assigned. All raw materials should be issued to production on a first in/first out (FIFO) basis. The oldest materials should be used first. Some materials (i.e., drug substances) require more precise identification and control. For these materials, a receiving date, manufacturing date, vendor I.D. number, and expiration date should be recorded, as appropriate. The maximum amount of information available should be incorporated. Raw materials or in-process materials sometimes originate from a production area within the plant. Complete documentation and traceability also must be maintained for these articles.

Materials should be received covered or in closed containers. All containers should be inspected for signs of damage that may indicate that the contents may have been subjected to conditions that could possibly affect quality, identity, strength, or purity. All signs of apparent damage should be properly recorded both on internal and carrier records. Redundant labeling on containers should be avoided. It should be removed or defaced if confusing or no longer valid.

D. Storage/Quarantine Areas

All raw materials associated with the final drug product—containers, closures, drug substances, and the like—must be sampled, distributed to laboratory functions, and tested for conformance to written specifications. These tests may be of a physical, chemical, or biologic nature. During the testing interval these materials are to be held in prescribed quarantine areas that are caged or segregated. Dividing areas with fencing or distinct aisles is an acceptable method for separating released raw materials from unreleased and rejected materials, provided that each area and the status of each material in that area is clearly identified. Caged areas must be

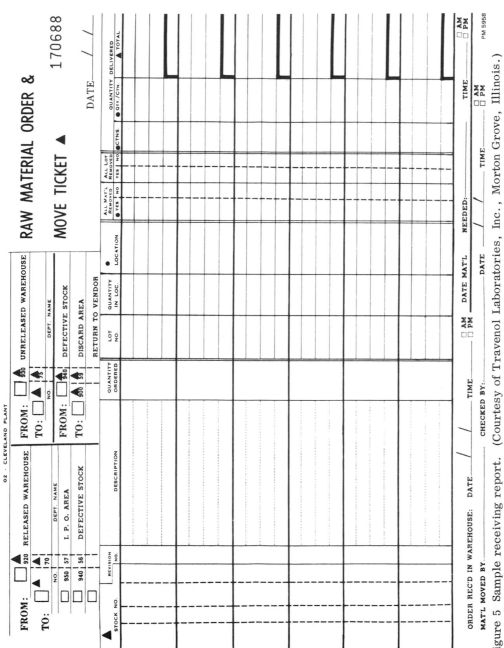

Figure 5 Sample receiving report. (Courtesy of Travenol Laboratories, Inc., Morton Grove, Illinois.)

provided for label storage segregated into released and unreleased sections. This secured area should be locked when not in use. A similarly caged area must be provided for rejected raw materials awaiting disposition. All raw materials should bear the release date, in addition to the stock number, location code, lot number, quantity, conditions for storage, and expiration date, if required. Efforts should be made to group similar items and numbers.

E. Distribution and Inventory Control

The manufacturing environment with its many operations is usually quite varied and complex. Sound material control and distribution systems are essential to good operations and production planning. The identity, traceability, and accountability of all materials must be ensured. Further, the identity of all materials in inventory, along with their quantity and location, must be known. Receiving reports (Fig. 5) should identify each item by stock number, name, vendor, manufacturer's lot number, unit of measure, and net weight per container. An accountability tag or sticker containing the same information is fixed to each container or pallet load. As the contents are used, the operator should record on the form the date used, destination (batch number, laboratory use, etc.), the quantity withdrawn, unit of measure, and the container balance (Fig. 5).

　　When a container is emptied, the accountability tag is removed and sent to a raw material accountability function for reconciliation. This function will have been provided with a copy of each receipt. The materials consumed can then be recorded for each item from the accountability tags. Periodic inventories are then made indicating the quantities remaining for each lot of raw material. Reasonable reconciliation should be expected. Significant discrepancies should be investigated to determine the problem and corrective measures should be taken.

IV. BATCH MIXING

Examination of the definition of an LVP and the raw materials (drug substances) they contain in the concentrations employed will lead the perceptive reader to the correct conclusion that the typical LVP is a clear aqueous solution. A present-day exception is an emulsion of vegetable oil in water with the addition of a lower-molecular-weight substance (e.g., glycerol) to enhance tonicity. Such a lipid emulsion is designed to provide calories in a minimum volume.

Example 1. <u>Typical LVP, Lactated Ringer's 5% Dextrose Injection</u>

　　Each 100 ml contains

Dextrose, hydrous, USP	5 g
Sodium chloride, USP	600 mg
Sodium lactate	310 mg
Potassium chloride, USP	30 mg
Calcium chloride, USP	20 mg

　　Approximate milliequivalents per liter:

Sodium	130
Potassium	4

Calcium   3
Chloride   109
Lactate   28

The solution is hypertonic with approximately 524 mOsm liter^{-1}. It is used for fluid, nutrient, and electrolyte replenishment.

Example 2. <u>10% Intravenous Fat Emulsion</u>

     Each 100 ml contains

Safflower oil   10 g
Egg phosphatides   1.2 g
Glycerin, USP   2.5 g
Approximate pH 8.0 adjusted with sodium hydroxide

The emulsion has 1.1 kcal ml^{-1} and 300 mOsm liter^{-1}. It is sterile and nonpyrogenic.

    Although not common, there are specialized LVPs that contain active ingredients that are not adequately stable in solution or compatible with the container to be supplied as aqueous solutions. Two examples are trisamino, a physiologic buffer, and urea, an osmotic diuretic. In these instances, the active ingredient is provided as a sterile, nonpyrogenic solid with a separate companion diluent (e.g., sterile urea for injection with a carbohydrate diluent). Sterile solids are most typically prepared by sterile filtration followed by lyophilization.

    With the exceptions noted, LVPs are primarily solutions and their manufacture must be performed in a disciplined manner. Stainless steel tanks with agitators to provide a uniform and common pool are routinely employed for batch mixing. Jacketed tanks are not uncommon for they provide a measure of temperature control. Elevated temperatures (40 to 50°C) can accelerate the solution rates of the drug substances.

    All LVPs are formulated on a weight per unit volume basis employing the metric system. Each catalog list number (product code) should have its specification setting forth the formula indicating the weight of each drug substance per unit volume and any special requirements (i.e., pH adjustments). In today's technology this information may be computerized so as to calculate the raw material requirements for the intended batch size (Fig. 6). The product code information is provided to the chemical weighing room where each ingredient is identified and weighed as specified. Scales with tape printers are useful in large operations. The printed tape expedites operations, serves as a convenient, permanent record for the batch history, and minimizes human recording errors. The remaining component for mixing a batch of product is Water for Injection. Water being delivered to the tank may be measured by metered valves to ensure volume control. Volume control can also be exercised by tank calibration or weight.

    The usual practice is to fill the tank with 50 to 80% of the required volume of water and add the drug substances with agitation. In-process assays may be performed for one or more key ions or other substances and adjustments in solute concentrations made as required before dilution to final prescribed volume. Batch sizes vary. They can be small (several hundred liters) or large (20,000 liters or more). The size of a batch must be integrated with the capacities of the filling line and the autoclaves. This is to ensure control over the elapsed time from beginning the preparation of a batch by addition of the drug substances to the water in the mixing tank to the start of the sterilization cycle for the packaged units.

MIXING RECORD

REF. SPEC. 20-8-2-100   MBR16

DATE	BATCH NUMBER	TIME FIRST WATER DRAWN
1-20-80	06588L5	
INITIAL VOLUME		TIME MIXED
5000 L	CODE NUMBER	TANK NUMBER
FINAL VOLUME		
		SOLUTION TEMPERATURE

SPEC. NO.   ISSUE DATE   DESCRIPTION

03-15-04-093   5-DEXTROSE-INJ USP

LAST FORMULATION CHANGE DATE : 02/27/79

COMPONENT NO.	LOT NO.	DESCRIPTION	EXTENSION	U/M	ADDED TO TANK BY 1	2
1) 02-02-04-008		DEXTROSE ANHYDROUS-USP	227.25	KG		
2) 03-15-23-001		WATER FOR INJ USP	QS			
2 COMPONENTS		EXTENSION TOTAL: 227.25				

WEIGHING & MIXING APPROVED BY	DATE	VERIFICATION OF CALCULATION/ASSAY BY	DATE

DISPOSITION	TIME RELEASED	CHEMIST	DATE	REVIEWED BY	DATE

953E

Figure 6 Sample mixing record. (Courtesy of Travenol Laboratories, Inc., Morton Grove, Illinois.)

The basis for this concern over the elapsed time is bioburden. Bioburden is the accumulation of various kinds and numbers of microorganisms contributed by the nonsterile drug substances (including the water), the equipment, the container components, the environment, and the workers. Each segment of the production sequence must be known, understood, and controlled to ensure a minimum effect on bioburden. Bioburden may be unique both as to the individual product and the environment in a particular plant location. Water for Injection and Sodium Chloride Injection support and promote the growth of microorganisms at different rates than Dextrose Injection and Amino Acids Injection do. Thus elapsed time can be varied depending on the product as well as the manufacturer. Time periods of 16 hr or greater are not uncommon. The chapter on Industrial Sterilization in Volume 2 also addresses this subject, but with emphasis on the microbiological aspect.

How does bioburden specifically affect batch size? A 20,000-liter batch may require 2 hr to mix, perform in-process assays, and make final adjustments. The filling operation, assuming a rate of 100 1-liter bottles per minute, takes 200 min (3 1/3 hr) to fill 20,000 bottles. At this point, 5 1/3 hr have passed. Let us further assume that an autoclave can accommodate 2000 bottles and that each autoclave cycle requires 2 hr from heat up to cool down. A total of 10 autoclave loads are required to sterilize the batch resulting in a total of 18 hr prior to the last load.

Elapsed time now totals 23 1/3 hr. The two options available to control elapsed time to an assumed 16-hr maximum are either to reduce the size of the batch or to increase the capacity or number of autoclaves to permit the production of additional batches during a workday and target for maximum utilization of the plant capacity and productivity of the work force. Thus all sequences of the element in production are interrelated and must be integrated to ensure control and compliance with the specified lapsed time. All production that exceeds this specified time must be discarded. This becomes an expensive proposition.

Another concern is that the raw materials used in the manufacture of a LVP are not free of particulate matter. Fibers, lint, metal, glass, paper, cardboard, plastic, and a miscellany of airborn dirt and dust particles may be present. These particles are now in the liquid bulk preparation and should be eliminated at this point in the manufacturing sequence by appropriate filtration before pumping the bulk product through the remaining processing equipment and lines enroute to the filling machine.

V. FILTRATION

Filtration may be defined as the separation of undissolved particles from a liquid by passing a solution through a septum or porous medium that allows the liquid to pass but retains the particles. Gases may be filtered using a similar procedure. Filtering gases is relevant to the production of LVPs when considering filters used as controller air vents.

The filtration of liquids is one of the most important operations in pharmaceutical technology. Originally, liquid products were filtered to improve their clarity and pharmaceutical elegance. Pharmaceutical elegance remains as important as ever, but in the case of LVP solutions, products are filtered to remove as much particulate matter at defined size ranges as possible. In general terms, a solution is filtered to remove:

1. Visible particles (50 μm and larger in diameter or length)
2. Invisible particles (less than 50 μm to approximately 1 μm) that contribute to the overall particulate burden and reduce the optical "brightness" or "sparkle" of the product
3. Particles as small as 0.2 μm, which includes the bioburden of fungi and bacteria

Filtration is not an absolute process by which all particles above a specified size can be totally removed. Nevertheless, it is realistic to anticipate that particle burden can be considerably reduced within specified size ranges. Tests are specified in both the United States Pharmacopeia and the British Pharmacopoeia to limit the particulate burden in LVP solutions to less than 50 per milliliter at 10 μm and 5 per milliliter at 25 μm, or 1000 per milliliter at 2.0 μm, and 100 per milliliter at 5 μm, respectively. These limits apply to the products through their expiration dates. In practice it is usually possible to reduce the counts in solutions by filtration initially to levels well below the official limits. Particle counts increase on packaging and often during storage of the product.

Filtration through the appropriate medium will remove bacteria, and a product may be sterilized during the process. A 0.2 μm, porous membrane filter, for example, is theoretically capable of retaining all bacteria. However, membrane filtration may not be totally reliable as a sterilization process. Filtration sterilization is used for thermally labile materials, but the main use of filtration of LVP solutions at the 1.0 μm level or less is to remove the majority of particulate matter and many viable microorganisms. By reducing the bioburden to low levels, the statistical probability of a heat sterilization process being successfully carried out is considerably enhanced. This is consistent with current concepts which recognize that thermal sterilization is not an absolute process. Sterilization can be regarded as an operation in which the chances of viable organisms surviving are reduced to levels where there is unlikely to be growth in any container in the batch. From this consideration it follows that the lower the initial bacterial count in a solution immediately prior to heat sterilization, the better the probability of achieving true sterilization and producing a solution completely free of viable organisms.

Although filtration in the submicrometer range removes viable microorganisms from a solution, there are few filtration processes that remove viruses (except, possibly, the larger adenoviruses). This is unlikely to be important when considering most LVP solutions, but becomes a consideration when dealing with proteinaceous or other solutions that can support viral growth. If a virus may be present and must be removed, considerable care must be taken in the selection of the filtration medium as well as the method of validation. Basically, the smaller the particle, the more difficult it is to remove from a liquid. The filtration processes themselves are by no means simple and have not been worked out theoretically in all their complexities. However, broad principles have been established that are useful in understanding the process as a whole.

A. Classification of Filtration Operations

The separation of suspended solids from liquids by filtration can be divided into three basic mechanisms: screen filtration, depth filtration, and cake filtration. These categories are by no means rigid. Separation by one process also may involve other mechanisms.

1. Screen Filters

A screen (or sieve) filter can be visualized as a plate with holes in it. These holes enable particles with dimensions larger than the holes to be retained on the surface. Instead of a plate, a woven sieve can also be used. The passage of fluid through the filter causes it to become less efficient as larger particles block the pores and reduce the flow.

2. Depth Filters

Depth filters are frequently used when small quantities of suspended matter must be removed from large volumes of liquid. The filtration medium consists of fibers or granular particulate solids arranged in a bed that allows the liquid to pass through. The path the liquid takes should be large in comparison to the size of the particles to be removed from the liquid. The particles are much smaller than the interstices between the fibers or granules of the filter bed so that they are not removed by straining or screening. The particles are trapped by gravitational, hydrodynamic, or electrical forces that are acting in the environment of the bed or, more likely, by a combination of these forces. A particle requires sufficient time of contact with the bed to leave the main stream of the liquid flowing through the bed and approach close enough to the solid granules or fibers to be captured by van der Waals forces at the surfaces. This type of particle/solid interaction is very complex and the theoretical analysis of a given system may often become somewhat unprecise.

Filters using depth filtration principles are widely used for "roughing" or prefiltering pharmaceutical solutions. Such filters remove most but not necessarily all of the particulate burden before terminal filtration in a final or polishing filter. Prefilters are almost invariably required when using membrane filters, especially if the membrane has an average pore diameter below 1 μm. Depth filters are often made from compressed fibers such as cellulose, cotton, or wool. More recently glass, metal or carbon fibers have been used. Ceramic filters made from unglazed porcelain have been used for manufacturing pharmaceutical solutions for over 100 years, but the preparation of drinking water by passage of water through pottery vessels dates back to ancient times. Sintered beds made by heating metal or glass powders until the particles just begin to fuse or sinter together have also been employed. Characteristics of screen and depth filters are compared in Figure 7.

3. Cake Filters

A filter consisting of a coarse woven cloth may be ineffectual because the holes in the cloth are likely to be much larger than the particles to be removed from the suspension. However, if the cloth is presented with a concentrated suspension of rigid particles that bridge the holes and form a bed on the upstream side of the cloth, the particles will be held back while the liquid passes through the small interstices that are formed. The properties of the filter bed or cake are dependent on the shape and size of the rigid particles from which it is made. For example, one of the most useful filter cakes can be made from diatomite that consists of irregularly shaped particles of around 100 μm diameter. A cake made from a suspension of diatomite removes submicrometer colloid particles with high efficiency from a product that is passed through the bed.

B. Theories of Filtration

The mechanisms that have been discussed are by no means exclusive and it is likely that several different mechanisms operate within any one type of filter. The various theories of filtration are often qualitative explanations and are rarely quantitative. The concepts are useful and enable empirical relationships to be drawn. The simplest model considers a packed bed of powder, granules, or fibers as a bundle of

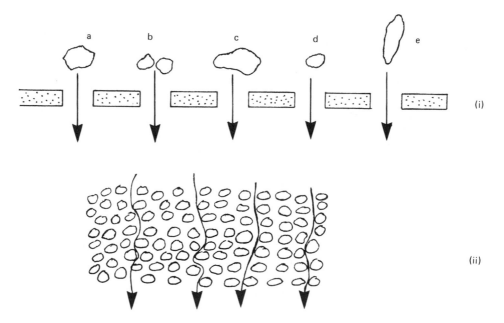

Figure 7 Screen and depth filters. (i) Screen filter with direct passage of the car-rier liquid: (a) particle too large to pass; (b) two (or more) smaller particles forming a bridge; (c) particle too large for aperture; (d) particle passing screen; (e) elongated particle capable of passing end-on. (ii) A depth filter illustrates a greater thickness and a more tortuous liquid pathway.

parallel capillaries. The basic rate equation for fluid flow through this type of sys-tem is derived by analogy with the flow of heat and is applicable to all types of filters:

$$\text{Rate} = \frac{\text{driving force}}{\text{resistance}}$$

The rate of filtration can be measured as the volume (or mass) of fluid passing through the filter in a unit of time (i.e., dv/dt). The driving force is the difference in pressure measured upstream and downstream of the filter. However, the filtra-tion process is not in a steady state because its resistance to flow increases with time as deposits of suspended solids are built up on the surface of the separating medium and by changes within the deposit as the fluid pressure compresses it. The resistance to fluid movement offered by a clean filtration cloth is only a fraction of that offered by a cloth in which most of the pores have been plugged by particles in the suspension. Nevertheless, the latter system is the more effective separation medium (Fig. 8).

Resistance to flow (R) is related to the viscosity of the liquid (η), the thickness of the porous medium (L), the area of the cake (A) in the direction normal to the liquid flow, and a property of the cake called the permeability (K). This relation-ship is shown in the equation

$$R = \frac{\eta L}{KA}$$

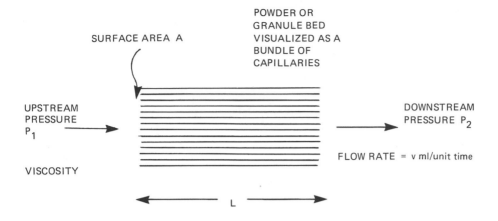

Figure 8 Resistance to flow through a filter bed.

If the flow rate is considered in terms of the familiar Hagen-Poiseuille relationship derived for a bundle of capillaries the flow rate becomes

$$\frac{dv}{dt} = \frac{Nd^4}{128\eta} \frac{dp}{dL}$$

where N is the number of capillaries of diameter d and dp/dL is the pressure drop across the bed. The permeability K depends in turn on characteristics of the cake such as the porosity, specific surface area, and the compressibility. Permeability may be defined quantitatively as the flow rate of a liquid of unit viscosity across a unit area of cake thickness under pressure gradient of unity. This is usually known as Darcy's law and is written as

$$K = \frac{L}{A(\Delta p)} \frac{dv}{dt}$$

where Δp is the pressure difference and v is the volume of liquid passing in time t.

      This simplified model enables the importance of viscosity on the filtration rate to be appreciated. In a practical situation the filtration rate of a high concentration of dextrose could be increased by heating the solution to decrease its viscosity. At its best, this and other models are empirical. There is a clear need for more information on the geometry of bed packing and a better understanding of the effect of pressure on the rate of buildup of deposit and the subsequent structure. The model obviously relates to filter beds or cakes but also applies to other types of depth filters. Thin membrane filters behave in a slightly different way and will be considered in a later section.

Simple models are usually inadequate to explain all variables encountered in practice. Other factors that may be influential in controlling flow rates through filters are:

1. Swelling of the filter medium by the solvent
2. Compressibility of the filter medium under pressure
3. Size and size distribution of the suspended particles
4. Tendency of the particles to flocculate or adhere together
5. Effective or relative viscosity of the suspension
6. Temperature of the suspension
7. Rate at which the filter cake is formed, especially in the early stages of the process

A simple straining or sieving process does not provide a complete description of how particles are removed from suspension. A particle passing through a bed of granules or powder is exposed to a number of forces, including gravity or electrical fields. In addition, there are drag forces, diffusional forces, and inertial forces that depend on the mass and the acceleration of the particle. A particle must be captured by the filtration medium, and this involves the short-range electrical forces at the solid surface. A particle may not actually have to strike the surface to be captured, but it must move close enough to encounter the surface forces. This means that the particle must cross the fluid streamlines that move around the solid surface of the filtration medium.

Depending to some extent on the particle density, it is likely that particles with diameters larger than 20 μm will cross fluid streamlines by inertial and gravitational forces, whereas particles with diameters of less than 1 μm will diffuse by Brownian movement. This is illustrated in Figure 9. If a filter bed is deep enough, submicrometer particles will inevitably be captured which may account for the use of sand beds to filter out bacteria and viruses. Electrolytes or surface-active materials in the solution will affect the magnitude of the charge on either or both the opposing surfaces, thereby affecting capture efficiency.

C. Advantages and Disadvantages of Screen and Depth Filters

Fibers or sintered materials collect suspended particles passed through them throughout their depth. The porous structures are neither regular nor strictly definable. The efficiency of particle retention depends on the flow rate, the fluid viscosity, the type and quantity of contaminant, and the complexity of the spatial arrangements within the filter matrix. In practice, these factors can be determined only by empirical observation of the filtration process. For example, an increase in thickness of the filter increases the resistance to flow but results in an increased capacity for particulate collection before becoming saturated. Depth filters collect particles that are much smaller than the pore through which the fluid passes. This means that characterization of the pores of the filter matrix bears little relationship to the likely performance of the filter when exposed to a particulate suspension.

On the other hand, a screen filter has its efficiency defined in terms of the mean or maximum pore size. These parameters may be measured by some related physical property such as the pressure required to force an air bubble through the wetted filter under standardized conditions. Assuming that it acts as a screen, any suspended material larger than the largest pore in the filter structure will be retained on the upper surface. Screen filters such as the cellulose membrane type have a much lower load capacity than depth filters and offer an increasing resistance

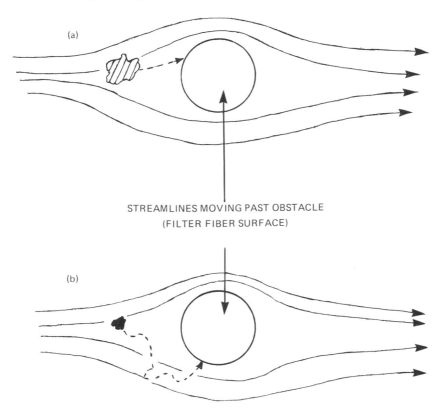

STREAMLINES MOVING PAST OBSTACLE
(FILTER FIBER SURFACE)

Figure 9 Particle capture by a screen or filter surface. (a) The particle is heavy
enough to be carried across streamlines moving around the surface by inertia.
(b) The particle is too small to cross streamlines by inertial forces, but Brownian
movement results in a collision with the surface.

to fluid flow as progressive plugging occurs. Because the pores do not interconnect
to any marked extent, very little lateral diffusion occurs within a screen filter.
Screen filters lack mechanical strength and must be supported by sintered glass
beds, polymeric matrices, or stainless steel mesh in order to provide a large
enough surface area beneath the filter. Special edge clamps are also required to
prevent bypassing of the filter. Because the screen filters are thin, the clamps
require engineering to much finer tolerances than those required for the compressible and thicker depth filters made of fibrous material. The special requirements
result in much higher costs for the ancillary equipment used with screen or membrane filters.
     Many of the features of screen and depth filters are complementary. For ex-
ample, a depth filter has a high capacity but is less predictable in terms of the size
of particle retained. A screen filter, on the other hand, has a lower capacity but
is more predictable, to the point where it can be relied upon to remove most particles larger than a specified size. To obtain the maximum filtration effectiveness,
it is possible to design systems in which most particles are removed by a depth
filter. This is then followed downstream by a final or polishing screen filter that
removes the remaining particles. Although adding to the cost, a prefilter usually
enhances the performance of a filtration system. The choice of filter combination

is made from a knowledge of the characteristics of the particulate material and the requirements in terms of end product usage, flow rate, and acceptable pressure differentials.

D. Ideal Filter Criteria

To some extent, the criteria selected for the definition of an ideal filter depends on the nature of the product to be filtered. When considering large volume parenteral solutions, it is possible to draw up a list of desirable characteristics.

1. A filter should be "absolute" in that there should be a known limit to the size of particles passing through into the filtrate.
2. There should be a means of independently checking the efficiency of the filter.
3. The filtration process should not be materially affected by the pressure differential.
4. The filtration medium should not interfere with the product being filtered, and should not impart toxic or pyrogenic substances or particles to the solution.
5. The filtration system should be sterilizable by heat, radiation, or gas.
6. The filtration process should be economical. The unit cost of the process should not contribute significantly to the overall cost of the final product.

E. Utilization of Filters

Difficulties can arise when attempting to filter suspensoids that either have properties of colloids or particles that are shaped in such a way that they form a readily compressible cake. It is common practice outside the pharmaceutical area to pretreat the system to change the nature of the suspensoid and help make it more readily filterable. This practice is less favored in the pharmaceutical industry because the products concerned are such that manipulations are not always possible. If a solution can be more easily filtered by a pH adjustment that changes the colloidal nature of a precipitate without damaging that product, or if a filter aid such as charcoal can be added to remove small amounts of colored materials from a dextrose solution, pretreatment is obviously beneficial. Other forms of pretreatment involve the heat coagulation of finely divided proteinaceous precipitates or the addition of filter aids such as paper pulp, talcum powder, bentonite, or diatomaceous earths. Each of these additives has the characteristic of forming open porous structures as an incompressible cake on the filter surface. In effect, filter aids act by forming an alternative filtration bed to provide additional depth or cake characteristics. Filter aids can be regarded as being inert, but in reality are often the source of trace contaminants such as soluble iron salts, which can provoke degradation reactions in sensitive products. Some medicants such as alkaloids are adsorbed by the solid. Another disadvantage of filter aids is that liquid is retained in the pores of the filter cake and lost in the manufacturing process. Should the filtered pharmaceutical product be expensive, the material lost may form an appreciable part of the overall cost of the operation. This is less likely for LVP solutions that in the main are simple solutions of salts or sugars. In this situation, an appropriate filter-aid system is often useful.

1. Choice of Filtration Medium

There is no ideal filtration medium for all purposes. However, there are a variety of media from which to choose. Some of the filters currently available to a producer of LVP solutions include:

Cellulose papers
Glass fibers
Sintered glass
Sintered metal
Sintered plastic
Unglazed porcelain
Sintered silver membranes
Cellulose ester membranes

Cellulose fiber and glass fiber papers have been in use for many years. They are inexpensive and may be employed as roughing filters or as supports for filter beds made of diatomaceous earth. However, solutions passed through a fibrous filter should have at least one further filtration through a nonfibrous medium.

Standard glass, metal, or plastic filters are used for roughing filtration or as supports for membrane filters. These types of filters have advantages since they are made from closely controlled sizes of classified spherical particles. This enables manufacturers to produce filter materials with pore sizes suitable for specific purposes such as clarification or sterilization. Metal filters made from sinters or fibers are usually employed for filtration of steam to remove particulates such as rust and scale, inevitably present in a boiler. Bacterial growth may occur inside sintered filters, but silver has a natural antibacterial activity. Silver sintered filters are thin and may be reused, which reduces the use cost of these materials.

Unglazed porcelain filters were first employed by Louis Pasteur as a bacterial filtration medium and are still employed in some processes. Porcelain candles are reusable but become chipped on cleaning so that the performance on reuse deteriorates. Disposable microporous porcelain tubes have been introduced (Selas Corporation), although the thin walls of the tube limit their application as depth filters.

Hollow fiber filters have been introduced in recent years that are physically smaller versions of a filter candle but made of cellulose or similar material. Hollow fibers have the advantage of a vast surface area for filtration for a relatively small volume of container and will undoubtedly be more widely employed in the future.

2. Membrane Filters

Described as the biggest single advance in sterile filtration technology, the introduction of cellulose membrane filters on a large scale produced a considerable change in the filtration of LVP solutions. The concept was described by Zigmondy during World War I. Sartorius sold membranes in Germany in the 1930s. However, the commercial development that followed after World War II introduced membrane filtration technology on a large scale. Currently, similar filters and filtration technology are available from a number of competitive suppliers.

Preparation of a Membrane Filter. The most common membrane filter is a thin, three-dimensional, porous system made of cellulose ester material. The esters are usually nitrates or acetates but membranes also have been made from rayon, cellulose, nylon, polyvinyl chloride, polypropylene, and even gelatin. A general method of production of cellulose nitrate filters involves gelling cellulose in a mixture of methyl acetate, ethanol, water, and glycerin, often with a suitable wetting agent such as Triton. The gelled mass is poured as a thin layer and the volatile solvent allowed to evaporate under carefully controlled conditions. As the solvent evaporates, spherical droplets of the cellulose come together to form aggregates, eventually drying as a continuous vacuolated structure. The size of the pores is controlled by the environmental conditions during production and the mixing process. The glycerol provides flexibility and aids in forming the pores but is washed out during the manufacturing process, as is most of the wetting agent, if it is added.

The detailed structure of a membrane filter has been demonstrated by scanning electron microscopy. The pore structure (Figure 10) shows large and small pores interconnected with each other. By taking sections through a membrane a progressive increase in pore diameter can be seen moving from the top to the bottom of the matrix. The key factor in filtration performance is the size of the largest pore. However, pore size is not the only factor because it is known that membrane filters also have some depth (i.e., adsorption characteristics). Small particles may therefore be held at pore surfaces by electrostatic bonding. Because membranes are relatively thin, there is little room for lateral communication between pores. Principal movement of fluid is from the front to the back; in that sense, the screen model of membrane filtration is realistic.

Etched Track Membranes. Unlike cellulose and other plastic membranes, etched track polycarbonate membranes do approximate a two-dimensional screen filter reasonably well. Originally, these filters (Nuclepore Corporation) were prepared by holding 5 or 10 μm thick sheets of polycarbonate in contact with sheets of uranium metal bombarded by thermal neutrons in a nuclear reactor. Fission products from the ^{235}U passing through the film leaves tracks of damaged polycarbonate, which can be dissolved with aqueous sodium hydroxide. This leaves uniform cylindrical holes through the film. The density and number of holes per unit area is controlled by the contact time in the reactor, and the size of the holes is controlled by the etching conditions, in particular the length of time the sheet is left in the caustic solution. By careful collimation it is possible to ensure that the holes or pores pass vertically through the surface. However, the tracks are not truly parallel. This is fortunate since two or more pores sometimes appear to overlap at the surface or a pore appears to be larger than the normal size. In fact, detailed examination shows that overlapping pores actually diverge from the overlapping point and make individual contributions to the filtration process (see Figure 11). Being made from polycarbonate, the membranes are flexible, strong, and not easily broken. The membranes are soluble in alkaline solutions but have the inherent chemical resistance of the parent plastic. They are also transparent and nonhygroscopic. The flow rate of liquids through etched membranes is similar to that through the corresponding cellulose membrane because although the etched membranes have fewer pores, they are thinner. Like other membranes, they clog but, in some applications, the increased strength of etched membranes enables material collected on the surface to be removed by applying a reverse flow. This allows an assembled filtration system using an etched membrane to be used for a longer time.

F. Testing and Validation of Filters

With the exception of the filter used to sterilize a liquid product terminally, the efficiency of a filtration process is rarely critical. Two types of tests may be employed: first, a direct challenge of a filter to ensure that it has the appropriate performance claimed for it, and second, a test that gives reasonable assurance to the user that a filter has the desired performance in actual use.

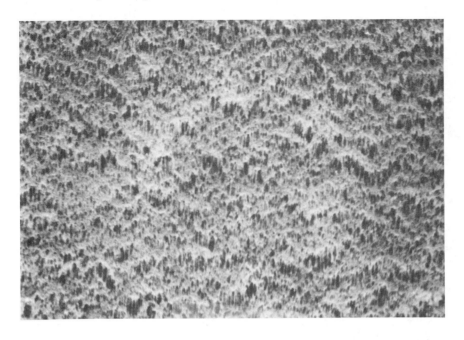

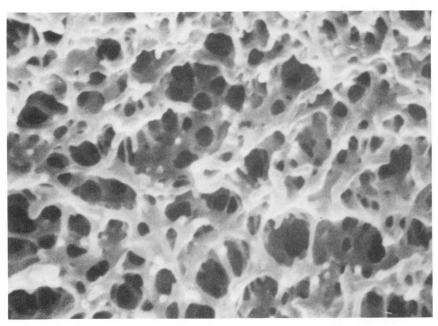

Figure 10 Surface (upper) and magnified cross section (lower) of Accurel 0.2 μm polypropylene filter. (Courtesy of Membrana, Inc., GHIA Division, Pleasanton, California.)

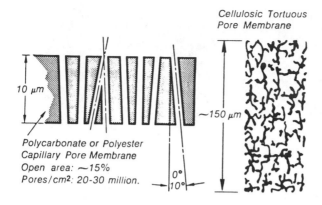

Figure 11 Cross-sectional comparison of Nuclepore capillary pore membrane and cellulosic tortuous pore filter thickness. (Courtesy of Nuclepore Corporation, Inc., Pleasanton, California.)

Because the major critical application of filters is the removal of viable bacteria from a solution, bacterial challenge tests are widely used by filter manufacturers. The passage test consists of filtering a culture of a suitable test organism in a liquid growth medium and incubating the filtrate to determine if any viable organism passed the filter. The usual test organism is <u>Bacillus subtilis</u>, because it is representative of a common small microorganism. However, <u>Chromobacterium prodigiosum</u> is preferred because the cells are smaller with a diameter of approximately 0.7 μm, and the colonies are a bright red color, which aids in identification. <u>Pseudomonas diminuta</u> is also a favored test microorganism, ellipsoidal in shape (0.75 to 1.0 μm long and as narrow as 0.25 μm in diameter). However, the actual size changes with the nutritional state of the organism and is influenced by the growth medium and incubation conditions.

Wallhauser [2] demonstrated that a nominal 0.2 μm pore-sized membrane filter could pass <u>P. diminuta</u> cells in direct relation to the challenge. Because such filters previously had been regarded as absolute in sterilization, this demonstration prompted a reevaluation of the concepts and the test methods. Reti and Leahy [3] discussed the background to a suitable validation protocol and suggested the following as being key factors influencing the performance of any test:

1. The test organism itself, and maintenance of the culture
2. Organism size and state of aggregation
3. Concentration/total challenge level in terms of number per unit volume
4. Effective concentration, viability after the challenge, and downstream sample size
5. The hydraulic challenge conditions, especially the pressure across the membrane, and any flexion caused by pulsing
6. The duration of the test

The complexity of the interrelationships between factors that affect the passage of this microorganism through a membrane means that the validation of such filters as sterilizing media is a difficult process. Wallhaus filtered large volumes of naturally contaminated water, not culture media. In any situation designed to mimic an actual requirement, it is better to use a medium that is closest to the production solution. It is obvious that microbial challenge tests are not useful as process integrity tests to ensure that a filter, and its related supporting equipment, is free of pinholes or breaks because the test organism would contaminate the system and, possibly, even the work environment.

The most common form of in-use integrity testing is the bubble point test. This consists of applying gas pressure to the upstream side of a wetted filter to determine the minimum pressure required to force bubbles of gas through the wetted filter. This test measures the size of the largest effective pores in the filter but also provides a useful safeguard against leaks in the filtration system as a whole (Fig. 12).

If the gas pressure is allowed to build up slowly until there is a slow steady stream of bubbles, the maximum effective pore diameter d is given by

$$d = 4\sigma \frac{\cos \theta}{P}$$

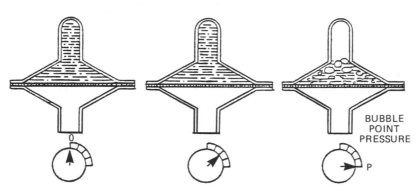

WHEN THE AIR PRESSURE AGAINST A WET MEMBRANE FILTER IS INCREASED, THE PRESSURE AT WHICH THE LARGEST PORE BEGINS TO PASS AIR IS THE BUBBLE POINT.

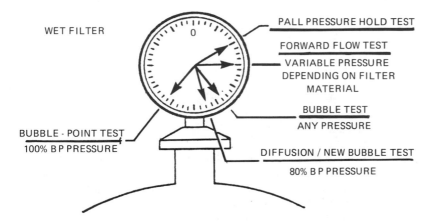

Figure 12 Filter pressure tests. [From J. Parenter. Drug Assoc., 33:273 (1979); by permission of the Directors of the Parenteral Drug Association.]

where

P = minimum displacing pressure
σ = surface tenison of the liquid used in the test
θ = angle of wetting of the solid surface by the liquid

This equation has been shown to be applicable to a number of different-shaped holes punched into plastic or aluminum sheet, the first continuous passage always occurring through the pore with the largest size. When different liquids were used, different maximum pore sizes were calculated, demonstrating the importance of the wetting action of the liquid. For most filtration media, water is satisfactory as a test vehicle unless a hydrophobic filter is involved, in which case a wetting agent must be added to the water.

Problems with the bubble point test began to appear when the large industrial type of membrane filters came into use, particularly in cartridge form. Bubbles could be produced at pressures well below the anticipated bubble point. This was found to be due to gas dissolving in the liquid-filled pores, diffusing through the filter and coming out of solution on the side where the pressure is lower. Essentially, the test measures the volume of air that diffuses through water-filled pores in a given time under standardized pressure.

The new diffusion test is carried out on nonsterile filters in the manner illustrated in the lower part of Figure 12. For a sterile assembly, two alternative methods are suggested. The first uses a soap film flowmeter to measure the flow rate through the filter. The second method uses an automatic diffusion tester. This is simply an electronic digital flowmeter that determines the rate of flow.

At best, these various tests indicate that the filtration system is in place correctly without any gross imperfections, pinholes, or punctures. There is as yet no certain correlation between the bubble test or the flow rate tests and the likelihood of bacterial passage.

G. Advantages of Membrane Filters

From the point of view of an LVP manufacturer, membrane filters, including etched track membranes, do have a number of advantages over the older depth and cake filters and filtration systems. These advantages include:

1. Efficiency (defined by a mean pore size) is nearly absolute.
2. The filtration media are nonhygroscopic.
3. Particles are captured mostly on the upper surface of the filter or at least within a thin upper surface layer.
4. Pores are slowly clogged and, especially with etched track membranes, may be cleared by back-flushing.
5. Most membranes have a considerable thermal stability and may be sterilized by wet heat before use.
6. Most membranes have considerable mechanical strength, provided that they are adequately supported. This allows high pressures to be applied across them.
7. Membranes are resistant to many acids or bases as well as organic solvents.
8. Unlike paper filters, membranes have low ash values, very high wet strength, and may often be easily rendered transparent, properties that are useful for a number of analytical procedures.
9. Because the particles are essentially collected by a sieving mechanism, there is less danger of solids being forced through the filter by pressure fluctuations during pumping operations.

10. The membrane matrix material is generally considered to be biologically in-
    ert. Thus, even if fragments are detached into a final product, this does not
    represent a biological hazard.

Membrane filters do have some drawbacks. The method of manufacture and the
thinness of the membranes require high engineering quality standards in the ancillary support equipment. This means that there is a relatively high initial capital
expenditure with appreciable production costs. The filters have limited capacity so
that to remove all but the finest particles from a solution a system of prefilters and
backing filters is essential. When setting up a filtration system, great care is required, because most of the cellulosic membrane filters lack dry strength and are
easily damaged. For this reason it is generally advisable to carry out some form
of integrity testing on the assembled filtration system before carrying out a critical
operation.

H. Membrane Support Systems

Membranes of all types are prepared in sheets and manipulated according to whether
or not the material is brittle in the dry state. One common form of membrane filter
is a flat disk mounted on a perforated metal plate or sintered glass disk for support.
The disks vary from 13 to 293 mm in diameter and are held in place with annular
disks or O-rings at the edges. Because prefilters are also usually required, a disk
membrane filter is often mounted with appropriate prefilters cut to the same diameter and separated from the membrane by plastic grids or meshes. A typical
142-mm filter holder is illustrated in Figure 13. This is suitable for batch sizes
up to approximately 100 liters.

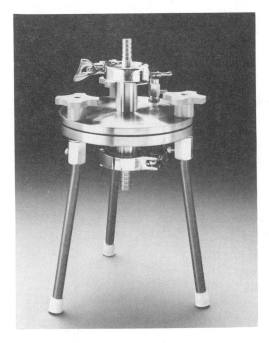

Figure 13 Typical 142 mm industrial membrane filter holder. (Courtesy of Millipore Corporation, Bedford, Massachusetts.)

Membrane disks also may be stacked together to increase the surface area and improve the flow volume. Stacking also enables a solution to be passed through a sequence of membranes of decreasing pore size to improve efficiency. However, the capacity of disks is limited and large volumes above 400 liters are passed through filter cartridges. Filter cartridges are now the main filtration configuration used because they have a much higher capacity. In the case of the brittle cellulosic membranes, these are made from strips of medium wound around a porous core. Other membrane cartridge filters may be made from flexible materials such as acrylonitrile-polyvinyl chloride copolymer. In this case, advantage is taken of the flexibility to pleat the membrane to increase the surface area (Fig. 14).

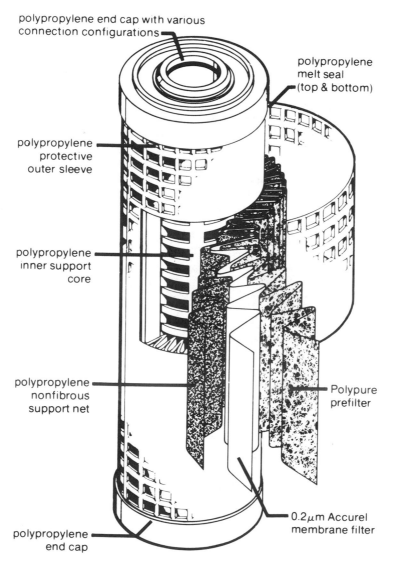

polypropylene end cap with various connection configurations

polypropylene melt seal (top & bottom)

polypropylene protective outer sleeve

polypropylene inner support core

polypropylene nonfibrous support net

Polypure prefilter

polypropylene end cap

0.2 μm Accurel membrane filter

Figure 14 Accurel cartridge filter showing construction. (Courtesy of Membrana, Inc., GHIA Division, Pleasanton, California.)

Cartridge filters come in a wide variety of sizes, types, and configurations, and may be connected in series or in parallel. The assemblies also may be supplied by the manufacturer in a sterile condition. Some cartridges are also disposable. Connections are made with appropriate accessories. A difficulty at present is that a number of manufacturers provide the components but these are generally not interchangeable between suppliers. However, in some cases, adaptors and accessories can be used to enable mixed systems to be assembled.

Because the success or failure of a batch may be critically affected by a single filter failing, a practice generally used by manufacturers is to pass the solution through two or more filters in series (i.e., redundant filtration). Each filter is individually checked for integrity so that the chance of a batch being rejected because a filter has failed is considerably reduced. Economically, this procedure does not materially increase the cost of processing a batch of solution.

VI. CLEANING PROCESS EQUIPMENT AND LINES

A. Water Systems

The drug substances, water, and the environment in a manufacturing facility are not sterile. Although filtration technology continues to improve and is employed for the removal of particulate matter, filtration alone cannot be depended on or resorted to for the control of microorganisms (bioburden) in the product or intermediate stages of its processing. Other measures must be employed and these are primarily directed to the water.

Target microbial limits should be imposed on the source water entering the plant, whether from a municipal supply or a private well. Limits of approximately 50 colonies per milliliter with no coliforms are common. Microbial quality should be monitored as this water is processed through the appropriate stages: filter beds, water softeners, carbon filters, deionizers, reverse osmosis, and compression stills. The target limits may vary but water for cleaning or initial rinsing may be set in the neighborhood of not more than 50 organisms per 100 ml while final rinsing and product water may have limits in the order of 10 organisms per 100 ml.

Growth of microorganisms is suppressed by recirculating the water hot (80°C) through the water system. Free-flowing steam can also be employed and is a more effective sanitizing agent, but it is more hazardous to the plant personnel and increases the relative humidity of the work environment if not adequately confined. Protective equipment and training to avoid burns from hot equipment or direct steam exposure should be provided to employees. Care should be taken to ensure that the steam is free-flowing. Air pockets can occur in complex equipment and piping systems, which can obstruct the free flow of the steam and result in incomplete sanitization.

Microbial plate counts of the water should be performed on a regular basis during its various phases of treatment. Product water should be tested daily. The coliform bacteria (Escherichia species) in the raw water entering the plant are of concern as they are indicators of the level of sanitation. Other waterborne organisms that can proliferate in deionized and distilled water are the gram-negative organisms, particularly from the species Pseudomonas, Xanthomonas, and Flavobacterium. Organisms from all of these species are quite easily destroyed by autoclaving. However, although they are viable, they give rise to endotoxins (lipopolysaccharides). Endotoxins are the fever-causing agents (pyrogens) in an LVP, which may be modified by heating in an autoclave but are not destroyed. Thus it is possible to have a sterile preparation that is pyrogenic. Endotoxin levels of about 150 pg ml^{-1} may induce a pyrogenic response.

Sanitation programs are designed to ensure a reduced microbial load and greater assurance that the final product will be sterile and nonpyrogenic. Lines, valves, and gaskets should not be ignored as foci for microorganisms. On a periodic basis, as dictated by plate counts and plant experiences, these component parts should be disassembled. Preferably, Water for Injection storage and distribution systems should be closed systems made with continuous stainless steel pipe. High counts can be brought into control by treatment with alkaline sanitizing chemicals (sodium hypochlorite or special organic chlorocompounds) followed by mild detergents. Anionic detergents (e.g., sodium alkyllauryl sulfonates) are preferred, for they do not leave residue. Most of the commercial detergent formulations contain alkaline agents or alkaline bulking agents (sodium tripolyphosphate, trisodium phosphate, sodium metasilicate, and the like). For this reason calcium hypochlorite should be avoided to prevent the formation of insoluble calcium salts with these complex anions. All parts should be thoroughly rinsed and inspected before reassembly.

After any interruption in production exceeding 1 day, the system should be recommissioned. It should be thoroughly flushed to overflow conditions with deionized water. All outlets should be opened for a period of time. After this initial flushing, the system should be inspected to ensure absence of leaks. When this sequence is complete, the system should be drained, secured, and the flushing operation repeated with distilled water. Water samples can be monitored by pH and conductivity to ensure removal of all chemical residues. Following this, the system should be sanitized by recirculating hot water or free-flowing steam as previously described. Confirmation of the adequacy of cleaning and sanitization can be made by plate counts made from water samples taken at strategic locations in the system.

Thorough and complete records should be maintained on the frequency and adequacy of the cleaning program. The record should include who performed and supervised the cleaning, date, cleaning agents employed, pH, conductivity, and plate counts. It should be emphasized that pH and conductivity are indirect but instant and necessary monitors for water quality. Plate counts require 24 to 72 hr of incubation for colonies to develop.

B. Mixing and Filling Equipment

The water system carries only Water for Injection and the primary concern is the suppression of microorganisms by cleaning and sanitization as previously described. However, mixing tanks, lines, filter housings, and filling equipment may be employed to produce a variety of products over a given period of time. Therefore, care must be exercised to avoid between-batch contamination. Fortunately, with the exception of fat emulsion, most products are clear aqueous solutions and copious flushing with Water for Injection can be employed between batches of product to avoid between-batch contamination. If the products between batches are qualitatively and quantitatively dissimilar, it may be necessary to disassemble the filter housing.

C. Production Planning

Intelligent production planning can minimize the risk of between-batch contamination, reduce the extent of flushing required, and reduce the need to tear down the filter housings. One way this can be accomplished is to start with the simpler product first and gradually process those that are more complex. An example of this approach is to schedule the following products in the sequences indicated: 0.9% sodium chloride, 0.9% sodium chloride with 40 mEq of potassium chloride, followed by 5% dextrose in 0.9% sodium chloride with 40 mEq of potassium chloride. Another scheme would be to schedule products with a concentration gradient from the lesser to the greater concentration. An example of this approach would be to schedule the following products in the sequence indicated: 2.5%, 5%, 10%, and 20% dextrose. Obviously, compositions from the simple to complex and concentration gradients can also be employed in production scheduling.

D. Cleaning and Sanitization

In all instances, at the end of the production day, all equipment is routinely dismantled. Filter housings and filling machines are disassembled. Tanks, pipes, valves, filters, and filling machines are thoroughly rinsed with tap or distilled water. Hot water may be employed to ensure removal particularly of those product residues that avidly support microbial growth (e.g., carbohydrates and amino acids). All parts are cleaned by the cleaning and sanitizing agents previously described. Pipes should be cleaned by brushes of a length adequate to traverse the entire length. Metal parts of brushes should be protected with plastic tubing to avoid scratching equipment surfaces. Wooden handles are difficult to sanitize, may shed splinters, and should be avoided. Troughs with pumps at the distal end may be employed to permit detergent and rinse water to be circulated at a high velocity through submerged parts (Fig. 15).

 Parts should be cleaned on a routine schedule and at a minimum every 24 hr. Over weekends and holidays the parts may be kept submerged in the cleaning and sanitizing solutions. Before reassembly, the parts must be thoroughly rinsed, and

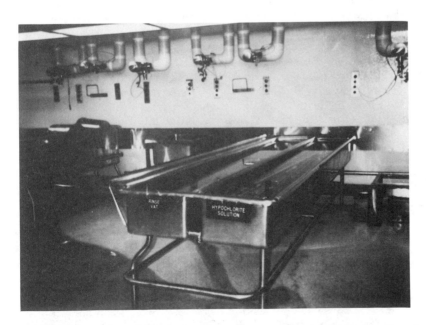

Figure 15 Cleaning troughs. (Courtesy of Travenol Laboratories, Inc., Morton Grove, Illinois.)

after reassembly the system (lines and filling equipment) should be sanitized by circulating hot Water of Injection.

Some installations are designed and constructed in a manner that does not require disassembly. These installations may be cleaned in place (CIP) by the use of high-pressure spray devices within the equipment. A primary design criterion for the CIP facility is minimal occurrence of nooks, crannies, and crevices. Welded, seamless piping that has a minimum of flange connections and valving is important. The sequence of cleaning and sanitizing these CIP installations is as described above.

E. Compressed Gases

Nitrogen, carbon dioxide, and air may be used during the processing of an LVP. Nitrogen is most frequently used to protect a product from air (oxygen) in the bulk stage or in the final container. Carbon dioxide may be employed to displace air or for pH adjustments. Compressed air may be employed to drive equipment, to clean and air-dry parts, and to provide overpressure in an autoclave.

Nitrogen and carbon dioxide are usually of high quality and most often purchased. Compressed air is economically generated in-house and should also be of an assured quality. It must be assumed that all gases will have contact with the solution, equipment, container, closures, and other product contact surfaces. Most compressed gases are discharged into the work environment. Therefore, these compressed gases should be processed so that they will make a very minimum contribution to particulate and microbial loads of the final products. Because the quality of the compressed gases is so important to the ultimate quality of the LVP, it appears appropriate to discuss a compressed air system.

Compressed air is the gas most routinely generated in-house and is the simplest system to describe. The controls exercised on air are equally applicable to the other gases, particularly the requirement for final filtration. Compressed air can be a dirty commodity unless it is generated by a suitably designed and maintained system. Clean compressed air is usually generated by an oil-free compressor. When oiled compressors are employed, adequate preconditioning must be imposed to ensure removal of oil to prescribed and tolerated limits. The air intake to the compressors would have a prefilter to remove large particulate matter and associated microorganisms prior to compression. During the compression phase, temperatures in the range 150 to 160°C are generated for fractions of a second. These are sterilizing conditions for most viable vegetative microorganisms.

After compression, the air is passed through a chiller and a dryer to remove residual moisture. Final treatment may include passage through chemical desiccants. More important, the air is passed through coalescing and microcoalescing filters for more complete removal of oil and moisture. The final treatment is filtration through a 0.22 or 0.45 μm hydrophobic filter system. These systems are usually constructed to withstand steam, hot water, and chemical disinfection and sterilization. Nooks, crannies, and crevices should be kept to a minimum, as these can accumulate oil and water and serve as foci for microbial growth and contamination. Once commissioned, if properly designed and maintained, these systems can stay very clean, almost sterile. The high temperatures and drying conditions are hostile to the vegetative organisms. High airflows are also cleansing. Surviving spores should be very low in number. All this will be realized provided that all filter systems are serviced on a routine basis. No prescribed service schedule can be specified. This must be developed from in-house data on air sampling for particulate matter and plate counts.

VII. CONTAINERS AND CLOSURES

A. Materials

The intent of this discourse is to present briefly the various systems and materials employed as containers and closures for LVPs as background for the handling and cleaning of these items.

Classically, glass containers have been employed for LVPs. Type II glass (sulfur dioxide-treated soda-lime glass) is routinely employed. Type I glass (borosilicate) is much more expensive and is usually reserved for specialty products with a high pH. Glass containers with screw-cap closures are no longer employed as containers for LVPs but are still used as pour containers for irrigation fluids.

Solid or open-hole rubber stoppers are used for the container-closure system. These are molded from either natural or synthetic elastomeric compounds. The open-hole system usually contains an air (vent) tube, which permits equalization of pressure as the fluid is withdrawn and indentations to receive the set spike or to introduce supplementary medication. The open end of the vent tube is sealed by means of a rubber disk, which is removed at time of use. Solid closure systems may be of several varieties. Again one may encounter a closure with an air tube sealed to the atmosphere by the rubber closure with a companion indentation to receive the set spike. A special device is required to open the vent tube. Another version is a closed-hole stopper with a single bull's-eye to receive the spike of the intravenous set. In this instance the spike is specially designed with an air inlet channel which permits introduction of filtered air to equalize the pressure as the liquid is dispensed (Fig. 16).

During this past decade, plastic has made substantial inroads as container materials for use in LVPs. These plastic containers are varied, being semirigid or flexible and fabricated from polyolefin or plasticized polyvinyl chloride. There is more freedom and latitude in design than with glass. Plastic containers may not

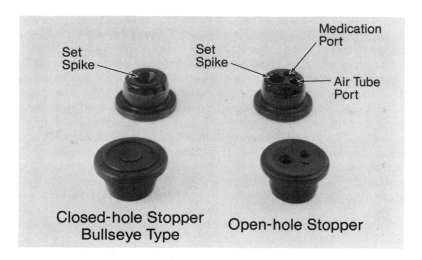

Figure 16 Rubber stoppers. (Courtesy of Travenol Laboratories, Inc., Morton Grove, Illinois.)

require the typical rubber closure. Ports or inlets for the introduction of other medications and for the insertion of the intravenous set spike are integrated into the design.

B. Glass Bottle Handling

Glass is both brittle and fragile. It must be handled with care in the manufacturing operations. The primary concern is not for a bottle that is cleanly broken, although this destroys its physical integrity. This type of broken container can easily be removed from the conveyor line. The greater concern is for glass particles, which may be sprayed around the area contaminating other bottles and be a hazard to the employees. Of further concern is a bottle that is subjected to the more subtle star and chip damage to the lip, neck, thread areas, wall, indented area provided for the band and bail, and the base. This subtle damage is more difficult to detect. If present, it could result in leakage and a nonsterile bottle during the product's shelf life. Every care should be incorporated into the design of the bottle and into bottle-handling procedures to prevent such occurrence. Bottles should not be stacked without suitable supports between layers, and they should not be rammed or banged about. Wet bottles are somewhat more resistant to this subtle damage.

Bottles with such subtle damage may not withstand the internal and external pressures generated in autoclaving. They may implode or explode during sterilization and destroy other units in the autoclave load, leading to a loss of product and a formidable cleanup. Equally serious is the bottle with subtle damage that survives autoclaving. This unit could lose its integrity and allow the introduction of nonsterile air during its commercial life, resulting in a nonsterile unit. Appropriate quality control inspection procedures are required to sort out this kind of product defect.

C. Glass Bottle Washing

There is no single system for washing bottles. The older and most typical procedure was to employ an alkaline (1 to 2% caustic) soaker cycle followed by multiple water rinses, progressing from tap or deionized water to distilled water or Water for Injection. More contemporary systems employ high-pressure water rinses. To conserve energy and costs, potable water is employed at the front nozzles in a conveyor sequence with distilled water reserved for the final nozzles. The final rinse water should be membrane-filtered (0.45 μm) to minimize the introduction of particulate matter into the container.

Most bottles will be new, arriving at the plant in cardboard (corrugated) boxes. To reduce the shedding of particles into the bottles, the cartons should be handled with care and in an inverted position. Discarded bottles from the filling room may be drained, rinsed, rewashed, and used, or recartoned for later use provided that the total elapsed time from initial use is controlled. This is to ensure that microorganisms are not allowed to grow in the nonsterile solutions and contribute to bioburden. Although not a common practice, bottles from a rejected or out-of-date batch have been reused. This may be more routine in countries where glass is both scarce and expensive. Extra care should be taken to ensure that the lips and necks of the bottles are not damaged when removing the outer closure and rubber stopper. Once in-process, the bottles should be expeditiously processed to completion to minimize the bioburden. Hot (65 to 75°C), dilute caustic can be employed to sterilize and depyrogenate if required.

Ordinarily, the liquids employed in the washing and rinsing cycles are at ambient temperature. The one critical control is water pressure; a low-pressure alarm should be present on all water lines. Periodically, the water supply pressure should be lowered by closing down the valves to ensure the pressure alarm is functioning. With the same frequency, the spray nozzles should be inspected visually to ensure that there is no blockage.

D. Rubber Closures

These components differ both in composition and design. Compositions range from natural to synthetic rubbers with a large variety of additives. Designs may range from the simple solid uniform stopper to a complex stopper containing holes, depressions, wells, and undercuts. Both composition and design can influence cleaning approaches. Cleaning of these parts is primarily directed to the removal of surface contamination, including the mold-release agents. Other surface contaminates include rubber particles from the cutting and trimming operations and particles contributed by the packaging and work environment. Harsh conditions, such as autoclaving, elevated dry heat, and strong alkali as a part of cleaning, are to be avoided if possible. Calcium soaps are frequently employed as mold-release agents, and these can be difficult to remove. Dilute isopropyl alcohol or dilute mineral acids (e.g., hydrochloric acid) are effective in removing these calcium soaps but are difficult to routinely employ in the work environment. Hydrochloric acid presents a hazard to the plant personnel, equipment, and environment (floor, drains, etc.).

A generalized scheme for washing rubber closures may be as follows. Parts are cleaned by placing in boiling or nearly boiling water (87 to 100°C) containing a mildly alkaline, anionic detergent. Stainless steel, jacketed kettles with screened overflow capability are preferred. Initial heating should be of 10 to 15 min duration to ensure that temperature of the closure is attained. Water (tap or distilled) is introduced by a bottom inlet to overflow conditions, assuring that the surface debris will be floated away and not deposit on the closures. After overflowing for a period of time (about 5 min) the kettle may then be dumped, refilled, and the cycle repeated as required.

A final step is to fill the kettle with clean water (preferably Water for Injection), heat to 87 to 100°C, and follow by overflow rinsing with Water for Injection. Depending on the part and the thoroughness of the initial washes, it may be necessary to repeat this final rinsing step several times. Washed parts should be protected by transferring them to covered stainless steel or polyethylene tote pans. Stoppers should be maintained wet and used promptly. Dry stoppers may abrade when inserted, generating particulate matter.

Suppliers can share important information relative to composition, mold-release agents, and recommended cleaning procedures. Close relations should be maintained with suppliers.

E. Air Tubes

These air inlet tubes are fabricated of glass or plastic (polyolefin). Like all component parts that have constant product contact, it is prudent to manufacture these tubes in the cleanest environment possible and to protect them adequately during shipping and storage. The tubes are cleaned before use by immersion in a mild anionic detergent. Tubes are thoroughly rinsed by introducing distilled water through a bottom inlet and allowed to overflow. Tubes are inserted into the closure as a subassembly and maintained in a wet condition until inserted into filled units. Because of the concern for bioburden the subassemblies are not stored for use at a future time.

F. Aluminum Caps

Three-piece cap assemblies are most common for LVPs. They are employed to secure the rubber stopper and do not have product contact. Usually, they are not washed but blown dust-free in a suitable work area. Aluminum-lined screw-cap closures are encountered in pour bottle containers. In this application, they represent the primary seal and have product contact. These parts may be washed before use, employing the same procedures used for rubber closures, or blown clean with compressed air.

G. Plastic Containers

Semirigid plastic containers have a physical structure similar to glass, and can be moved by a conveyor system without additional support. This class of bottles is washed and processed in the same manner as glass containers described above. Flexible plastic containers lack sufficient physical rigidity to be transported on conveyor belts through the washing and filling procedures and must be subjected to special handling. Their manufacture should be in a clean environment. Electrostatic cleaning devices have been found helpful in cleaning plastic surfaces. These devices function by neutralizing the electrostatic charges of particles permitting them to be blown or vacuumed away. Good environmental controls should be employed in the area used to fabricate the container to minimize contamination.

   Particle counts should be performed on representative samples of containers on a periodic basis as a measure of the adequacy of the environmental controls. When particle counts exceed established action limits, washing of the containers may be achieved by multiple injections of warm, filtered, distilled water in specialized assembly sections.

H. Epilog

Washed parts usually have a finite use time. Parts not used within a specified period (e.g., a work shift) may be dried or left in distilled water with continuous overflow. The dried parts must be rewashed before use unless other appropriate protective measures are imposed. Washed, wet, cleaned parts may also be held at a minimum of 70°C to suppress microbial growth.

   Cleaning procedures should be devised that are appropriate for each component part, dictated in some measure by its chemical composition and previous handling and storage history. Filtered air (0.22 μm porosity filter) and ionizing air guns are receiving attention as means for dry cleaning less critical components.

   The adequacy of the total cleaning procedure should be evaluated by appropriate means. No cleaning chemical residues should survive. The parts should be substantially free of all particulate matter. Microscopic/membrane or electronic counting procedures on eluates from washed parts will provide excellent guidance as to fulfillment of specifications for level of cleanliness.

VIII. FILLING

Because highly accurate fills are not necessary with LVPs, filling is generally un-complicated. The USP recommends that parenterals with a volume of 50 ml or more contain a 2% excess for mobile liquids and 3% excess for viscous liquids. In general, LVPs exceed this minimum recommended excess. The percentage excess may typically run higher for the small volume than in the large volume containers. Because from 5 to 15 ml of fluid may be required to fill the intravenous set and pro-vide for the undrained residue in the container, the intent of the excess is to ensure that the labeled volume is available for delivery to the patient.

Rigid glass and semirigid plastic containers are typically filled to a predeter-mined level on a high-speed conveyor system. The fill level is established by ad-justing the height of a fill and vent tube. Container shape and size, plus the fill level, determine volume. Pipet fillers and volume transfer cup systems may be employed in slower speed or lower production volume operations. Some fillers use a weighing principle, but accuracy is often compromised as speed is increased. Flexible plastic containers are usually filled by volumetric displacement systems consisting of a cylinder and piston assembly, which draws in a fixed volume of fluid that is then discharged into the container. The piston stroke, which is adjust-able, determines the volume. Weighing systems and volume transfer cup systems are sometimes employed. Another method is to place the flexible container in a conformal mold, which determines volume, and to fill the container in much the same manner as a bottle.

Regardless of the type of filler used, the fill volume must be checked period-ically by inspecting the volume against the graduations molded or printed on the container or by weight. This control is usually done after sealing.

IX. SEALING

The sealing operation, which establishes the integrity of the container, is typically as varied as the design and composition of the container itself. Glass intravenous containers typically require an elastomeric closure. The headspace above the fluid may be flushed with a gas (nitrogen or carbon dioxide) if required by the formula-tion. A partial vacuum can be created by filling warm or hot solution and sealing promptly. A higher vacuum is created by mechanical means immediately prior to seating the closure. Aluminum caps are then applied and crimped around the neck finish of the bottle. This is a very critical phase of the sealing operation in that too much crimping force can result in a damaged seal, whereas too little force can result in a weak seal. Both head (downward) and side pressures must be controlled during this crimping process to ensure a sound seal without damage to the lip or neck of the glass.

The closure system for glass containers employing open hole stoppers is composed of three parts: a rubber disk to maintain the seal under high vacuum, an aluminum disk to provide additional security, and an aluminum ring, which holds both disks tightly against the rubber stopper. The outer ring is crimped over the neck finish of the bottle by rollers, which apply force to the top of the closure as well as the side. Sufficient head pressure must be applied to the top of the bottle to seat the closure fully. The side pressure must be just enough to crimp the clo-sure fully without damaging it.

Glass pour bottles do not employ a rubber closure. These containers have threaded neck finishes. Lined aluminum screw caps with outer seals are rolled and crimped on the container. Precautions relative to head and side pressure indicated above must again be observed. Semirigid plastic containers may employ a rubber closure as a primary seal with a plastic overcap. All-plastic seals are also encountered. Final seals on flexible plastic containers will be as varied as the designs and compositions they employ. Inlets (ports) for the introduction of supplementory medication and for insertion of the intravenous spike are easily integrated into the design. Spin welding, heat (radio frequency or thermal), and solvent seals probably prevail.

The final step in the processing of an LVP is sterilization. This subject is treated in the chapter on Industrial Sterilization in Volume 2.

X. NEW DIRECTIONS

This chapter has attempted to present the fundamental concepts and methods associated with the manufacture of the traditional LVP. One must be aware that although the traditional LVP was designed to provide water, electrolytes, and nutrition (carbohydrate, amino acids, or fat), it also serves as a vehicle for the administration of drugs.

Liquid concentrates of important drugs packaged in ampules or small vials are frequently added to LVPs. There are several reasons for this. The drug additive may not be sufficiently stable or compatible to be a component of the prepackaged LVP, but may be added shortly before administration. In addition, the use pattern may be too varied or specialized to justify and support a fully manufactured product. Insulin, heparin, multivitamins, calcium salts, and buffers are examples of this class of drug additive. When the additive is stable and used frequently or in emergency situations new LVPs have resulted. Potassium chloride in various concentrations is now available in a variety of LVPs. Lidocaine hydrochloride in dextrose injection has recently been introduced into the U.S. market. The antiinfective drug metronidazole, dopamine, and heparin have also been introduced in ready-to-use intravenous dosage forms.

Antibiotics are usually presented as sterile powders because they are not stable in solution, but special LVPs have been designed to facilitate their reconstitution and delivery.

A completely formulated manufactured product has several advantages over extemporaneous compounding. The manufactured product is more cost-effective in that one does not have to employ two or more separate manufactured products, the costs associated with compounding are eliminated, and the risk of touch contamination associated with compounding is reduced or eliminated. Because of these very important advantages, one may expect to see this new and improved form of drug packaging and delivery receive increasing attention.

The increased interest in parenteral nutrition has also caused a reexamination of the packaging of nutritional materials: carbohydrates and amino acids. Presently, these products are packaged separately as liquids. Carbohydrates and amino acids are compatible when compounded for short-term storage but not as manufactured products. Plastic containers with separate compartments have been introduced. The compartments are connected by a membrane that can be pierced or ruptured. One compartment contains the amino acid preparation, while the other contains the carbohydrate, and the entire package is processed by steam sterilization. At the time of use, the membrane is ruptured to result in the compounded product without the risk of contamination.

It is probable that these two areas—drug delivery and parenteral nutrition—will result in further innovations in the design, packaging, and manufacturing of LVPs. It is expected that this area of activity will be exciting and innovative far into the future.

REFERENCES

1. Akers, M. J., Attia, I. A., and Avis, K. E., J. Parenter. Drug Assoc., 33:195-202 (1979).
2. Wallhausser, K. H., J. Parenter. Drug Assoc., 33:156-171 (1979).
3. Reti, A. R., and Leahy, T. J., J. Parenter. Drug Assoc., 33:257-272 (1979).

Following are additional sources of information on the manufacturing of large volume parenterals.

Groves, M. J., Parenteral Products, William Heinemann, London, 1973.
Orr, C., Filtration: Principles and Practices, Parts I and II, Marcel Dekker, New York, 1977.
Svarovsky, L., Solid-Liquid Separations, Butterworth, Woburn, Mass., 1977.
Technical literature from manufacturers of filtration materials and equipment (e.g., Millipore, Gelman, Pall, and Membrana).

8

Records and Reports

DAVID C. FRY

Bristol Laboratories
Division of Bristol-Myers Company
Syracuse, New York

The documentation prepared during the production and testing of pharmaceutical products is the most complex and extensive of any industry that produces a consumer product. Furthermore, the production standards for parenteral drugs are the most demanding of any dosage form because of the need to avoid contamination, be it chemical, particulate, or biological. The records generated during the course of production of these drugs are exceedingly important because it is from the completeness and accuracy of these various documents that the true quality of the product is determined.

I. PURPOSE OF RECORDS AND REPORTS

There are many individual records and reports which, when put together, tell the story of how a drug was processed and what quality attributes it possesses. Each of these individual documents has a fundamental reason for being prepared and retained for future reference.

A. Scientific Purpose

When any scientific experiment is performed, the experimenter makes a great effort to keep detailed records which document the materials used, the conditions, the observations, the test results, and the conclusions drawn. These same steps and rigors of documentation are followed in the evaluation of new drug substances for safety and effectiveness. A written protocol is prepared which identifies the materials to be used, the conditions of testing, and the nature of the data to be obtained. From analysis of the data collected, a conclusion is drawn concerning whether or not the product has therapeutic merit. If the decision is favorable, the product is suitable for marketing. All future material that will be marketed is expected to have the same characteristics of quality, purity, safety, and effectiveness just as if it were subjected to the same extensive testing. In order to provide a basis for realization of this expectation, records of the production and control of drugs attempt to show that today's product is a reproduction of that which underwent extensive testing. These records basically indicate:

1. The identity and quality of the raw materials and packaging components
2. The performance of each step and the equipment used in manufacturing and packaging
3. The laboratory data establishing the achievement of physical, chemical, and biological quality characteristics

If this information conforms to established standards, the material can be released for sale with the expectation that it will have the desired pharmacological effect.

B. Regulatory Purpose

The maintaining of certain records is a legal requirement mandated by the U.S. Food, Drug and Cosmetic Act [1]. Documentation generated during the manufacture of a drug constitutes legal evidence which may be used to decide the question of how well a firm fulfills its legal obligations. After an activity has been concluded, the records documenting the performance of the act may be the only evidence that remains. If the records of that event are nonexistent, inaccurate, or incomplete, a defendant may have no other option than to concede a contest over what actually transpired because the documentation is unable to provide a clear picture of the events that occurred or the conditions which existed at that time. In a legal situation, the regulator can take the position that if the record does not accurately reflect what was done, then in essence, the action was not performed. The quality of data is directly proportional to the quality of evidence that records are able to provide in a regulatory setting.

The quality of data in records providing regulatory evidence has special meaning to the parenteral drug manufacturer. FDA investigators routinely raise the question of validation data for sterilization processes without the discovery of nonsterile products in the marketplace. The quality of the data in the records can be the difference between total recall of affected products and continuation of marketing. In the former case, the plant may be required to close until data suitable to FDA can be obtained. This can cause severe economic hardship to the firm involved. In the latter case, minor deficiencies can be corrected with virtually no adverse economic impact. Information contained in written records must be able to answer questions of regulatory officials and withstand close scrutiny so that there is reasonable assurance that the processing and testing performed demonstrate that the drug in question conforms to established standards of identity, strength, quality, purity, safety, and effectiveness.

C. Business Purpose

There are several records and reports generated in conjunction with the production of drugs which are neither required by law nor needed to demonstrate the quality of the product. Such records and reports are supplementary to the processing of a batch of drug and may be prepared from the raw data generated during the manufacture of individual batches. As successive batches of a product have been shown to conform to established standards, it is customary to review applicable standards and processes with the intent of improving efficiency or obtaining some cost savings. Such reviews may be performed at specified intervals or on an ongoing basis. The information accumulated is useful for providing reports of production status and for determining labor standards, overhead costs, and the degree of success in meeting standards of quality. Such reviews can be used to tighten or loosen limit ranges, to

determine what tests or examinations are most suitable, or to identify the most
appropriate points during processing to perform sampling. Process improvements
and changes in test methodology can also result from such review.

Certain reports to management are required by federal regulations concerning
drug manufacturing [2]. Recalls of drugs from the marketplace, written observations provided by Food and Drug Administration (FDA) investigators at the conclusion of an inspection, and regulatory letters or any legal action relating to violations of good manufacturing practice brought by the FDA must be brought to the
attention of responsible officials of the firm. Furthermore, certain types of investigations, such as those involving complaints, returned goods where there are
questions of the quality of associated batches, and salvaging of drugs following possible exposure to adverse conditions which may affect the quality of the products
must be brought to the attention of management. In all cases, if the responsible
officials are not personally involved in or aware of such situations, they must be
notified in writing, thus documenting the situation as well as the notification.

II. RECORD CONTENT

The records and reports required by the Food, Drug and Cosmetic Act and supporting regulations extend from development of a dosage form with testing for safety
and effectiveness to routine batch manufacturing, testing, and distribution and subsequent information on patient experience. This chain of events in the life of a drug
product affects various disciplines and levels of personnel education and training;
however, the one common thread running through all of these events is the subject
of written records and reports. Regardless of individual format, length, or subject matter, there are basic elements found in all records and reports which are
complete. Whether the document pertains to research, any aspect of production or
quality control, records associated with pharmaceutical processing will contain the
elements shown in Figure 1.

A. Who?

The person or persons performing and reviewing the activities that the record is
documenting must be identified. The identification must be specific to the people
involved. The identification may be a name, signature, or initials; however, initials may not be adequate in cases where specific identity is required. In certain
cases, such as master formula records, full signatures are mandated by federal

---

1. Who did the work?

2. When was the work done?

3. What work was done?

4. Where was the work done?

5. What conditions prevailed during performance of the work?

6. What conclusions can be drawn from the work?

Figure 1 Elements contained in pharmaceutical processing
records.

regulations [2]. Other devices, such as time clock numbers, are used by some firms as a means of identifying personnel. This is helpful when using computers or other mechanical means of data handling which also have the need to indicate the performer and reviewer of the work.

Identification of persons performing specific duties during the course of processing a batch of drug must be included in certain documents. Regulations [2] require that the individuals performing the following activities be identified in the official record documenting the work:

1. Sampling components, drug product containers, and closures
2. Dispensing components for manufacturing
3. Cleaning and maintaining equipment
4. Preparing master production and control records
5. Approving the labeling to be affixed to the drug product
6. Performing any significant step in the entire operation
7. Performing any testing
8. Reviewing laboratory records for accuracy, completeness, and conformity of the material tested to established standards
9. Determining that an investigation of a complaint is not necessary

Although one specific case of identifying the person reviewing a record is cited above, regulations [2] generally require that the person supervising or checking any work performed be identified in the record.

By identifying specific individuals who performed the work and those who reviewed or approved it, individual responsibility is established. Thus, if the FDA believes that regulatory action is necessary to correct deficiencies, culpable individuals are identified. The regulations [2] clearly state at the outset (Sec. 210.1) that persons responsible for failure to comply with the regulations shall be subject to regulatory action.

B. When?

Performance of work must be fixed at a point in time. For most duties, this can be the month, day, and year; however, when a process requires a certain time sequence for the performance of an activity (such as mixing) for a designated length of time, hours and minutes may need to be indicated.

Because microbial contaminants multiply as a function of time, Section 211.111 of the regulations [2] has special interest to the parenteral manufacturer. This regulation requires that where it is necessary to assure the quality of the drug product, time limits must be established and followed for each phase of production. The phases of production where time limits are to be specified are at the discretion of the individual firm. Deviation from established limits are permissible provided that such deviation does not compromise the quality of the drug; however, such deviation must be justified and documented.

The regulations proposed in 1976 for large volume parenterals [3] contain some specific time requirements. These regulations are not final and have no official standing. Examples of time constraints proposed by the FDA are:

1. Static water lines must be flushed for at least 5 min.
2. Time elapsing between addition of water to the batching tank and exposure of the last filled unit to the sterilization process shall not exceed 8 hr.

3. Sterilization parameters such as vent time, product come-up time, and cooling time must be determined.
4. The length of exposure of heat-liable products to the sterilization process to provide a specified microbial lethality should be based on studies indicating degradation as a function of time.

To establish that these activities were performed, written records of accomplishment would be required.

C. What?

This element is the heart of the record, for without describing the work performed there would be no need to prepare the document. In parenteral drug manufacturing, work that must be documented includes:

1. Receiving, sampling, and testing components, containers, and closures
2. Dispensing designated quantities of the correct components, containers, closures, and labeling
3. Processing the drug, including compounding, filling, sterilizing, and packaging
4. Sampling, inspecting, and testing the batch at specified intervals
5. Preparing and cleaning equipment
6. Performing auxiliary testing such as environmental monitoring and stability testing
7. Reviewing all production and control records
8. Preparing master production and control records, including specifications
9. Monitoring information from outside sources such as product complaints or returned goods

This information must be as detailed as possible so that when individual records of the various processes and operations are combined, they provide a clear picture of what events transpired. From this combined information, one can judge whether or not and how well prescribed activities have been accomplished. This compiled information is reviewed in its entirety before the product to which it pertains can be released for sale. If any unexplained discrepancies are detected, they must be thoroughly investigated and a record of the investigation included with the batch production records. This investigation must extend to other batches, whether or not already marketed, if they have been implicated by the discrepancy.

D. Where?

Not only is the location, such as a manufacturing plant, identified in records, but such specific identification as the line on which the processing took place is also recorded. Additionally, the major pieces of equipment used during the processing of the batch must be recorded. This is needed so that investigation of possible mix-up or cross-contamination can be facilitated when necessary and the scope of the problem determined.

Chronological records of equipment cleaning, maintenance, and usage are also to be maintained. Such records must show the date, time, product, and lot number of each batch processed. Entries must be made in chronological order. The maintenance to be recorded is that above and beyond routine lubrication and adjustment. Therefore, to comply with these requirements, it is necessary that all major pieces of equipment and production lines having stationary equipment be identified with some specific name or number.

E. Conditions

Specific information should be provided describing the limitations of the parameters or circumstances under which the work was done. Certain criteria may be necessary to enable the work to be accomplished as desired. For example, to achieve satisfactory solubility of ingredients, specific temperatures or pH ranges may be required. The filling of a powder may necessitate certain relative humidity conditions to ensure flowability. The aseptic filling of parenterals dictates that microbial contaminants in areas of product exposure to the atmosphere be established and that they be limited in number.

The regulations governing manufacturing operations [2] dictate certain conditions for aseptic processing:

1. Floors, walls, and ceilings must be easily cleanable.
2. Temperature and humidity must be controlled.
3. Air must be filtered through high-efficiency filters and have a positive pressure differential relative to certain surrounding areas.
4. Environmental conditions must be monitored.
5. The area and equipment must be cleaned and disinfected.
6. Equipment used to control the aseptic conditions must be maintained.

The proposed LVP-CGMP regulations of 1976 [3] went even further in that specific conditions were proposed as industry standards. Certain classes of water were to be established, and the quality of each varied depending on its use. The FDA proposed that:

1. Water used for equipment washing be potable, subjected to some process for controlling microbial contaminants, and contain not more than 50 organisms per 100 ml
2. Water used for compounding or final rinsing of equipment conform to USP requirements for Water for Injection, contain not more than 10 organisms per 100 ml, and either be stored at a temperature of 80°C or more or, if stored at ambient temperatures, be held for not more than 24 hr
3. Water used for cooling terminally sterilized product be treated to eliminate organisms and contain not more than 1 organism per 100 ml

Other standards were proposed for air, compressed air, and operating conditions of sterilizers. Adherence to all of these proposed conditions at this time is not mandatory. However, such guidelines suggest the need to establish and then document the conditions which do exist so that the relationship of these conditions to product quality can be assessed.

F. Conclusions

Conclusions can be drawn only after gathering all necessary facts. Decisions should be based on the performance of work to justify proceeding with the next step or operation. Regulations [2] require that all production and control records, including those derived from packaging and labeling, be reviewed by the quality control unit to determine compliance with all established procedures before the batch is released for distribution. The conclusion of the review is the decision of whether the records indicate that conformity with procedures has been accomplished and whether testing indicates that the material meets established standards of strength, quality, purity, and identity. The conclusion is indicated in the report by some definitive statements such as "release," "reject," "approved," or "meets requirements." This is followed by the signature of the person making the decision and the date of the decision. The regulations [2] require that only those materials found to meet established requirements may be used in production or released for sale.

III. RECORD MAINTENANCE AND RETRIEVAL

Many sections of the U.S. Food, Drug and Cosmetic Act require that written records and reports be prepared and maintained. The terms "records" and "reports" are not clarified in that there is no indication of the content, extent, or depth of detail required. For example, research-intensive firms are thoroughly familiar with the new drug section of the Act, which states that applications submitted for approval must contain "full reports of investigations" which have been conducted to demonstrate the drug's safety and effectiveness. To determine what "full reports" are and the extent of the investigations that must be conducted, regulations that the FDA has promulgated must be reviewed.

A. Records Subject to Inspection

The factory inspection section [704-(a)] of the Act [1] contains general requirements concerning the records which are to be maintained and which are subject to inspection by FDA investigators. The inspection of a drug manufacturer may extend to records, files, and papers as well as processes, controls, and facilities to determine whether or not the drugs are adulterated or misbranded, but the right to inspect such records and papers is limited to those documents associated with prescription drugs. For parenteral drug manufacturers, this may not be significant since virtually all drugs administered by injection, with the possible exception of insulin, are prescription drugs. However, if one chooses to define parenteral drugs as drugs that are administered by a route other than oral, this limitation could have some importance.

When any drug manufacturing establishment is being inspected, no inspection may extend to financial data, sales data, pricing information, personnel files (except to determine qualifications of technical and professional personnel), and basic research data (except that for new drugs or antibiotic drugs). Although the law speaking to inspections does not specifically describe what records are to be maintained, it is clear that documentation must be prepared by drug manufacturers to establish that the drugs produced are not adulterated or misbranded.

B. Good Manufacturing Practice Requirements

Since specific records and reports that must be maintained to document the manufacturing process are not defined by the Act [1], the key section of the Act must be located to identify the applicable regulations to be reviewed to obtain this information. In Section 501 (a) (2) (B), Congress expresses the concept that to assure that drugs have designed characteristics of strength, quality, purity, and identity, they must be manufactured and packaged in facilities and under a system of controls both of which conform to current good manufacturing practice (CGMP). This term, establishing some nebulous goal, was not defined, but Congress did provide the authority to promulgate regulations for the efficient enforcement of the Act (Sec. 702).

Regulations specifically defining those methods, facilities, and controls for drug manufacturers which constitute current good manufacturing practice have been adopted. They were first published in 1962 when the so-called GMP requirement was enacted by Congress and have been revised with the passage of time. The current revision became effective on March 29, 1979. These regulations apply to the manufacture, processing, packaging, and holding of finished drugs (dosage forms), and therefore they apply to all drugs, including parenterals.

In the mid-1970s the FDA had the goal of preparing regulations defining those activities and procedures constituting current good manufacturing practice for individual operations of the industry, such as the manufacture of such dosage forms as tablets, capsules, and parenterals. A proposal pertaining to the manufacture of large volume parenterals was published for public comment in the Federal Register of June 1, 1976 [3]. Shortly after that publication, the FDA requested comments on extending those proposed requirements to all parenteral products and their manufacture. Neither proposal has been finalized by the FDA as of this writing.

1. Record Availability

The CGMP regulations [2] speak specifically to manufacturing and control processes for drugs. They also contain the specific requirements concerning records and documentation. Subpart J of the regulations states that records which are required therein must be available for authorized inspection at the site where the activities described in the records occurred. The records shall be subject to photocopying or reproduction as a part of the inspection. Because of this requirement, it is well to remember that the goal of any record is to transmit or record factual information so that the reviewer can make an intelligent decision. Therefore, unsupported opinions or conclusions, as well as gratuitous comments on related issues, have no place in official records.

The 1979 revision was published as substantive regulations. This means that failure to comply with the regulations is a violation of law; the regulations have the force and effect of law. Therefore, if a record required by the regulations is not maintained or prepared, the law has been violated and both the drug product involved, as well as the persons responsible, can be subjected to the penalties of the law. This is the first time that these particular regulations have been so regarded.

2. Record Retention

Section 211.180 dictates that records directly pertaining to the production, control, and distribution of a specific batch of drug must be retained for a specific period of time which is dependent on the expiration period for the batch of drug in question. For parenteral drugs, such records must be maintained for 1 year in excess of the assigned expiration date. Furthermore, records pertaining to the components, containers, closures, and labeling must also be retained for 1 year after the expiration date of the batch in which they were used.

3. Retrieval Requirements

Because of the need to maintain voluminous records on the testing of raw materials and the processing of them into a batch of drug product and the requirement to store these records for an appreciable period of time, the filing and retrieval of such records for review upon request can be a formidable problem.

Paragraph 211.180 (c) of the CGMP regulations [2] requires that production and control records be available for review and inspection during the entire time period for which they are to be maintained. In order to do this, a defined system must be employed which minimizes mix-up by filing records of similar but different material and which allows for ready retrieval upon request.

Manual Systems. Manual filing systems consist of individual file jackets for each batch of drug product, containing various documents indicating all of the work done on that specific batch of product. The jackets are identified with the batch number and contain all of the records (generally the originals, although copies are permissible) associated with the production, testing, and release (or rejection) of that batch. These are generally filed consecutively by batch number in a central location under the jurisdiction of a specifically identified organizational unit so that the control and retrieval of the documents can be facilitated. Such systems require a considerable amount of space depending on production volume and product-line variation of the firm. To conserve space, microfilming or other reduction photocopying of such records may be performed. When this is done, equipment for reading and copying must be available to government inspectors. Original records, if not microfilmed, must also be available for reproduction by FDA representatives. Thus all records in the jacket must be clear and legible. It is customary that even when microfilming is performed, original records are maintained until they have served their usefulness.

Automated Systems. Automated filing systems vary according to individual firms, but most have some degree of computerization associated with laboratory testing and the storage, calculation, or retrieval of laboratory data. Certain parts of the manufacturing process, such as weighing of raw materials or the issuance of production records, can be automated; however, there is no totally automated system of record keeping which does away with the human element and manual input of data. The 1979 revision of the GMP regulations [2] speaks to the role of computers in record maintenance. According to Section 211.180(c), if records are maintained at a site other than where the documented activities occurred but can be retrieved by computer or other electronic means, the requirement is met. When such automatic, mechanical, or electronic equipment is used in data or information handling, it must be routinely inspected or checked according to a written program which is designed to assure proper performance of the equipment. Records of such checks or inspections must be maintained.

When computers or related systems are used to generate batch production or control records, controls must be exercised over the use of the system to ensure that changes in master records are instituted only by authorized personnel. Input to and output from the system of formulas or other information must be checked for accuracy. A backup file of data entered into the system is also mandated except where certain data, such as calculations performed in connection with laboratory analysis, are eliminated by computerization. However, in these cases, a written record of the program used to perform the calculation is to be maintained together with data validating the program. Hard-copy data must also be maintained to assure that information is accurate in the event of alteration or accidental erasure of data in the automated system.

IV. RECORD SYSTEMS

A. Production Records

In order for consecutive batches to be as nearly identical as possible, certain acts must be reproduced with a measurable degree of uniformity. One prerequisite necessary for this achievement is a complete set of master production records. These records include (1) the batch formula and (2) the manufacturing directions. Another cornerstone upon which reproducibility of a process is built is performing specified actions according to written procedures. This includes checking and verifying, normally with signatures of the two persons involved, that the actions have been accomplished as directed. This applies to the preparation of the master production records, as well as the individual steps associated with the production of the drug.

1. Master Production Records

For each specific quantity of drug to be produced, written master production records must be prepared. Information to be contained therein, according to Section 211.186 of the regulations [2], includes:

1. Name and strength of the product, together with a statement of the dosage form.
2. Name and weight or measure of each active ingredient per dosage unit and a statement of the total weight or measure of the dosage unit.
3. Complete list of names and quantities of all ingredients used in the batch.
4. Statement of any calculated excess amount of any ingredient.
5. Statement of the theoretical weight or measure at appropriate points of manufacturing.
6. Statement of theoretical yield, including limits which, if not met, require an investigation to determine the cause.
7. Description of the container, closure, and packaging materials, including a sample of the label and labeling used. The samples are to be signed by a person responsible for approving such materials.
8. Complete manufacturing instructions, sampling procedures, and special notations or precautions to be followed.

2. Batch Production Records

From the master records that describe the model after which all successive batches are patterned, the production records for the processing of individual batches are prepared. These documents provide the complete history of the manufacture and control of a specific quantity of material. According to Section 211.188 of the regulations [2], these records must include:

1. A reproduction of the appropriate master record. This is checked for accuracy and then signed and dated by the person performing the check.
2. Documentation showing that each significant step prescribed for the manufacturing and packaging of the batch has been performed. The documentation includes:
    a. Dates on which events took place.
    b. Identity of major equipment and processing lines used.
    c. Identity of each specific batch of ingredient used.
    d. Weights or measures of each ingredient used.
    e. Any laboratory data and test results.

     f. Results of inspection of packaging and labeling area before and after use.

     g. Statement of actual yield and conformance to limits prescribed in master records.

     h. Complete records of labeling, including specimens of all labeling used in the batch.

     i. Description of the container and closure used.

     j. Records of any sampling performed.

     k. Identity of persons performing and directly supervising or checking each significant step.

     l. Any investigation arising from problems discovered during review of completed records, yields not meeting specified limits, or established specifications not being met.

    m. Results of any examination or inspection conducted on product during processing.

The records of labeling and sampling mentioned above may be separate from those associated with other processing activities. Records of labeling would identify the specific lots of materials used, the persons performing the work, the amount of work produced (both acceptable and waste), an accurate count of the individual labeling materials issued for use, amount of labeling used, amount of labeling wasted and amount of labeling remaining (these quantities must be reconciled within narrow preset limits), the dates and places where the packaging took place, and the results of any inspection of the labeling process. Sampling records should identify the amount of sample, the material sampled, the location of the material sampled, the person taking the sample, and the date of sampling. Generally, such sampling records accompany the sample to the laboratory.

B. Control Records

Just as production requires master records in order to reproduce drug products, the measurement of drug product quality must be done according to master requirements. The master tools for analytical determination are (1) product specifications and (2) analytical procedures. The specifications detail the characteristics of product quality and the limit ranges of test values that constitute acceptable quality. Products meeting all these requirements may be released for sale; products not meeting one or more requirement may not be released for sale. Analytical procedures detail the equipment and techniques for performing each test or examination. The procedures also include the method of calculating the result from the data obtained.

These documents do not need to be reproduced for each batch of product produced. The analytical records generated identify the procedure used by referencing it. The test results obtained are compared with the appropriate specification. The result of this comparison is recorded in the records.

1. Batch-Related Information

Production records must be complete and accurate and reflect exactly what took place during fabrication and packaging of the product. How well these activities were performed and how successfully the batch imitates the master material is measured by laboratory testing and evaluation of the results against written standards. In order to produce reliable results, testing must be controlled just as tightly as the manufacturing process. Data and information required by regulations (Sec. 211.194) to demonstrate that the test results are reproducible include:

1. A description of any sample identified with the location from which it came, the amount of sample, the identity of the batch which it represents, the date on which it was taken, and the date on which it was received by the laboratory for testing.
2. A statement of the method used in testing or examining the sample. (Prior to using the method, other data must be generated to establish that the method is accurate and reliable for the product tested; such reliability or suitability of the method must be verified under actual conditions of laboratory use.)
3. Amount of sample used for each test.
4. All information developed in the course of performing each test, such as observed results, graphs, charts, and spectra. Such records are to be identified to show the material tested.
5. All calculations performed, including units of measure, conversion factors, and equivalency factors.
6. Statement of test results and an indication of how the results compare with established standards and specifications for the material tested.
7. Identity of the person performing each examination or test and the date on which such work was performed.
8. Identity of the second person reviewing the records for accuracy, completeness, and compliance with established standards or specifications.

On occasion, it may be necessary to change or modify an existing test method. If this is done, records indicating the reason for the modification and data verifying that the modification is accurate and reliable for the material tested must be established and maintained.

2. Reference Standards

To quantitatively measure an unknown, one must have some material whose characteristics are thoroughly known. Reference standards must be characterized according to written procedures and stored under known conditions to preserve their integrity. In order to prove the authenticity of a reference standard, complete records of all testing performed must be maintained. This also applies to reagents and test solutions. The records maintained should clearly identify the source of the material, its purity, its potency, and the expiration period.

3. Instrument Calibration

Since laboratory testing requires a high degree of precision, it is important that laboratory instruments, apparatus, gages, and recording devices be calibrated periodically. To demonstrate that such work is performed as prescribed, written records of such work must be established and retained. Such records must also be reviewed to determine if the conditions of calibration conform to the conditions of use and to establish that specified criteria or limits of sensitivity are met. Such records indicate the person doing the work, the date the work was done, the standard used for calibration, the measurements made against the standard, any repairs or adjustments required, new readings made following repair or adjustment, and the decision of acceptability of the instrument for use including the identity of the person making the decision.

4. Stability Testing

Not only must the drug be shown to meet criteria of quality, but the ability of the container-closure system to preserve the characteristics throughout the shelf life of the product must also be established. The designated expiration date on the labeling of the drug product is established by testing designed to ascertain the stability of the product under its specified conditions of storage. Such testing is done according to a written program intended to assess degradation or physical change as a function of time. The data may also be used to establish storage conditions. Since stability testing is done on each product, the documentation establishes adherence to the program, which specifies:

1. The sample size and test interval.
2. Storage conditions for samples (certain conditions of elevated temperature and/ or relative humidity can be used to predict product stability).
3. Reliable, meaningful, and specific test methods (such methods should be stability indicating, i.e., able to measure the concentration of degradation products).
4. Testing of the product after storage in the same container-closure system as that in which the product is distributed.
5. If the product is reconstituted prior to administration, testing of the reconstituted product.

C. Validation Records

The term "validation" has never been officially defined by the FDA. The word is used in several places in the CGMP regulations [2]; however, it is not explained nor is any indication given as to the nature of the records to be maintained to show that something has been validated. In public speeches FDA compliance officials have indicated that validation is the process of proving that something (a piece of equipment or a process) does what it is supposed to do. To establish proof of performance, one must first define the nature of the operation as well as its limitations and then test it. When the testing is done, the tests and how they were performed must be identified. The data gathered and any analysis of results must be recorded.

Validation of pharmaceutical processes is just like scientific testing performed to prove or disprove a hypothesis. First the hypothesis is defined; then in turn a testing program is defined, tests are performed, and data are gathered. Finally, the data are evaluated to enable a conclusion to be drawn as to whether or not the hypothesis has been proven.

1. Protocol

The testing program or experiment should be described in a written protocol. An outline for a typical protocol is shown in Figure 2. The objective should be a statement of what the experiment is designed to do (i.e., the hypothesis). The purpose explains what the equipment or process does. The section on design characteristics explains how the process or equipment is designed to perform a certain function by specifying the key aspects and the limits of operation (e.g., speed, temperatures, etc.). The prevalidation or qualification aspects delineate those matters that must be accomplished in order for the tests to be valid. This would include documentation that the article functions properly or its integral parts have the designed sensitivity (e.g., calibration). The testing program defines the tests to be performed, including the frequency of sample collection, the duration of the test run, the methods of analysis of all samples, the challenges applied to the system, and the number of replicates to be performed. The section of the protocol concerning data analysis defines how the data are to be evaluated and what applicable

---

1. Objective

2. Purpose

3. Design characteristics

4. Prevalidation/qualification parameters

5. Test procedures

6. Data analysis

7. Acceptance criteria

Figure 2 Outline of a typical testing protocol.

statistical treatment is to be given the data gathered. The acceptance criteria indicate the conditions that must be met in order for the validation efforts to be considered successful. Among the criteria may be limits on the variability measured.

The preparation of the protocol is generally an effort combining the disciplines of manufacturing, engineering, and quality control. Therefore, the protocol should reflect approval of these groups by means of signatures of responsible officials. The documentation of the work performed toward satisfying the validation requirements is extensive, as much raw data in the form of calibration records, manufacturing records, and analytical records are generated. All documentation should be filed as a complete package, together with the protocol and evaluation of the data so that the reviewer can readily determine what was to be done, whether the specified activities were accomplished, and how successful the efforts were. The data should be reviewed by responsible officials of the affected department as well as quality control personnel, indicating approval of the system or article validated. These files should be treated with the same respect as batch records and filed with the intent of routine retrieval.

2. Change System

Once validation has been accomplished, changes to the system, equipment, or process should not be made without prior review to evaluate the impact of the action on the validation data previously gathered. This review process should be formalized and documented. Specific forms can be devised for this purpose. The form should provide space to characterize fully the nature of the planned alteration. Review of the written request must be performed before any mechanical work is performed. In order to facilitate the rapid circulation of the written request, there needs to be close communication among manufacturing, engineering, and quality control management. A copy of the written and approved change order can be incorporated into a dynamic chronological historical file maintained on a given piece of equipment or a process. The performance of the work should be recorded in appropriate log books. When the work is completed and revalidation is required to document the effect of the change on product quality, a new protocol should be generated and new data gathered, evaluated, reviewed, and approved.

3. Process Validation

The CGMP regulations [2] indicate that not only are certain manufacturing processes to be validated but that certain aspects of analytical work must be validated (Sec. 211.165). The only mention of validation of manufacturing processes in these regulations is in Section 211.110 and 211.113. The former section states that procedures must be established to monitor production output and to validate the performance of processes that may be responsible for causing variability in the characteristics of in-process material as well as the drug product. The latter paragraph mandates that procedures designed to prevent microbiological contamination in products purporting to be sterile include validation of any sterilization process. Figure 3 lists some typical processes and systems used in parenteral drug manufacturing which should be considered for validation.

The proposed regulations [3] concerning processing of large volume parenteral drugs do not specifically mention validation. However, they do indicate that records should be maintained documenting the testing performed by and approval of the quality control unit regarding design, engineering and physical facilities of the plant, the equipment, process and control procedures, and the container-closure system used. Furthermore, the proposal included a new section, subpart M, which provided specific information on the design and testing of sterilization processes employing steam or water. Described in this section are specific studies (heat distribution and heat penetration) which characterize the sterilization vessel and the lethality of the process used and aspects of controlling the sterilization process. All of the work described must be recorded.

Validation testing is performed to prove that defined operating limits are uniformly achieved and that the operating control limits chosen result in a product that meets established specifications. These data, suitably recorded and evaluated,

---

1. Mixing (bulk product)

2. Filling

3. Filtration

4. Sterilization of product

5. Sterilization of equipment

6. Washing and sterilization of product containers

7. Washing and sterilization of closures

8. Dye testing—leaker testing

9. Compressed air

10. Environmental air (including laminar flow)

11. Water treatment

12. Water distillation, storage, and distribution

13. Other water systems (deionized or reverse osmosis) used for container or equipment washing

14. Cleaning/disinfection of equipment/facilities

15. Steam used to sterilize product contact surfaces

16. Integrity of container-closure system

Figure 3 Typical processes and systems to be validated.

provide a firm with knowledge of process capability as well as a record of those conditions that result in the achievement of product quality.

4. Supplier Validation

The general CGMP regulations have long required testing of components, containers, and closures prior to their use in a batch of product. The 1979 revision [2] included an exemption from this requirement for the manufacturer of the dosage form. If a report of analysis for each lot is provided by the vendor and the reliability of the supplier's analysis is established through appropriate validation of the test results, testing of each shipment is not required. In order to establish the reliability of test results and validate a vendor's performance, a written program must be developed defining how often lots of components, drug product containers, and closures are to be sampled and tested by the dosage form manufacturer. Obviously, the program should provide for comparison of the dosage form manufacturer's results with those of the supplier. Furthermore, the tests to be performed and the allowable limits must be specified. Written records of these tests must be maintained together with the evaluation of the comparison of the results.

5. Analytical Validation

A clue to an official definition of validation, at least insofar as the use of the term as applied to analytical testing is concerned, is found in Section 211.165(e) of the CGMP regulations [2]. This paragraph dictates that the accuracy, sensitivity, and reproducibility of test methods employed are to be established and documented. It then states that such validation and documentation may be accomplished in accordance with another regulation. The referenced paragraph requires that laboratory records indicate the source of data, which establishes that the method used in the testing of a sample meets appropriate standards of accuracy and reliability for the material tested. Thus validation of an analytical method is the development of data that demonstrate the accuracy, sensitivity, specificity, and reproducibility of the method tested under actual conditions of use. To demonstrate that this has been accomplished for each different method used, complete records must be prepared delineating the testing program used to establish each of these characteristics.

Validation of analytical methods and personnel can be performed on an ongoing basis by submitting samples of known materials (unknown to the analyst at the time) to the same tests. Plotting results from these samples can indicate bias or other internal laboratory problems. The records of this work must be kept separate from other laboratory data so that no mix-ups occur. Personnel need to know of the existence of the program, but the documentation they prepare in the course of testing is the same in format and content as would be used for any work they are required to do.

D. Standard Operating Procedures

The result of controlling pharmaceutical processing is precise duplication of material subject to clinical testing. In addition to formulas and manufacturing instructions for each batch of drug product, specific written instructions are required to perform related operations reproducibly. A list of such activities mandated by CGMP regulations [2] as requiring written procedures is contained in Table 1.

Table 1 Operations Requiring Written Procedures

Regulation	Operation
211.56(b)	Sanitation of buildings and facilities
211.56(c)	Use of rodenticides, fungicides, insecticides, fumigating agents, cleaning and sanitizing agents
211.67(b)	Cleaning and maintenance of equipment
211.80(a)	Receipt, identification, storage, handling, sampling, testing, approval or rejection of components, containers, and closures
211.84(d)(3)	Testing of containers and closures
211.94(d)	Methods of testing, cleaning, sterilizing, and processing containers and closures to remove pyrogenic substances
211.100(a)	Production and process control operations, including: Charge-in of components Calculation of yield Equipment identification Sampling and testing of in-process materials Time limitations on production Control of microbiological contamination Reprocessing
211.101	Charge-in of components, including: Formulation to provide 100% of the labeled amount of active ingredient(s) Weighing/measuring of components Supervision of weighing/measuring components Addition of components to batch
211.110(a)	Controls, tests, or examinations conducted on samples of in-process materials
211.113(a)	Control of objectionable microorganisms in nonsterile products
211.113(b)	Prevention of microbiological contamination of sterile products, including validation of the sterilization process
211.115(a)	Reprocessing of batches
211.122(a)	Receipt, identification, storage, handling, sampling, and examination/testing of labeling and packaging materials
211.125(f)	Controls for issuance of labeling
211.130	Controls to assure that correct labels and labeling and packaging materials are used
211.142	Warehousing of drug products, including quarantine and storage conditions
211.150	Distribution of drug products
211.165(c)	All sampling and testing plans, including method of sampling and number of units of batch to be tested

Table 1 (continued)

Regulation	Operation
211.167(a)	Testing for sterility and pyrogenicity
211.167(b)	Testing of ophthalmic ointments for the presence of foreign particles and harsh or abrasive substances
211.167(c)	Testing of controlled-release dosage forms for rate of release of each active ingredient
211.180(e)	Annual review of laboratory data for evaluating quality standards
211.180(f)	Notification of responsible officials of investigations of discrepancies, recalls, returned drugs, inspectional observations, or regulatory actions
211.186(a)	Preparation of master production and control records
211.198(a)	Handling of written and oral complaints
211.204	Holding, testing, and reprocessing of returned drug products

1. Preparation

The dictionary indicates that a procedure is a course of action. A complete set of procedures (one for each discrete operation) defines the actions to be taken to perform a job. In order to define the course of action to be taken to get raw materials into a marketable product, one must start with written policies. By working from the top down to individual departments, actions that cut across divisional and departmental lines can be identified. This enables writing efforts to be related and coordinated. A written course of action should be prepared by the group that will be carrying out the action. It should specify what action is to be performed, when it is to be done (schedule), and who is to do it (responsibility). Procedure writing can become extremely cumbersome and overly detailed if the "what" turns into a description of "how." There are many instances where the "how" of accomplishing a job is just as important as the job itself. However, details are better placed in another set of internal departmental procedures or work instructions, so that changes, when necessary, can be instituted more readily. The "what" of a course of action details the work flow and describes the pathway of a system, indicating interdepartmental relationships and responsibilities. The "how" of a procedure describes for each action point of responsibility the individual steps taken to accomplish the work.

2. Procedure Review

Because the majority of procedures written have a very real impact on the quality of the product or on the firm's compliance posture, many firms have designated an organizational group within the quality control department as having responsibility for review and approval of all written procedures. The approval of procedures is mandated by the CGMP regulations (Secs. 211.100 and 211.160) as a responsibility of the quality control unit. Furthermore, after a batch has been produced, the records documenting that production activity must likewise be reviewed by the quality control unit to assure that all appropriate written procedures have been followed (Sec. 211.192). During the stage of preparing or revising written procedures, the appropriate organizational units affected by the procedure or responsible for implementing the procedure must review and approve the procedure. Thus the final document issued for use should contain the signatures and dates of responsible persons reviewing and approving the procedure. The final review is that of the designated quality control official. The process for drafting, reviewing, and approving written procedures should be a formalized system which itself is a written procedure. Included in this system should be periodic review for revision, distribution of procedures, and identification of departments affected by changes in procedures.

3. Procedure Distribution

The regulations [2] require that procedures be written and that the procedures be followed. In order to follow procedures, the persons carrying out the duties must be trained in the requirements of the procedures. Procedures must be written so they can be understood and then they must be circulated for reading by the user. Written procedures accomplish nothing if they are prepared only to fill a manual which sits in a bookcase! Once written and approved, the procedure must be distributed to all persons affected by it. To do this, an up-to-date listing of recipients must be maintained for each procedure. When a new procedure is issued, the system should also provide for retrieval of the previous edition. Having a person place the new document in the manual and remove the old copy is of no value if the person holding the manual is not informed of the change and the change is not communicated to other affected personnel.

The procedure system should also provide for periodic review of all procedures, even if no revisions in text are required. Frequently, due to the press of work, procedure review is not accomplished as often as it should be. When it is done, the reviewer should carefully compare the text against what is actually done. With the passage of time, small changes can creep into practice until the work done no longer resembles the written procedure. If the organizational unit responsible for procedure issuance and distribution requests a review of all procedures on a scheduled basis, procedures can be kept current to reflect current practice. To show that this review has been performed and that procedures are current, some firms choose to reissue procedures at designated intervals. Each procedure should bear a date of revision which indicates the time at which it was placed into effect. Each revision should be signed by persons approving the procedure; signatures should not be affixed until the reviewer reads and agrees with the text.

4. Procedure Conformance

As stated above, procedures must be followed as written. However, occasions arise that necessitate change. If such change is isolated or temporary, it must be documented in affected records together with a statement of justification. One cannot make a change in established procedure on a whim simply because it seems convenient. There must be a sound, logical reason for doing something other than what is required. If the change or deviation is likely to continue for a time or become permanent, consideration should be given to official revision of the written procedure. Deviations are recognized in the regulations [2] as being necessary on occasion. For example, distribution of stock which is not the oldest is permitted (Sec. 211.150); however, such an occurrence should be temporary. In any event, the reason for the change must be documented. To prove that conformance with a procedure has been achieved, the procedure should identify the documentation system or record in which information is to be placed. Furthermore, the nature of the information to be recorded should be stated. Thus a review of completed records enables one to determine if the procedure has been followed.

E. Raw Materials

The raw materials used in pharmaceutical production consist of components (active and inactive ingredients), containers, closures, and labeling. The regulations [2] are quite specific as to how these materials are to be handled by dosage form manufacturers. For each shipment of each material, the following operations must be documented:

1. Receiving
2. Sampling
3. Testing, including decision of acceptability
4. Usage/disposition

1. Receiving

Upon arrival of a shipment at the manufacturing plant, the material must be inspected for correctness of labeling on the shipping containers identifying the contents. The container is inspected for evidence of damage, and the contents may be examined for appearance or gross contamination. As part of checking the material into the plant, a receiving report is completed to document the receipt of the shipment. This form may also be used to record the results of the visual examinations. The form generally bears a discrete number which is used as a receiving number. All shipments must be broken down to individual vendor's lots so that each can be received independently. Information recorded on the receiving document includes:

1. Identity and quantity of each vendor's lot
2. Name of supplier
3. Supplier's lot number
4. Date of receipt
5. Receiving number (or other internally assigned lot number)
6. Purchase order number
7. Identity of person receiving the material
8. Identity of person performing any visual examination
9. Results of any examination performed for appearance, condition of containers, or condition of material

2. Sampling

Before any material can be used in a batch of drug, it must be representatively sampled, examined or tested, and released for use by the quality control unit. To obtain samples of these materials, a written sampling plan must be used which describes the number of containers to be opened and the amount of material to be withdrawn from each. Special precautions required to protect the health of the person performing the sampling should be included in the sampling instructions. Furthermore, equipment and sample containers should be specified. The containers opened for this purpose must be marked as having been opened for sampling. Records documenting the performance of sampling contain the following information:

1. Identity of material sampled
2. Lot number (receiving number)
3. Number of containers in the lot/amount of material in each container
4. Identity of person performing the sampling
5. Date of sampling
6. Amount of sample taken
7. Location from which sample taken
8. Location to which sample sent for examination or testing
9. Notes on the condition of material observed during sampling (e.g., unusual appearance, contamination, etc.).

3. Testing

No material may be used for production of a drug unless and until it has been found to be suitable for its intended purpose. Written specifications are prepared for each material describing those aspects and conditions of suitability. In order to demonstrate that these characteristics are possessed by the material, records of all tests and examinations performed must be prepared and maintained. These records should contain all the information described earlier in Section IV.B. In the event that such testing is not done by the dosage form manufacturer, a certificate of testing performed by the supplier may be used to demonstrate the satisfactory nature of the material. In the case of ingredients, the manufacturer must perform at least one specific identity test.

After the shipment of material has been judged satisfactory for use, it may be stored for some period of time until entirely consumed. Since storage conditions may affect the identity, strength, quality, or purity of such materials, retesting for appropriate characteristics must be performed (Sec. 211.87). Sampling and testing for this purpose must be documented as stated above. The decision resulting from such retesting, as well as the original testing, must be recorded, together with the identity of the person reviewing the results and making the judgment on the acceptability of the material for use. The performance of retesting is required prior to use when any storage condition (such as heat or exposure to air) may adversely affect the usability of such material. If this reveals that a designated specification is not able to be met, an investigation must be performed in an attempt to determine the cause. Such investigation must be documented reflecting the scope of the investigation, the persons performing the investigation, the data and information collected in conjunction with the review, and the conclusions drawn.

4. Usage

Individual inventory records are required (Sec. 211.184) to be maintained for each lot of each component, drug product containers, and closures. In the case of components, the usage of each lot must be reconciled against the quantity of material received. Minor discrepancies are normal, but limits should be established for the degree of variation permitted. Occasions on which the limits are exceeded necessitate an investigation of the cause of the discrepancy. This investigation should be documented as outlined in Section III. The inventory records must contain sufficient information to permit determination of any batch of drug product associated with the use of each lot of component, drug product container, and closure. Such inventory records generally consist of an individual file card for each lot of material received and released to stock. On the card is listed:

1. Name and lot number of material
2. Quantity of material
3. Date of release/date of required retesting
4. Date of each usage
5. Quantity withdrawn, including any samples
6. Batch number against which material is charged

5. Vendor Approval

In addition to testing raw materials purchased from vendors, most firms make it a practice to purchase only from "approved" vendors. These are suppliers whose performance has been established and proven over a period of time. This may be accomplished on the basis of testing programs (see Sec. IV.C.4) and repeated success in the ability to meet specifications.

Vendor approval may be required for materials not previously purchased from the specific firm in question. Samples of the material to be purchased may be subjected to more scrupulous testing than would be routinely done upon receipt of a shipment. The vendor's manufacturing site may also be inspected. Records of the testing done, including test methods, results, and comparison to any intended specification requirements, should be maintained.

If a site visit is performed, a written report should be prepared. Inspection reports should indicate who did the inspection, when it was done, the equipment and processes examined, the identity of the material to which the inspection applies, and the status of the firm's facilities, systems, and documentation relative to CGMP compliance. Checklists may be prepared to aid in assuring that critical aspects of the vendor's process are reviewed. Such records may include contracts and purchasing agreements or guarantees of quality or delivery. If approved vendors are designated in material specifications, approvals should be reviewed periodically. In other cases, lists of approved vendors should be provided to receiving personnel so that a check of the supplier's name can be performed immediately at the time of receipt of the material, together with checks of material condition.

F. In-Process Controls

The documentation of parenteral manufacturing processes depends on the complexity of the product at hand. The manufacturing process generally consists of formulating a therapeutic ingredient into a homogeneous mass of designated strength, filling the material into a container, closing the container, and removing microbial contaminants. These activities are conducted according to specific written plans and directions. The production and control records have been described previously, but during the time over which these events occur, there is opportunity for the process to vary. The extent of this variation must be measured and documented to establish that the overall process is controlled and that each individual unit in the batch will have quality characteristics that meet established limits. The following subsections describe documentation of some of the major activities occurring during parenteral processing.

1. Material and Equipment Verification

In order to control quality, one must start with the correct materials and use the correct equipment to manufacture the product. Therefore, before any process begins, special effort must be made to check the labeling of the materials to be used against that which is specified on the formula card or other official listing

prescribing material identity. Furthermore, examination should be made of designated equipment to verify that it has been properly cleaned from its last usage and
adjusted for the current process before the process begins. Performance of such
checks should be directed from official manufacturing instructions. Documentation
of accomplishment may be indicated by signature of the person performing the check
and date of performance. These checks are so important that they should be independently checked by a second person who also verifies this performance by signing
and dating the record. Equipment verification should also extend to review of appropriate logs which attest to the cleaning of the equipment. Material verification
may also extend to a second weighment of the components. If performed, these
weights should be independently recorded. Similarly, when ingredients are added
to the mixing vessel, the addition should be marked in the record. Thus the completed manufacturing record reflects that not only were specified ingredients issued,
but the correct quantities were also added to the batch. All of the checks performed
should be recorded in the manufacturing record as separate, independent steps in
the manufacturing process.

   2. Filling

   After batching has been completed according to written directions and specified control tests have been satisfactorily completed, the material is designated as
being suitable for further processing (i.e., filling). Subdividing a large volume
into many units of small volume on high-speed equipment is difficult to do with a
high degree of uniformity. To document the degree of uniformity achieved, individual containers from each filling head are selected periodically for measurement of
the weight or volume of the contents of the container. These results are plotted
on control charts which indicate upper and lower limits of acceptable variability.
The range of individual values and the mean of the values obtained at each time
interval may similarly be calculated and plotted. Since the charts are ultimately
filed with the batch record, they are identified as to the drug processed and the
batch identification number. Other information recorded consists of the identity of
the line or equipment on which the batch is being processed, the date and time of
measurement, the measured weight or volume from each filling head or nozzle, the
control limits for the range and mean of individual values, and an indication of acceptability. If excessive variation is detected, machine adjustments may be required. When such action is taken, it should be identified on the charts and new
measurements should be taken and recorded after the adjustment.
   During filling of parenteral solutions, examination may be made for particulate matter to evaluate the cleanliness of the containers, the product, and the sealing operation. Control charts can be prepared for examination of such attributes.
These charts indicate the fraction defective in the lot. The data are drawn from
independent evaluation of random samples. In addition to recording the routine
identification of product, batch, line, time, and personnel, information concerning
the number of units inspected, the number found defective, and the ratio of the two
is documented. This information is subsequently used to compare the performance
of a specific batch with a series of batches by computing the average fraction defective. This is calculated by dividing the total number of defective units by the
total number of units inspected in the series of batches. This record of comparison
is kept by control personnel separate from the data on a specific batch and is not
filed with batch records. Such data indicate trends and are used to judge the overall effectiveness of the process.

3. Sterilization

Steam Sterilization. The LVP–CGMP regulations [3] proposed in]976 contain the most specific requirements for terminal sterilization of pharmaceuticals ever published by the FDA. The data specified should be obtained for each and every sterilizer load. Records of sterilization identified as to date, product, batch, and chamber number should contain:

1. Temperature data from a mercury-in-glass thermometer located in the sterilizing medium, including the time of reading
2. Time and temperature data from automatic temperature recorder indicating the temperature of the product being sterilized
3. Documentation that overpressure (when used) is established prior to initiation of cooling
4. Information on action taken if automatic alarm activates during processing
5. Results of checks made to determine that bleeders are operating satisfactorily during processing

Records of steam sterilization should include information on any biological indicators if such are used. Such information would include the relative heat resistance of contaminants in the product being sterilized, the expected number of microorganisms in the load, the concentration of biological indicators in the load, the heat resistance of the indicator, the location of the indicators in the load, results of microbiological testing for surviving biological indicators, and a calculation of the lethality of the sterilizing conditions employed for the time of exposure.

Ethylene Oxide Sterilization. Records of ethylene oxide sterilization should indicate the times and temperature of the material subjected to the process, the length and amount of presterilization humidification, relative humidity maintained during sterilization, gas concentration during the cycle, and concentration, location, and type of biological indicators used. Results of testing performed for sterility, surviving biological indicators, and residuals of ethylene oxide, ethylene glycol, and ethylene chlorohydrin should be prepared and maintained.

Sterilizing Filtration. When sterilization of liquid parenterals is accomplished by means of filtration, the user of the process must document the specific type of filter material used, the porosity of the filter, and results of tests performed to indicate that the filter was intact, both before and after use. The filter assembly used must be sterilized by steam or gas before use. Records of this sterilization process must also be prepared and maintained as indicated above. If filters are changed during the filtration process for any reason, the time of such change should be recorded in the batch record together with results of integrity tests and the reason for the change. Any action taken during filtration with regard to the filter must be thoroughly explained in the batch record so that any subsequent question of possible nonsterility or excessive particulates can be investigated as necessary.

4. Leak Testing

Flame-sealed ampuls are generally subjected to a process for testing the integrity of the seal. This process invloves immersion of the ampuls in a highly colored solution in a pressure vessel and rapidly changing the pressure differential between the inside and outside the ampul. This change causes solution to enter ampuls having defective seals. Vials sealed with a vacuum may be subjected to a "spark" test which indicates the quality of the seal and the ability of the container-closure system to maintain the vacuum. Defective units can be removed from the batch in both cases by physical examination. The defectives are tallied and recorded for the purpose of accountability. Rates of defects in individual batches are recorded similarly to the examination for particulates in filling previously described.

Records of dye testing should indicate the identity of the vessel used, date of test, identity of the batch of solution used, pressures employed, and duration of exposure to each pressure. Batch records should also be prepared for the manufacture of each batch of dye solution. Records of vacuum testing of vials should indicate the voltage applied.

5. Lyophilization

The freeze-drying process is sophisticated, not only because of the degree of control required to produce a satisfactory product, but also because of the need to maintain aseptic conditions. The records must be highly detailed, indicating the cleaning and disinfecting of the chamber, when these activities were performed relative to use, the cleaning and sanitizing agents used, and the parameters of the freeze-drying cycle. Records of processing must be clear as to time, pressures, and temperatures. Calibration of the recording devices and sensing instruments are also important and must be thoroughly documented.

G. Environmental Monitoring

One of the most important aspects of process control for parenterals is the determination of the environmental conditions that existed during the time of manufacture. Prediction of contaminants in the product is based on knowledge of the various vectors to which the product is exposed. The umbrella CGMP regulations [2] touch upon environmental control in a very general fashion. They indicate that there must be procedures for process control which assure that the product possesses the quality and purity it purports to possess. The only reference to environmental control during the processing of parenterals speaks to facilities for aseptic processing. Section 211.42 simply requires that there be a system for monitoring environmental conditions.

The proposed regulations [3] dealing with the production of LVPs are uniquely different in that the FDA proposed finite standards for specific environmental systems. Even though the products affected by this proposal are terminally sterilized, the FDA advanced the concept that in order to ensure the biological quality of the finished product, one must control all of the factors affecting microbial contamination at each stage of processing. To produce a contaminant-free product, one takes all reasonable steps to avoid contamination of the product wherever possible, regardless of subsequent steps such as filtration which are designed to remove contamination. The proposed regulations for LVPs speak very clearly to documenting the conditions prevailing during production and identify specific aspects of the environment that must be controlled. Table 2 contains the parameters and control limits proposed for environmental control during LVP manufacturing.

Records of environmental monitoring must first describe the sampling program, what systems are monitored, the frequency of monitoring, and the parameters monitored. Table 2 also indicates the frequency of monitoring designated by the proposed LVP-CGMP regulations. The records must also indicate the results of the testing and conformity with established limits. The results should be reviewed retro-

Table 2 Features of Environmental Control for LVP Production

Environemntal system	Parameter	Frequency	Limits
Air in controlled area	Particles	Not specified; monitor	Not more than 100,000 per cubic foot 0.5 μm and larger
	Temperature		72° ± 5°F
	Relative humidity		30–50%
	Pressure differential		0.05 in. water gage relative to less clean adjacent areas
	Changes		Minimum 20 per hour
Air over filling line and microbial test sites	Particles	While filling is in progress	Not more than 100 per cubic foot 0.5 μm and larger
	Filtration		HEPA filters certified for efficiency
	Velocity		Laminar flow 75–105 ft min^{-1}
	Illumination		Minimum of 100 fc at work surface
Compressed air (points of use)	Particles	1 per day, covering all points weekly	Not more than 100 per cubic foot 0.5 μm and larger
	Purity		Free of oil and oil vapor
	Moisture		Dehumidified to prevent condensate in lines
Water for cleaning	Microbial purity	1 per week, covering all points monthly	Meet PHS standards; not more than 500 organisms per 100 ml
Water for manufacturing, final rinse	Chemical purity	1 per day, covering all points weekly	Water for Injection, USP
	Microbial purity		Not more than 10 organisms per 100 ml
	Storage temperature		Minimum of 80°C or dispose after 24 hr at ambient temperature
Water for cooling the product	Microbial purity	Every sterilizer cycle	Not more than 1 organism per 100 ml

spectively to determine the norm for a given parameter. From this review one can determine the need to change sampling frequency or to revise specifications.

Section 211.188 of the regulations [2] requires that the batch and control records which are prepared for each batch of drug include complete information relating to the production and control of the batch. Environmental monitoring records pertaining to the environment in which a batch was processed may be considered as being batch related. Such records provide completeness relative to the control of the batch. The information contained in these records can be used, together with other data, to evaluate the situations indicating potential product contamination. For example, to judge the impact on product of an environmental parameter having an unusual result, one considers the result collectively in light of all data available. Thus an effective monitoring program can enhance the ability to make sound decisions on product quality.

Parameters other than those indicated in Table 2 are generally monitored by parenteral manufacturers. Surfaces of equipment, walls, and floors may be examined for microbiological contamination by swabs or Rodac plates. Samples of air may be taken for microbiological evaluation. Lubricants used for machinery in aseptic areas may also be tested for sterility. Records of such sampling need to indicate the site, and in the case of air, the volume sampled. If codes are used to designate sampling sites, the key to the code should be maintained with the records.

When test results exceed established limits, an investigation of the cause should be performed. Unfortunately, the time required to obtain microbiological results allows time for the routine cleaning of the sampling site and results may not be able to be corroborated. However, the potential of the site presumed to be contaminated must be evaluated for possible contribution to product contamination. Records of such investigations should, therefore, indicate the timeliness of follow-up sampling, the extent of the resampling, the test results, and an overall narrative description of how the data bear on the quality of the product. It is exceedingly important that the final conclusion be based on fact rather than hearsay or opinion. Part of the evaluation should include consideration of the lethality of the sterilization cycle used as demonstrated by validation. Batches of product may need to be quarantined until the investigation is complete. The records of investigation should be included in the appropriate batch records. Corrective action taken to prevent recurrence must be evaluated for effectiveness. Documentation of such action should be included with the investigational report.

H. Finishing Operations

Finishing operations are those activities that involve the placing of closed containers, together with labeling, into packages for shipment and ultimate sale. These activities include the receipt, identification, storage, handling, sampling, examination or testing of labeling and packaging materials, placing of labeling on containers, accounting for quantities of product and labeling used, examination of labeled product during fabrication of the completed package, and reviewing records of these operations to determine the conformity of actions with established procedures. The records maintained for these operations are similar to those prepared for the handling of raw materials and the fabrication of them into a dosage form. They may be briefer because the processing is less complex and detailed. This is not to diminish the importance of these records since labeling of unmarked containers is one of the most critical steps in the overall process. The FDA has stressed the importance of control of packaging and labeling operations in the preamble to the

1979 revision of the CGMP regulations. The Commissioner stated that "labeling mix-ups are one of the major reasons for recalls."

1. Material Examination and Usage

Just as for components, drug product containers, and closures, packaging materials and drug product labeling must be subjected to a written program detailing the process of receiving, handling, identifying, sampling, testing, or examining these materials (see Sec. IV.E). Similar records of the handling of these articles must also be prepared and maintained to document the sampling, examination, or testing of each shipment prior to use. Since these activities must be documented as occurring before the materials are used, accurate recording of dates to verify the chronology of events is a necessity. In order to render a decision on the usability of packaging and labeling materials, written specifications must also exist for these materials. For labeling and other printed materials, a copy of the text in the form of original artwork, press proofs, or other documents verified for accuracy should be used as the standard against which the sample of incoming material is compared. Documentation establishing the authenticity of the standard by indicating the individual approving it should also be maintained. The importance of reviewing the standard for accuracy cannot be overemphasized. Product recalls have occurred because decimal points were missing in the declaration of product strength or dosage statements. In other cases, small spots that could be mistaken for a decimal point were present at places which significantly altered the meaning of the statement.

Once labeling and packaging materials are found to be satisfactory for use, records continue to be necessary. Storage locations need to be reflected to document that these materials are properly stored to avoid mix-up or to document that their suitability for use is protected. With the advent of roll labels employing special plastics, adhesives, or coatings, temperature and humidity during storage may be important to maintain the quality of the article so that it will adhere to the container at the time of use. In such cases these parameters should be continuously recorded. Once text changes occur or for other reasons the packaging or labeling material becomes obsolete, existing stocks should be promptly destroyed. Records of inventory should be updated to reflect this action when it occurs.

If on-line printing of the drug product container or labeling is performed, the devices used for printing should be controlled as described above. This is regardless of whether the device prints the full text or only a few characters, such as the lot number and/or the expiration date. The device may be examined physically or a specimen of the printing may be prepared for review to verify that the print conforms to the standard. These devices must also be controlled through storage and issuance for use not only to protect the quality of the article but also to prevent misuse. All of these activities must be documented to reflect what happened to each device from the time of receipt to the time of use and ultimate destruction.

Labeling and packaging materials should be issued for use just as carefully as ingredients dispensed from the pharmacy. Records attesting to the specificity and quantity of material issued for use should be prepared. Those items selected for use should also be verified at the line prior to use for conformance to that material specified by the batch production record. This examination should be recorded in the batch record identifying who did the check and when it was done. It is wise to record the material identification on the batch record rather than visually comparing the material against the designation specified in the record. Records should also indicate who dispensed the materials from stock and the lot number or receiving number on the material dispensed.

Labeling should be counted. Any printed material that is product specific must be held in special esteem. Once packaging begins, all labels and labeling consumed must be recorded, whether these materials are placed on product, defaced, or rejected as waste. Any remaining material is also tallied. Remains and material consumed (including waste) must be reconciled with the total quantity issued for use. Records must be prepared showing these quantities and reconciliation, including calculations. Narrow preset limits must be established from experience against which the reconciliation is compared. If the specified quantities of labeling are not found as defined by the limits, an investigation must be conducted to determine where the missing labeling is or why there is an excess of labeling remaining. Such investigation must be recorded and the document included with the production records. It is mandatory that the reconciliation be done promptly upon completion of packaging so that an investigation, if required, can be effectively performed. In some cases, the packaged material may need to be reopened to verify that the material in question was used as designated. If so, records of this rework (reexamination) must be prepared to indicate where it was performed, who did it, when it was done, and the results or findings. It is difficult to record too much information concerning the receipt, examination, storage, and issuance of packaging and labeling materials because this information can become vitally important when attempting to investigate a mix-up or a labeling accountability discrepancy.

2. Packaging Operations

The essence of controlling a packaging operation is to assure that the correct packaging and labeling materials are used on the correct batch of filled product. To do this, the regulations [2, Sec. 211.130] require that sufficient space be used to separate operations, that a lot or control number be used to identify the product, that materials be examined for suitability and correctness prior to use, and inspection of the facilities before and after use. Records of packaging and labeling operations must therefore identify where the work was performed, the equipment and personnel used, and the materials employed specific as to batch.

The verification of materials has just been addressed. Records of inspection of facilities can take two forms. The objective is to verify that materials unsuitable for use are not present. This includes foreign material from previous processing which may be hidden due to machine jams or spills. Some firms choose to specify how the inspection is to be conducted in a written procedure. Articles and locations (waste bins, interior of machinery) to be examined, persons responsible, when the inspection is to be done, and the action to be taken in the event of any type of finding is all specified in the procedure. The record of inspection may then be a positive statement of performance followed by a signature indicating that such inspection was accomplished. If foreign material is found, it may or may not be documented since the signature may be withheld until the facility is judged suitable. The other method is to use a checklist for each packaging line specifying the points of examination and having the inspector record the findings at each point. In either case, some documentation system must be devised attesting to the fact that any foreign materials were removed from the line prior to use. In cases of sequential runs of different batches on the same equipment, the inspection following completion of packaging of the first batch may also serve as the inspection preceding the subsequent batch. Documents should then identify the previous batch so that an investigation of discrepancies, if needed, can be facilitated. A decision as to when two distinct inspections are needed is made at the discretion of the individual firm and depends on the control system employed. Variations in time between processing of batches, changes in equipment to handle container sizes, changes in packaging materials and the ability to restrict personnel access to packaging lines are all factors affecting that decision. When two separate inspections are performed, documentation should be separate and filed with the records of the batch to which it belongs.

Records of packaging must reflect any samples removed from the batch for laboratory analysis, permanent retention, or stability testing. Not only must the product be accounted for, but the labeling components must also be reconciled. Sampling records should reflect who took the samples, when they were taken, how much was taken, and where they were sent. Samples of labeling materials taken as specimens of the material used and included in the batch record should also be included in the reconciliation.

In manufacturing and filling a parenteral into a container, the control of the process is accomplished by periodically examining the process, recording the results, and taking action to adjust the process as necessary based on the findings. Similarly, in packaging and labeling, since it is mandatory that the container bear the correct label and not be defaced or damaged by the packaging equipment, similar actions of sampling, examining material, and data recording are performed. Checks are usually performed by both manufacturing and quality control personnel. Records of these checks are independently maintained. The sampling performed by production is generally done on a spot-check basis at specified time intervals. The items checked (such as component correctness, lot number, expiration date, package content correctness, pallet stacking) are recorded, together with any necessary adjustment or corrective action taken, such as when defective product or components are found. Such corrective action must include documentation of where the defect first occurred and the action taken to remove the defect produced during the intervening time. The sampling by quality control may be done during processing or upon conclusion of packaging. The sampling is statistically based to predict the overall quality of the batch. Criteria for quality, such as definition of critical, major and minor defects, and the tolerable rate (accept/reject criteria) for the presence of such defects, should be included in the product specifications. The number of samples examined, the results of the examination, and conformity of the results to specified standards must all be recorded. The identity of the persons performing the examination and evaluating the results must be contained in the documents. If defects are found to be present at an unacceptable rate, the material may be reworked to remove the defect. In such cases, the lot should be subjected to another statistical sampling upon conclusion of the reprocessing. The rework, resampling, and results of the reevaluation should be recorded separately from the data from the original packaging to avoid confusion. However, the decision on material acceptability should be based on the data representing the status of the lot.

3. Record Review

Upon completion of packaging and prior to release of the batch for sale, all records bearing on the processing and control (testing or examination) of the material must be reviewed for conformity with established procedures and specifications [2, Sec. 211.192]. Insofar as packaging and labeling is concerned, this means that the final review must assure that documentation exists to verify that proper labeling was used, that the labeling and packaging was performed as directed, that the packaging and labeling areas were inspected prior to and after use, that specimens of labeling used have been retained, and that the packaged material was inspected and found satisfactory. Furthermore, if any discrepancy was found during processing, it was satisfactorily resolved. The review includes verification of the yield, a calculation comparing the amount produced (including accountable loss or waste) against the amount that could have been produced from the specified total quantity of ingredients. This calculation is important as a check to detect unidentified losses or mixups. Documentation of this review must indicate what records or parts of records were examined and what the findings were. If discrepancies are detected at this point, they must also be investigated and resolved before release of the batch for sale. The batch records must be amended or corrected and a report of the investigation and its results included in the official files.

I. Miscellaneous Records

   1. Calibration Records

Regulations [2] specifically dictate (Sec. 211.68) that where automatic, mechanical, or electronic equipment is used in the manufacture, processing, packing, or holding of a drug product, such equipment must be calibrated, inspected, or checked according to a written program which is designed to assure proper performance. It is also required that records of such work be maintained. Although this requirement is clarified with regard to laboratory instruments (see Sec. IV. B. 3), it also applies to equipment used in production or for environmental control. Items such as pressure gages, temperature recorders, timers, scales, and thermometers must all be calibrated periodically. Documentation must be prepared attesting to the suitability of the equipment for use. Suitability is based, in part, on the equipment having sensitivity or ability to measure parameters in a range commensurate with the measurements to be taken and recorded. For example, a thermometer required to measure temperatures at 1° intervals should not have only 2° markings on the scale. Furthermore, calibration should measure the accuracy of 1° changes in the range of use experienced in production.

The proposed regulations [3] for LVP production contain some definitive requirements for calibration records. Such documents are to include:

1. A description of the equipment
2. Dates of purchase and installation
3. Operating limits
4. Date, time, and type of test used to determine suitability for use
5. Results of each test or examination
6. Signature of person performing each test

If corrective action (repair or replacement) is required to bring the equipment into compliance with operating specifications, this information must be recorded in the appropriate equipment log, as well as in the record of calibration. To demonstrate that the action was effective, appropriate testing should also be performed and recorded. In addition to the foregoing information proposed by regulations, it is well for calibration records to indicate the identity of the standard against which the equipment or instrument was measured. It is preferable to provide traceability to standards set by an official standard setting body such as the National Bureau of Standards. Certificates of such traceability should be retained in permanent files. The time for retention of calibration data proposed by FDA was 2 years after the expiration date of the product produced on the equipment.

   2. Equipment Cleaning and Maintenance Records

The importance of documenting fulfillment of procedural requirements is seen in the detail required for records associated with the cleaning and maintenance of equipment [2, Sec. 211.67]. The procedures for such operation must:

1. Assign responsibility.
2. Delineate schedules for cleaning, maintenance, and sanitizing.
3. Identify the cleaning and sanitizing agents to be used.
4. Specify how protection of equipment from contamination after cleaning has been performed is to be accomplished.
5. Direct that inspection for cleanliness immediately prior to use be performed.

To verify that these actions have been accomplished as specified, logs are to be maintained for individual pieces of equipment which show for each batch processed:

1. Date of processing
2. Time of usage
3. Product manufacture with the equipment
4. Lot number of the product manufactured

This log may also be used to record the performance of the cleaning and maintenance dictated by written procedures. Such work must be independently checked by a second person and both must date and sign or initial the log as documentation of the work performed. Entries must be made in chronological order. Again, detail and specificity of records is of prime importance so that investigations of problems such as potential contamination of product can be facilitated when the need arises.

3. Sanitation Records

Just as the cleaning of equipment is important to drug processing, the sanitation and care of the overall facility is important to the entire production process and the potential for contamination. In aseptic operations, not only must the equipment be sanitized, but the facility surfaces (walls, floor, and ceilings) must also be disinfected. Therefore, the requirements for sanitation and documentation of such work are virtually identical to those described above for equipment. Since sanitation also extends to the exterior of the facility and the potential for the entry of vermin, documentation should extend to the identification of agents used as rodenticides, insecticides, and fungicides, how and where they are used, who applies them, when, and how much of the agents were used. Even if this work or any portion sanitation is performed by contractors or temporary employees, these activities must be documented.

4. Reprocessing Records

Reprocessing can be performed at any phase of production starting with rework of components. The objective is to take material that does not conform to standards or specifications or which otherwise may not be suitable for use and remove the defect or condition in a manner that will ensure the meeting of all standards and characteristics. Several types of rework have been described previously. Whatever the problem or the nature of the defect, full records of reprocessing must be prepared to identify the condition, the nature of the work done to remedy the situation, where the work was done, the materials and equipment employed, the identity of the persons doing the work, and measurements made to evaluate the success of the process. Because all reprocessing involves the quality of the product, it is absolutely mandatory that the records reflect the review and approval of quality control personnel. The review should occur initially prior to performing the reprocessing so that the potential of the process can be evaluated for expected success or other adverse effects. Upon performance of the reprocessing, the documents and product should be evaluated for quality, and final records should reflect that all standards and characteristics of quality have been met and that the material is suitable for further use or sale.

5. Distribution Records

Records of distribution of drug products must accurately reflect who received each batch of drug so that in the event of product recall, all units comprising the batch can be located in the marketplace. Such records must contain:

1. The name and strength of the product
2. A description of the dosage form
3. The name and address of each consignee
4. The date and quantity of material shipped
5. Control number of the material shipped

By strict adherence to a procedure of shipping all material on a first in/first out basis, some firms identify customers receiving a specific batch of product simply by chronological determination of when a lot was being distributed and to whom shipments were made during that period. This can be complicated by replacement into distribution of returned goods; however, such events must be readily identified.

6. Returned Goods Documentation

Drug products may be returned to the manufacturer for any of innumerable reasons. Virtually all of this material is destroyed, but there may be occasions when it is worthwhile to redistribute certain material. Regardless of the ultimate disposition, records must be prepared for all material returned. These records should indicate the identity (name and strength) of the material returned, its lot or control number, the quantity of material in each lot, the date of receipt, the person and location from which the return is received, and the reason for the return. If the drug is destroyed immediately, this should be noted on the record of return together with the date of disposition. If the drug is to be considered for subsequent resale, its quality must be reaffirmed. Therefore, the material must be sampled for laboratory testing. If the quantity of material returned is sufficient to make testing and redistribution feasible, but the appearance of the containers or packages casts doubt on the safety, identity, strength, quality, or purity of the drug, the material should be destroyed unless testing or an investigation can provide factual information which overcomes the doubt. For this reason, records of returns should indicate the condition or appearance of the goods. Reprocessing may be performed to bring the product into compliance with established standards for redistribution. Records of testing or reprocessing with subsequent testing must be prepared to establish the quality of the material. Should any return implicate the quality of this or other batches, an investigation must be performed. Information gathered from the investigation must be reduced to writing and placed in appropriate batch records.

7. Salvaging Documentation

Salvaging of drugs is concerned with determining whether products that may have been exposed to improper storage conditions may be distributed. When there is direct evidence of exposure to adverse storage conditions such as fire, water, or smoke, products may not be salvaged. When the picture is not so clear, laboratory testing must be employed to judge the suitability of the material for sale.

Records of salvaging must indicate the name of the drug, its lot number, and the disposition, as well as the test results and evidence used in judging the quality of the drug.

J. Administrative and Personnel Records

There are certain records which, aside from serving basic administrative purposes, have a bearing on the processing of drugs and their quality. Some of these are needed to comply with CGMP requirements and are described in the following sections.

1. Job Descriptions

Although job descriptions may generally be considered as serving a purely administrative need (and they certainly are not mentioned by CGMP regulations), they can serve a valuable purpose in CGMP compliance. One main thrust of the regulations is that there be written procedures for virtually all production and control activities. In order to perform these procedures, responsibility must be defined. By specifying responsibility in written procedures according to job title, a word processor can be used to define the duties of each position. By sorting out all of the duties of a specified position, an accurate job description can be prepared. Conversely, duties contained in job descriptions can be used to cross-check the responsibilities designated by written procedures.

2. Training Records

CGMP regulations [2] require that a person be trained in a specific job and in the regulations as they relate to the job function (Sec. 211.25). By having an accurate job description and a complete listing of procedures involved in the performance of a job, one can define the training required. To document that training has been received, a record for each employee should be prepared which includes the person's name, job function, specific training courses or instruction received, date of such instruction, person performing the training, and procedures governing the subject in which instruction was given. If the training program is formalized, additional records may be maintained. These would show the course content and further define the subject presentation by describing audiovisual aids used and outlining the instructional material. Any quiz or examination used to demonstrate the employee's comprehension of the material presented should be included.

3. Consultant Records

Since full-time employees must be demonstrated to possess adequate knowledge and experience to perform their job duties, the 1979 revision of CGMP regulations [2] extended this requirement to persons retained to provide advice in special matters. Records of such persons providing consultative services must be maintained and include the name of such persons, their addresses, and their qualifications. Furthermore, the nature of the service provided should be documented.

4. Health Records

The health of persons coming in direct contact with parenteral drugs during their manufacture is an important aspect of environmental control. Persons having an apparent illness or open lesion that may adversely affect the safety or quality of drug products must be excluded from direct contact with components, drug

product containers, closures, in-process materials, and drug products until the
condition has been corrected. Therefore, all personnel must be instructed to report to supervision any health condition that may have an adverse effect on the drug
product with which they are associated. Once reported, such condition should be
reported on official health records and work performance records to document the
exclusion from contact with the articles mentioned. The records should reflect
dates of reporting, the temporary work area to which the person is assigned, the
date the condition is remedied, and the name of the person (who should be medically
competent) making the decision that the person can return to work in the critical
areas. If a firm has the practice of screening all employees, especially those working in filling areas or other operations of direct product contact, health records
should reflect the nature of the screening tests (such as throat swabs for infectious
disease), the date of the test, and the test results.

V. REPORTS

The preceding section has identified several record systems and defined the information or data to be recorded. Virtually all of this data recording is mandated by
regulations [2]. The term <u>record</u> is considered to be somewhat indefinite since it
can be used to either describe an individual document or a set of documents which
vary in length and content as the need requires. However, all records are concerned
with the documentation of all details associated with the performance of work. The
information documented is quite specific as it relates to an event or series of events
occurring at a finite point in time. Reports are quite different in that they are secondary documents. Reports are usually prepared from raw data or information
contained in one or more records. Reports are a compilation of information from
one or more sources. Because CGMP regulations [2] are primarily concerned with
the documentation of work and the recording of data bearing on the manufacture of
a batch of drug, there are few references to the preparation of reports. Since reports summarize information or draw conclusions from other data, there are basically two types of reports. One type of report is based on information concerning
the work done by the drug manufacturer. This type is prepared by employees of
the firm. Other reports are prepared by persons outside the control of the firm
but have a significant impact on the quality of the product produced by the firm or
the firm's business.

A. Internally Generated Reports

1. Investigation of Deviations

The CGMP regulations [2] require that any discrepancy in batch records or
the failure of material to meet any specification be thoroughly investigated (Sec.
211.192). They also require that a written record of the investigation be prepared
and include the conclusions drawn and any follow-up work. Many examples have
been given in the preceding sections describing instances where such investigation
is necessary and the information to be recorded when such investigation is
undertaken. In all cases, the intent is to determine what went wrong, define the
action taken to correct the situation, and to provide data establishing that the corrective action taken was effective. To do this, it must first be determined that a
discrepancy exists or that the data indicating failure of material to meet specifications are valid. The verification or confirmation of the problem is where the investigation begins. It may then extend to work performed by other persons, such
as production personnel, by review of the records generated at the time of work

performance. By reconstructing the events that took place, systemic flaws or errors can usually be identified. A comparison of what was actually done is then made with what was supposed to have been done. The failure to follow established procedure, misunderstanding of what was required, or the failure to have a defined procedure are basic causes of discrepancies. If the cause can be located, effective corrective action can usually be defined. However, other investigations may be unable to reveal the cause. In any case, all of the matters studied or examined in an effort to define the cause of the problem must be reduced to writing in a single document (report) which is filed with the appropriate batch record. If more than one batch is involved, copies should be prepared for placement in individual batch files. The report should indicate all of the work done (samples tested, records reviewed, interviews conducted) and thereby delineate the factual situation. The facts gathered need to be placed in time so that the chronology is clear. The conclusion can be drawn only if facts are presented. By putting all the facts together, the real problem should become evident. The apparent problem represented by the failure or discrepancy at hand may only be a symptom of a larger or more significant situation. As a general rule, the report of an investigation should contain the following basic elements:

1. Description of the discrepancy or failure
2. Efforts undertaken to locate the cause
3. Factual statement of the results of the efforts
4. Conclusions drawn from the facts gathered
5. Action taken based on the conclusion

2. Reports of Analysis

Reports of analysis are used by manufacturers to supply requesting customers with an indication of the quantitative quality of a specific lot of material. This report summarizes the laboratory data by providing the results of the tests or examinations performed on the material. These reports usually identify the material to which it pertains, the tests performed on the material, and the results of each test. The report may also indicate the range of acceptable limits employed by the firm for each test.

One customer always requesting such information for the material it purchases is the U.S. government. Such requests are really performance requirements which are placed into procurement contracts. Manufacturers supplying material to the government are required to submit certificates of testing verifying that the material meets stated characteristics of quality. These certificates are statements signed by a quality control official, indicating that specified tests have been performed and that the results of such tests meet stated criteria.

Another way in which the government is involved with reports of analysis is the certification of antibiotics or insulin. Each batch is tested by the manufacturer and the results of specified tests are placed on a form sent to the FDA with samples of the batch for testing. Upon satisfactory testing of the batch, the FDA results are entered on the form and compared with those obtained by the manufacturer. If all are found to meet established criteria, the form is signed and returned to the manufacturer, thereby becoming the certificate for the batch.

3. Trend Analysis

The CGMP regulations [2] state that records must be used for evaluating on an annual basis the quality standards for each drug product (Sec. 211.180). This review is intended to indicate whether or not changes in specifications or manufac-turing/control procedures are required. To facilitate this review, firms may choose to prepare reports of trend analysis on an ongoing basis. Such reports may be a simple plotting of each test in the specification, indicating the result of each batch against product limits. Such plots are commonly known as P charts. By employing statistical calculations of process average and standard deviation, a nar-rative report can be prepared defining the status of performance of each product. From this, a decision can be made on the need to change specifications or controls. Such charts should include all batches, even those which are rejected. When speci-fications change or when changes are made to eliminate the cause of rejection, new process averages and charts should be prepared. Because of the loss of sensitivity associated with large numbers, the process average should be updated periodically by having a defined cutoff point such as the total number of batches produced in a specified time period.

4. Internal Audits

If management desires to have an independent evaluation of compliance status, audits of operational units, systems, or products may be performed. The investi-gation may be done by an outside consultant, a special corporate body, or by a des-ignated group within the firm. The designated group often is a section of the quality control organization; however, the success of the audit will be infinitely greater if the group reports directly to top management. The general mission is to assess the degree of compliance with company policies and regulatory requirements. When such investigations are made, reports are prepared. These reports indicate the areas or operating units evaluated and the findings, usually limited to deficiencies, in each area. Such reports should be considered confidential and have limited dis-tribution. Once the deficiency is identified to operating management, a plan of ac-tion and a schedule for implementation of the plan should be elicited. Appropriate follow-up investigation should be conducted to evaluate the success of the action taken. Audit files should contain reports in three basic areas: (1) identified defi-ciencies, (2) planned action and schedule, and (3) follow-up evaluation.

5. Recalls

Although there is no legal requirement that defective drug products in the marketplace be recalled, such events do occur with the encouragement of the FDA. Recent adverse experience with recall effectiveness has caused the FDA to rewrite its internal procedures defining the agency's role with respect to assuring effective removal of defective products from the market. In the future, some of the action to be taken by the FDA in evaluating the effectiveness of a firm's recall efforts will be based on records and reports prepared by the recalling firm. The need for FDA follow-up to a firm's efforts will be based on the medical hazard presented by the defect and the success the firm has in obtaining response to its recall notification.

When recall is undertaken, a firm is expected to maintain records indicating the persons or firms to whom notification is sent, the response of such firms, and the quantity of goods returned. As indicated in the procedures revised in January 1980, the FDA expects firms to expend their resources to determine the effective-ness of the recall request. Therefore, records of such effort must be maintained and the results periodically reported to the FDA. Records on effectiveness checks performed by the firm should indicate how many were performed, the names of the accounts at which checks were conducted, when the check was performed, and the identity of the employee(s) performing the checks. Based on information obtained, periodic status reports should be provided to the FDA district office. Such status reports should include:

1. Number of consignees notified and date and method of notification
2. Number of consignees responding and quantity of recalled material on hand
3. Number of consignees not responding
4. Quantity of material returned and quantity of material accounted for
5. Number of effectiveness checks performed and results
6. Estimated time frame for completion

When the defective material is recovered and the recall is considered complete, the material may be reworked or destroyed. To complete its records, the FDA will expect to be provided with a report indicating the disposition of the material.

B. Externally Generated Reports

1. Reports of Analysis

Just as a drug manufacturer may be requested to provide a report of analysis on its products, a supplier of raw material may provide a report of analysis to the dosage form producer. Such a report would contain the same information as that described previously. The report from the supplier cannot be taken solely at face value by the drug manufacturer. Rather, the data in the report must be validated on a periodic basis. For a fuller discussion of such reports, see Sections IV.C.4 and IV.E.3.

A manufacturer may also receive a report of analysis from the FDA. The factory inspection section of the Food, Drug and Cosmetic Act states that if an investigator obtains a sample of food during an inspection of a food processor, a copy of the results of analysis is to be furnished to management. Although this paragraph does not extend to drugs, the FDA has used the underlying concept as a basis for voluntarily providing firms with the results of testing performed on drug samples obtained during the course of inspection. With the advent of the Freedom of Information Act, the results of tests performed on samples of drugs by the FDA should be available to the manufacturer unless the samples were obtained for regulatory purposes and the proceeding has not been terminated. When samples are collected during the course of an inspection, it may be well to request the results of analysis from the FDA district office.

2. Complaints and Adverse Reactions

Whenever a customer reports any defect or the failure of a drug to produce its desired effect, the data and information must be evaluated. Every attempt must be made to get from the complainant a full and accurate description of the circumstances. All such information must be recorded as to who provided the information and when it was received. From the evaluation, a decision must be made concerning whether or not an investigation needs to be conducted. If the report indicates possible failure of the product to meet any specification, an investigation is required. Records of such reports and investigation must be established. These must contain:

1. Nature of the complaint
2. Name and address of the complainant
3. Name, strength, and lot number of the product involved

4. Reply to the complainant
5. Findings of the investigation and follow-up if performed; if an investigation is not performed, the reason and name of the person making such determination

Adverse reactions to drug products reported to the manufacturer should be considered in the same light as a complaint concerning a product defect. Similar procedures should be employed for evaluating the report of reaction as are used for product defects. The medical significance of the reaction may warrant a different degree of urgency to the investigation, but the key is that the report be verified and appropriate follow-up action initiated as indicated.

Information on adverse reactions and drug experience must also be reported to the FDA if the drug in question is the subject of an approved NDA. Depending on the seriousness of the reaction, reports may be required to be made within 15 days of receipt. Information on effects which are to be expected or which are not alarming are to be reported annually.

3. Inspection Results

Upon concluding an inspection of a drug manufacturer, the FDA investigator provides a report of observations listing those conditions which he or she believes constitute deviations from current good manufacturing practice. Depending on the seriousness of the observations, the report may be followed with a letter from the district office to management identifying those conditions that require prompt attention. This is the first step in the initiation of regulatory action. Both the report of inspection observations and any action brought by the FDA relating to CGMP's must be brought to the attention of top management if these persons are not personally involved in or aware of such actions.

REFERENCES

1. U.S. Food, Drug, and Cosmetic Act, Title 21, U.S.C. 321-392.
2. Code of Federal Regulations, Title 21, Part 211.
3. Fed. Regist., 41(106) (June 1, 1976).

9

Environmental Factors in the Design of a Parenteral Production Facility

A. MICHAEL KELLER

Syntex Agribusiness
Des Moines, Iowa

The facility in which parenteral operations take place is more than just a building to house the activity. It is, in fact, a complete set of conditions, carefully arranged and planned to provide an unnaturally clean production environment. The core of the facility is the clean production area. It is not only visibly clean from contaminants, but is as free from microscopic, viable and nonviable, contaminants as it is possible to make the area. To achieve such cleanliness and still provide for the entrance and exit of personnel, supplies, and products, a very complex system of barriers, buffer areas, traffic control, and environmental control must be developed. This development begins with the selection of a plant site, chosen to minimize in all ways possible inadvertent ingress of contamination to the plant itself. Then a series of zones are established in the floor plan (Fig. 1) to provide both a barrier to the ingress of contamination and a space allocation for activities requiring appropriate levels of cleanliness. At the same time, the zones maintain a buffer to the next, more clean area. Thus the areas within a plant progressively become more clean by design and by control until the cleanest critical area is achievable at the level required for the safe production of parenteral medications.

Therefore, the design of a parenteral facility requires giving careful attention to a variety of environmental parameters, such as site selection, area planning, space planning, design and construction features, traffic flow of personnel and supplies, and service features. This chapter deals with the impact of these environmental factors on facility design. It should be noted that many of these factors also apply to other types of pharmaceutical production facilities but with emphases that differ with the specific needs of the operation.

I. SITE SELECTION

The first step in producing a parenteral production environment is to choose the best possible site. Site selection is not a simple or straightforward task but in most respects does not differ from the site selection task for any production facility. The criteria for site selection can be assembled in two general groups: basic factors and pharmaceutically important factors. Basic factors such as land availability, land cost, construction costs, taxes, utility costs, labor availability, labor costs,

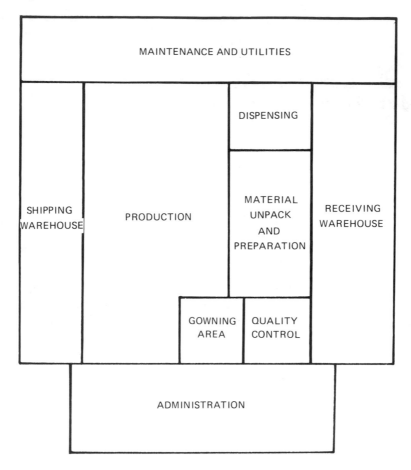

Figure 1 Typical layout of a parenteral plant.

and so on, although important, do not affect the provision of a clean production environment. Pharmaceutically important factors are those which require special consideration because of unique pharmaceutical needs.

A. Basic Plant Requirements

Basic plant requirements include an adequate supply of raw materials, transportation availability, market proximity, adequate utilities, and labor supply. Raw materials, transportation availability, and market proximity can be evaluated together, giving emphasis to each as the specific situation requires. A parenteral facility is unlike a heavy industrial plant, which must be located near the source of its raw materials to minimize freight, since most pharmaceutical raw materials are relatively small in volume and weight. But proximity to a source of a particular raw material may be of concern to a pharmaceutical facility for reasons of control. Minimizing shipping may aid in minimizing potential contamination, material degradation due to aging or lack of environmental control (e.g., temperature or humidity), or may ease the security problems associated with controlled substances. The pharmaceutical facility may utilize rail, truck, or air transportation, although truck is the predominant means. To minimize the potential for damage and contamination and minimize security risks if controlled substances are involved, the potential plant site should be served by several truck lines to reduce the number of interline transfers.

B. Energy

A parenteral facility is not a fuel-intensive operation, but does require a reliable source of energy for both domestic uses, such as heating, cooling, hot water, and lighting, and production uses, such as sterilization and distillation. Coal constitutes a vast energy source, but is seldom used in any but very large plants, even if it is readily available, due to the high cost of environmental control equipment required. When available, natural gas is usually the least expensive fuel but is especially susceptible to curtailment during peak use periods. Various grades of fuel oil are available in most areas. Electricity is also considered an energy source. Electricity is the usual energy source for lighting and equipment power but may also be used for heating, cooling, or steam production. If the electricity must be generated by burning coal, oil, or gas, it probably will not be an economical primary energy source. If the electricity is generated by another method, particularly hydroelectric, it may be an economically viable alternative.

The pharmaceutical concern about energy is that it be reliable. Steam used for sterilization and sanitation must be of consistent quality and must be continuously available. Two types of failure may occur: equipment failure and fuel shortage.

Protection from equipment failure can be obtained by redundant equipment installation. In a redundant system, critical items of equipment are duplicated and operated as standby equipment. In some cases, the standby equipment need not be the same size as the base equipment if noncritical steam uses, such as heating or humidification, can be curtailed during periods of emergency operation. Duplication of critical equipment has the added advantage of allowing routine maintenance on the idle equipment without scheduling production downtime.

Protection against fuel shortage is obtained by dual fuel capability. Fuel oil, natural gas, and propane usually can be burned in the same boiler with the addition of appropriate fuel systems. Electricity cannot be used for heating boilers made for burning gaseous or liquid fuel, so redundant boilers are necessary if electricity is to be used as a standby fuel source.

The selection of a fuel combination is not a pharmaceutical concern but an economic consideration. The pressure, temperature, and quantity of steam produced is a function of equipment design, not fuel type.

C. Water

Water is an ingredient common to most parenteral formulations and copious quantities are needed for equipment cleaning, container washing and rinsing, process and personnel cooling, and steam generation. A basic premise for the water system of a parenteral plant is that the water quality must be controlled. Given some range of supply quality, the in-plant treatment must be able consistently to produce water of a desired quality. Whether supplied through a municipal treatment plant or obtained directly, water is usually taken from either wells or a surface supply such as a river or reservoir. Well water has a more consistent temperature and quality than surface water, but may be of a higher hardness (mineral content). Surface water temperature will tend to vary seasonally, as will its quality, due to contamination by floods, industrial accidents, or even sabotage.

D. Waste Disposal

Waste disposal includes solid, liquid, and airborne wastes. Solid wastes normally pose little problem for parenteral facilities since most solid waste consists of paper or plastic film, all of which can be compacted and buried in a sanitary landfill or incinerated. On-site landfills may be considered, but are usually a poor alternative due to the growing complexity of environment concerns about landfill site selection and operation. Environmental concerns about the disposal of hazardous solid wastes are becoming more serious. Special attention must be given to facilities for the disposal of broken glass which may contain product residue, or product itself, which may have to be discarded either in total or by component. If laboratory animals are used, special disposal methods may be required, but normally, burial in a landfill or incineration are the best disposal methods.

Liquid waste disposal usually presents the greatest concern for a parenteral facility. Storm sewage, usually runoff from a roof, can be both a direct and an indirect problem. In a direct sense, a plant site should have natural drainage so that the plant does not risk flooding or being surrounded by swamplike conditions during wet seasons. The achievement of drainage artificially, by pumps, levees, and so on, is expensive, often difficult to maintain, and is subject to failure. Indirect problems can be caused by trace quantities of chemicals finding their way into storm sewage; for example, cooling tower water treatment chemicals, chemical spills in or around the plant, or airborne chemicals that settled on the roof. These amounts are normally quite small and can be controlled, but if the storm sewage finds its way to a stream that has a low or intermittent flow, the contamination may be significant.

The greater concern with liquid waste is process waste, including spills, sanitation chemicals, rinse water, and laboratory wastes. If the plant must treat its own wastes, an extensive project is indicated. Regulations covering sewage treatment plants are moving toward a zero-discharge concept; the treatment plant effluent will not increase the contaminant load of the stream into which it discharges. Having a municipal system to accept plant sewage does not solve all treatment problems. The Environmental Protection Agency is establishing pretreatment standards for various types of industries, and pharmaceuticals is one. In essence, these standards will make it mandatory, or at least economically prudent, to pretreat industrial sewage before discharge to public-owned treatment works (POTW). The general contaminants that the POTW cannot handle or cannot handle economically must be eliminated by pretreatment, which may require holding tanks, settling basins, or chemical treatment.

Site selection also may be strongly influenced by nontechnical factors. A company's philosophy may dictate that all facilities be built on a common site. In other cases, the parenteral facility may be an adaptation or expansion of an existing facility, or an existing facility may be acquired by purchase. In these situations, items that are normally factors in site selection become given characteristics, and attention must be turned to minimizing shortcomings and meeting the unique requirements for a parenteral facility site.

II. FACILITY AREA USE PLANNING

Planning for a production facility requires a determination of the functions necessary and the size and location for each function. A general assessment of the proposed plant operation will reveal the facility needs, the type of environment necessary, and the functions that must be integrated into a smoothly operating unit. After these needs are determined, a review of the functional needs will lead to a determination of area requirements and relative location for each function.

A. General Operational Assessments

A first step in the design of a parenteral environment should be to define needs. At least the following aspects must be analyzed:

1. Type of Production Line

Parenteral production may be done batchwise, continuously, or in an integrated semicontinuous manner. A batch operation is one where a discrete volume of product and its related assembly and packaging components are moved step by step through the production process, maintaining a tight accountability at each step. A continuous production operation is typified by a chemical plant "pipeline" process, where an operation is performed continuously, for example, in the mixing of hot and cold water. Accountability by comparison of input versus output is usually not possible, with emphasis instead being on process control. Integrated operations are those where continuous processes are utilized, but breaks in the process allow accountability checks after critical steps.

Batch Operations. Batch operation is suited to small production volume and a minimum financial investment is necessary. The equipment required may be glass carboys or glass-lined steel tanks with laboratory-style equipment for weighing ingredients. Product quality, consistency, and homogeneity are all relatively easily controlled in a batch operation. Production documentation can be complete since it is easy to define clearly the ingredients, the process, and the final product.

Since the scope of each individual process step in a batch operation is limited, little equipment and space are needed. Consequently, batch operations are usually done in a series of relatively small rooms, as illustrated in Figure 2. Environmental control for the individual steps of a batch operation is relatively simple, perhaps only a laminar flow hood.

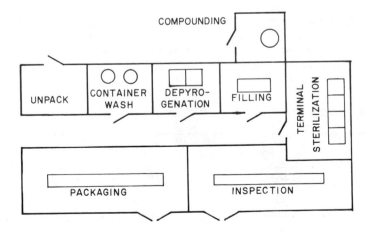

Figure 2 Batch production layout.

Batch operations are normally very flexible, permitting maximum utilization of equipment for a variety of products. Economically, the batch operation is undesirable because it is labor intensive and does not exploit the economies of volume. Although product accountability may be good for each step of a batch operation, it may be difficult to maintain during periods of storage between production steps, where there is always a risk of inadvertent mixing of two or more separate batches of in-process product. Similarly, although it may be relatively easy to provide a clean environment for a batch production step, it is difficult to maintain pharmaceutically clean conditions while the product is transported between production steps or while the product is stored between production steps.

Continuous Operations. Continuous production operations are suited to very high volume production requirements and minimize all the shortcomings of a batch process; labor, production time, and environmental exposure of the product are all minimized. Continuous operations have another unique set of shortcomings however. Most important is that product quality assurance is difficult. It is impossible to document the ingredients or process cycle for a product produced in a continuous process as well as one can for a batch process. Documentation for a continuous process emphasizes process control, whereas batch processes emphasize recording. Although the difference may seem insignificant, it may be important. For example, in a batch process setup each unit of product may be subjected to a particular operation such as sterilization, and this operation may be well documented by a chart record of the temperature and time for a group of units. In a comparable continuous operation, there will be a temperature record, but if, for example, a short temperature deviation was noted, it might be impossible to isolate the unit or units that were affected by the deviation, thus placing a much larger amount of production in question.

Environmentally, the continuous process has both advantages and disadvantages. Since intermediate material-handling steps are eliminated, the potential for product contamination during those steps no longer exists. Continuous processes usually require more space than batch processes and more complex equipment is required. An idealized continuous process might be as shown in Figure 3. It is readily apparent that the diversity of tasks being performed in a common area, for example, filling and packaging, would make it impossible to provide and maintain a clean environment such as would be required for filling. Pharmaceutical processes are composed of steps too diverse in environmental requirements to allow total use of continuous operations. Even compartmentalized steps, as illustrated by the dashed-line walls in Figure 3, are impractical because of the accessibility limitations and because of the relatively large openings necessary for product and personnel to travel between adjacent areas.

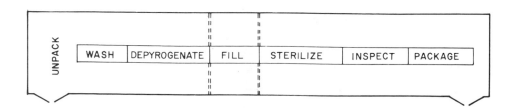

Figure 3 Continuous production layout.

Integrated Operations. To utilize the advantages of both types of processes, a parenteral operation may be broken into discrete steps as for a batch process, but then these small steps will be grouped or integrated into larger, more efficient process steps. Figure 4 illustrates how the batch process of Figure 2 may be integrated. The container preparation steps of unpacking, washing, and depyrogenation are done in a continuous manner but are separated environmentally so that debris from the unpacking operation cannot contaminate the washing. Immediately after preparation, the containers are transferred, either batchwise as in trays or continuously by conveyor, to a filling area which is adjacent to but not common with the container preparation area. The filling area can then easily be maintained as a cleaner environment. Following filling, sterilization is separated as a unique step. Finally, inspection and packaging are grouped into a continuous process requiring less rigid environmental control than that of the preceding steps.

2. Diversity of Product Line

Where the production is limited to only a few product lines, the layout can be "fine-tuned" for optimum efficiency. When the product line is diverse, more space may be necessary to accommodate a more flexible operation. Equipment that can run varied products, containers, and so on, will often be larger and require more storage space for change parts. Or, complete machines may have to be moved in and out of a line for a product change.

3. Container Size

Small volume parenterals (SVPs) and large volume parenterals (LVPs) obviously require different space considerations. All production equipment has container size limitations—large containers require large equipment and more space throughout the line. While a day's usage of small ampuls may be moved into the feeding position of a line in a single load, the supply of containers to a line filling 1 liter bottles will require continuous replenishment. If containers are packed in corrugated cardboard on wooden pallets, an additional unpack or load transfer area may be needed to prevent an unnecessary particulate load near the washing area, as was illustrated in Figure 4.

At the end of the filling line, the large and heavy LVPs will require more provision for mechanized material handling equipment, including accummulation and segregation areas. Door sizes, too, must be large enough to accommodate large carts. The relatively small bulk of SVPs often makes it possible to handle them manually without major problems.

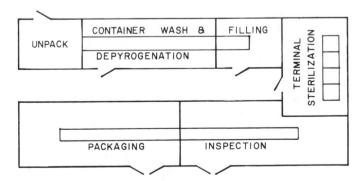

Figure 4 Integrated production layout.

4. Environmental Control Needs

Adequate space will be needed for both line equipment and support areas. For an aseptic filling process, provision must be made for sterilization and depyrogenation of containers before filling, normally by hot air ovens or tunnels. Then filling requires an aseptic environment with the attendant support rooms. After filling, the containers can be taken directly to inspection and packaging.

Nonaseptic filling, followed by terminal sterilization, normally requires less rigid environmental control. A well-controlled washing process may produce acceptably clean glassware and eliminate hot air sterilization prior to filling. Following filling and sealing, an accumulation and segregation area is required to accumulate the product for transfer to the next process step.

5. Product Characteristics

Liquids are probably the easiest products to handle, with consideration of batch size being necessary when a means of transporting the product to the filling line is determined.

Powders are difficult to handle. A batch-type process may be imperative to prevent loss and cross-contamination in material-handling systems. Dust control systems are absolutely necessary, and provision will be necessary for frequent cleaning of the systems.

Emulsions may require compounding areas close to filling lines to ease transfer problems. Pumping systems will be very critical. Overhead gravity feed to filling might be desirable.

Suspensions will require a means of maintaining a homogeneous mixture prior to filling. To minimize the time the suspension resides in the piping, reservoir, and pump system, filling rates should be kept high and the distance from compounding to filling should be minimized.

B. Area Planning

The design of a parenteral plant, not unlike any production facility, must carefully integrate an array of complementary and sequential activities—area planning. To aid in this integration, various means of grouping the separate functions of the proposed facility can be used. Since providing an exceptionally clean, perhaps sterile environment for filling is the most critical need, area planning may be addressed by designing functional groups around this critical area with particular attention given to maintaining cleanliness.

1. Environmental Control Zone Groupings

Section 212.222 of the proposed Current Good Manufacturing Practices for Large Volume Parenterals (CGMP-LVP) [1] published June 1, 1976, requires that "Air over filling lines and at microbiological testing sites shall:

(a) Have a per-cubic-foot particle count of not more than 100 in a size range of 0.5 micron and larger throughout the entire work area upstream of the work piece.
(b) Be supplied at the point of use as specified in Section 212.77."

Section 212.81 of the same CGMP requires that "The weighing, mixing, or filling of large volume parenteral drug products and transfer operations, as described in Section 212.3(b)(13), shall be performed in specifically designated areas that shall meet the requirements for a controlled environment area. . . ."

From these environmental condition requirements emerge the first two of a series of cleanliness levels which provide, together with the physical aspects of the facility, successive barriers to product contamination. These barriers form environmental control zones as illustrated in Figure 5.

Zone 7: Filling Line. The walls of the filling area are the last physical barrier to the ingress of contamination, but within the filling area a technique of contamination control known as laminar flow may be considered as the last barrier to contamination. This last zone is specifically required and defined in the proposed CGMP Section 212.222 and will be discussed later in greater detail.

Zone 6: Filling Area. Zone 6 is a distinct zone of the controlled environment area for an aseptic filling process, but may not be a distinct zone for nonaseptic filling processes. The proposed CGMP defines and requires controlled environment areas for any weighing, mixing, filling, or transfer operation. Whether aseptic or not, the filling area is usually the most highly controlled environment created by a structural barrier in a parenteral facility. Air handling system requirements are the same as for zone 5, but for aseptic filling microbiological control is also specified. For nonaseptic filling, the distinction between zone 6 and zone 5 may be the minimization of activity around the filling line to reduce contamination potential.

Zone 5: Weighing, Mixing, and Transfer Area. Zone 5 encompasses those activities of "weighing, mixing, filling or transfer operations" addressed by CGMP Section 212.81 which are not handled as zone 6 but which require a controlled environment. Air-handling systems are equipped with HEPA (high efficiency particulate air) filters capable of removing 99.97% of all particles over 0.3 μm in size and have temperature and humidity control. Microbiological load is highly controlled or eliminated and special measures are taken to aid sanitation.

Zone 4: Clean Area. Production areas immediately preceding or following a controlled environment area in the production flow are often controlled as an area intermediate between a general production area and a controlled environment area. Activities in these areas may include washing and preparation of equipment or accumulation and sampling of filled product. Air filters of slightly lower efficiency

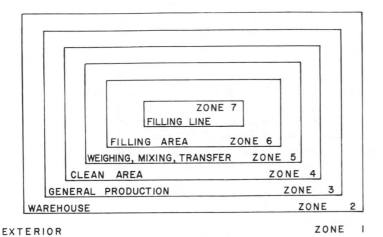

EXTERIOR   ZONE   1

Figure 5 Environmental control zones.

than HEPA filters may be employed to control particulate contamination in the sub-visible range. Some attempt is usually made to reduce or control the base micro-biological load.

Zone 3: General Production Area. The third zone of environmental control is formed by the periphery of the general production area. Openings into the area are usually well sealed and large enough for only essential material-handling equip-ment and personnel. Windows are either absent or sealed closed. Insects, crawl-ing or flying, and rodents should be absent, having been controlled in the general plant area. Air-handling systems remove most airborne contamination in the vis-ible range.

Zone 2: Warehousing. The second environmental control zone provides min-imal protection for materials and product. It is the first zone created by a struc-tural barrier. Exterior walls and roof are effective in stopping large objects such as people. Due to the fact that large openings are required for easy access (truck doors, etc.), this barrier may be only marginally effective against insects, rodents, and birds. Control of airborne contaminants is often little more than window screens or rough air intake filters.

Zone 1. Plant Exterior. The environment within which a plant is located is the first environmental control zone. It is largely a base point from which to work in determining the requirements for the various control barriers, but it is also a zone that can be controlled. This control can be affected through planning and man-agement. Planning may involve choosing a location that is free of objectionable air-borne contaminants such as may be present in heavily industrialized areas, or it may involve landscaping which will discourage the growth of objectionable insects. Management actions to control zone 1 might include the maintenance of "sterile" areas around the facility where weeds, insects, and rodents are controlled or elim-inated.

2. Functional Groupings

Another essential grouping necessary for area planning is the functional group-ing. As the name implies, similar activities are grouped together for the purposes of ensuring that all necessary functions are considered during the planning process and to aid in proportioning the available space efficiently. After the groupings are established and after initial concepts have been proposed, a table of space require-ments should be prepared. This table will list the various functional units being considered and the space or percent of space allocated to each. Initially, if no other guidelines such as comparison to a similar facility are available to establish the area relationships, assumptions may have to be made to establish a starting point. As operations in each area are finalized, the space allocations will be adjusted, but such adjustments must be made carefully, determining what effects there may be upon other related groups. For example, an increase in production area space may result in the need for additional warehouse or quality control space. Table 1 illus-trates how a table of space requirement can be started. As the facility plan becomes more complete, the table of space requirements, like an iterative mathematical solution to a series of simultaneous equations, will become more accurate and will help ensure that all important functions are appropriately considered.

Production Functions. Production space needs are directly related to pro-duction volume requirements. This does not mean that a fixed relationship can be found to indicate space needs as a function of production output. Rather, once

Table 1 Space Requirements

Function	Area	
	Square meters	Percent
Production Operations	11,094	45.1
Warehouse	7,606	30.9
Administration	1,018	4.1
Utilities	1,016	4.1
Quality Control	1,716	7.0
Engineering and Maintenance	1,104	4.5
Employee Services	1,014	4.1
Security	39	0.9
Total	24,607	100.0

production requirements are known or estimated, economic comparisons of various production concepts, layouts, and equipment can be made. If the premise is accepted that production is the purpose of a production facility, it follows that production needs are a valid basis, although not necessarily a complete one, for determining the needs for other functional units within the facility.

Warehousing. Basic warehousing functions include receiving, shipping, and in-process storage. Related functions that must be provided include storage of operating supplies and excess or surplus equipment. Receiving areas include unpacking, sampling, and incoming quarantine. Shipping includes quarantine prior to shipment. The storage of spare parts, air filters, change parts, water treatment chemicals, office supplies, laboratory supplies, janitorial supplies, production supplies, uniforms, and so on, may be handled as central storage or individually by department, but nonetheless must be provided for. The location of warehousing with respect to production areas should facilitate the holding of materials in a controlled manner convenient to the processing areas. The first and most basic warehouse function is to receive and hold incoming materials. To be most efficient, these materials should be held as near to the beginning of the production process as possible, but yet be isolated so that any contamination associated with warehousing can be contained. Warehouse space is usually of greater height than production areas, is less rigidly controlled from an environmental and sanitation standpoint, and usually has a relatively high density of flammable materials. Thus a separate, but adjoining area separated by a firewall is usually the best arrangement.

Administrative Areas. Administrative area planning requires careful analysis of the direct and indirect administrative requirements of a particular plant. Company policy regarding office space for the various levels of supervision and management must be determined. Successively higher levels of supervision are usually provided successively larger office areas. Some offices are individual, while some are grouped in an "open area" concept. Working supervisors often have work areas within the production areas, but some companies provide adjacent offices. Most important is an awareness of the close supervision and exacting documentation requirements for the production of parenterals. Storage of both in-process and historical records must also be considered. The relative location of administrative areas demands particular attention. For the direct supervision necessary to maintain production, a close proximity is desirable. Any other support offices should be separated from the production area because, first, production area contaminations can be related to people—the reduction of numbers of people will reduce the challenge to the plant cleanliness. Second, many of the "fringes" normally associated with administrative areas—plants, flowers, closets, outside windows—are potential contamination sources. Finally, the traffic of visitors, vendors, employment applicants, and so on, who are not particularly acquainted with pharmaceutical discipline can be reduced.

Indirect administrative requirements are related more to the relationship between the plant and company or corporate headquarters. These indirect administrative requirements will include functions not directly related to plant operation, such as company or corporate management and staff functions.

Utilities. Utilities within a pharmaceutical plant can become complex. Due to their diversity and the basic requirement for their control, utilities must be located in an easily accessible area. Piping systems, in particular, must be initially and often periodically cleaned and serviced. Exposed overhead piping is not acceptable from a cleanliness or contamination standpoint since they collect dirt, are difficult to clean, and may leak. Buried or concealed pipe may require unacceptable demolition for cleaning or repair. The choice of location for utilities can have important ramifications for the entire plant because of the amount or lengths of piping and wiring in, over, under, and around critical production areas.

Quality Control. Quality control serves several functions and therefore may be located in one or several locations. The sampling and testing of incoming raw materials is best done at the point of receipt, the incoming warehouse staging area. However, sampling can often be done in the staging area and be transported to another location for testing. Quality assurance, a production monitoring function, may be defined as a quality control subgroup. If separate facilities are provided, a midproduction location is ideal, but, as for incoming sampling, the area and equipment requirements are not so great as to preclude operation from a remote site.

The general laboratory function is such that it should be close by, but integration into the production area is not necessary and perhaps even not desirable in order to relieve quality control from undue production pressure. Generally, pharmacology laboratory facilities, if needed, should be remote because of contamination risk from animals. Microbiology may require conditions equal to the cleanest production area and should be adjacent to the general laboratory to utilize some of the same support services but must be effectively separated from production to prevent contamination crossover. A final discrete function of quality control is documentation. This is not a direct production support and might be located so as to utilize some of the facilities of the general administration area.

In summary, if quality control is considered a single entity in a single location, this function must be immediately adjacent to production. If split into operational units, incoming quality control and quality assurance would best function in production locations. General laboratory, pharmacology, microbiology, and documentation can be in one or more adjacent or remote locations.

Engineering and Maintenance. Engineering support will depend on the plant size, degree of sophistication, and the amount of support provided by the parent corporation. Engineering responsibilities and involvements tend to range widely— any location within a facility will have pros and cons. From an engineering stand- point, even a location outside the plant can serve well if access to the production area by engineers for fieldwork is not too difficult. Often, particularly in small or less complex plants, maintenance or other plant service functions such as util- ities are combined with engineering, making an in-plant location desirable. In these cases, a location near the maintenance or the utility area is usually chosen.

Although often associated with engineering, maintenance is a unique and dis- tinct function. Maintenance responsibilities cover all areas of the plant and can generally be grouped into two categories, plant maintenance and production main- tenance. Production maintenance is a direct production support function and includes all the routine and recurring operating maintenance work. Production maintenance facilities are usually minimal, often only a place to store a toolbox, and seldom have more than a small workbench. Personnel normally utilize the same employee services as the production personnel and seldom require any other special provi- sions.

Plant maintenance operations, in contrast, are more diverse. They vary from heavy maintenance on production equipment to cosmetic work on the building exterior and often include plant service functions such as sanitation, groundskeeping, or waste disposal. Facilities required are extensive and must include provisions for equipment cleaning, disassembly, major rebuilding of equipment, and painting. These operations are alien to pharmaceutical operations and must be isolated. Al- though maintenance requires access to all parts of a plant, it must be conveniently located to be able to receive and handle cumbersome and bulky goods. An absolute must is that the plant maintenance shop be located so that its personnel have easy access to major plant utilities and service equipment. A desirable location might be on an outside wall of the plant, near a loading dock and with access to the plant boiler room and air-conditioning equipment area.

Employee Services. Employee services that must be provided include cafe- teria, locker rooms, rest rooms, and personnel services such as interviewing, benefits, and health facilities. Of these, the cafeteria location and size are prob- ably the most difficult. A determination of its function must be made by consider- ing the following questions:

Will the cafeteria prepare hot meals, be catered, or be served by vending machines?
Will the cafeteria need to accommodate all employees at once, or will the lunch and
    break times be staggered?
Will the cafeteria be used for noon meals only, or will it also serve as a break area
    and employee assembly area?

The general problem associated with cafeteria facilities is sanitation, with security being a second important problem. With respect to sanitation, the presence of food creates a potential rodent and insect problem. If fresh food preparation is involved, the cafeteria must be isolated from the production area. With respect to size re- quirements for a cafeteria, cafeteria facilities are often efficiently utilized for coffee breaks and employee assemblies as well as for lunch breaks. In addition to deter- mining size, the answer to these questions indicate that the cafeteria should be lo- cated close to the production area to minimize travel time to and from workstations. In large plants, small lunch facilities are sometimes located throughout the plant, but because of the critical environmental control necessary in a parenteral facility, this system is difficult to control.

Locker rooms and their location must be considered in view of their role in the overall plant dress code. In some respects, locker rooms serve the plant as does a cafeteria: most employees use them, they are used for only a short period of time, and they may require servicing by outside vendors for collecting soiled and dispensing clean uniforms. The volume of people to be handled through a locker room will be determined by the number of personnel to be attired in plant uniforms.

Rest room facilities are usually considered in conjunction with locker rooms. For small plants, rest room/locker room combinations may be adequate. For larger plants, conservation of employees' time to and from rest rooms and OSHA requirements for rest rooms within 200 ft of work areas may require additional facilities.

Two closely related services to be planned into a facility are the personnel and employee safety and health offices. The personnel office must be located so as to be convenient to interview employment applicants, but also must be located to provide benefits service to employees. To minimize employees leaving the production areas and the possible need for uniform changes, and so on, these services should preferably be located in or near the production area. Similarly, employee safety and health services (medical, first aid, etc.) are necessarily located in or near the production area.

Security. Security is a plant service that also should be included in initial planning. If controlled substances are to be a part of the plant operation, then the production area, or an appropriate part of it, must include security in the planning. Access means should be limited so that monitoring of personnel is facilitated. The layout of the area should facilitate surveillance by camera or by visual means. Effective security is multileveled and utilizes electronic aids, but must always be backed by surveillance. From a physical planning standpoint, security requires space. Wherever personnel control is needed, such as at the various security zone entrances, facilities for security equipment or guards must be provided. Minimum requirements are for a desk and equipment console. Somewhere, as at the main entrance, a security "headquarters" is required. The complexity and sophistication of the security system will affect the space required but, in general, the space required for electronic systems, and so on, may be little different from the space required for guards. Functions that may be part of the security operation and thus require space consideration include:

Visitor control: Signing in and out, issuance of badges or passes, escorting visitors, information or instructions.
Emergency reaction: Monitoring alarm devices, issuance of emergency fire or police alarms, disaster alarms, weather alarms, directing emergency vehicles.
Critical system monitoring: Monitoring and reacting to alarms on process system or plant equipment.
Off-hours process control: Starting or stopping equipment or processes at predetermined times, logging of critical data.
Security response: Respond to or investigate security violations or alarm conditions.

3. Proximity Groupings

All plant support functions have reasons to be within, near, or adjacent to the primary production area. These needs are real, and it may be helpful and important to define a type of "proximity priority" to aid in choosing the optimum location for the various functions. Extensive use of this grouping must be avoided when making planning decisions since a seemingly valid argument can be made for locating any service function near the production area, depending on one's point of view.

4. Personnel Flow

The movement of personnel should be planned during the design of individual plant areas, but because of its importance, it should also be reviewed periodically during the planning process as a total facility need. Although each individual production area may have a smooth and efficient personnel flow pattern, a discontinuous or crowded pattern may develop when several individual production area plans are combined. Discontinuous or crowded flow patterns can decrease production efficiency, increase security problems, and increase the problems of maintaining a clean environment.

An evaluation of personnel flow should be made in terms of the Environmental Control Zone Groupings on page 362. Personnel flow paths from zone to zone must be such that access to higher levels of cleanliness is only through change rooms, gowning areas, locker rooms, or other areas as may be required to prepare the personnel for the cleaner area.

From an administrative standpoint, personnel should have direct and well-defined paths from the plant entrance to their usual work area. If possible, a central area from which work assignments are made is desirable. If several production areas exist, secondary assembly areas may be needed to control the assignment of personnel.

Security concerns about personnel flow may include minimizing access to controlled substances and minimizing the personnel traffic in or near work areas where controlled substances are handled. Employee safety, as defined by OSHA, the Life Safety Code, building codes or local requirements will dictate the number and size of egress means for a work area. The controlling factor usually is the number of employees concerned, but the types of hazards must also be considered.

The flow of material and personnel through a common corridor is usual. However, highly traveled personnel corridors are inefficient and unsafe paths for moving materials, particularly if heavy forklifts are required. Further, the use of dedicated material flow paths helps reduce the potential contamination of various packaging materials.

Parenteral plants, like any other plant, have visitors, and the degree of access to be granted must be determined. Planning for visitors and nonproduction employees in advance can prevent or lessen many future problems, particularly in critical areas. A glassed mezzanine or balcony provides absolute isolation, yet may give an excellent view of the process, but may not be adaptable for single-floor layouts. For single-floor, low-ceiling facilities, liberal use of windows along personnel corridors will minimize requests for access into the various production areas.

III. DESIGN CONCEPTS

The progression from operational concepts and floor plans to working drawings and then to a functioning plant requires grappling with the real problems of just how something is to be done. Often, the alternatives may differ little and the one chosen may depend on the personal preference of the engineer who will do the detail design work. In other instances, basic concepts are involved, dictated by parenteral needs or "state of the art."

A. Filling Suites

The filling area, being the most highly controlled plant environment and the most
critical site for potential product contamination, is a logical starting point for designing a plant layout. An analysis of production requirements and the selection of
equipment can determine the physical size, shape, and characteristics of a filling
area. In the design effort, experience is invaluable for the determination of working and access space required. Both materials—containers, caps, stoppers, etc.—
and product must be brought to the filling equipment by conveyor, cart, or hand.
Filled containers must be taken away and waste must be disposed of. Space needs
must be considered for filters, cabinets, stools, and operator or maintenance personnel access.

Design work can proceed backward from the filling area along the path(s) of
container, closure, and product supply. To minimize contamination potential,
these paths should be as direct as possible with a minimum of material handling.

In the direction of product flow, design can proceed from filling toward sterilization, inspection, and packaging. Design in this direction must provide for careful segregation of production by batch, perhaps requiring intermediate hold areas.

In addition to the incoming flow of containers and product and the outgoing
flow of filled product, the flow of personnel must be a part of the filling room design. Change rooms must be provided for each controlled area. To utilize change
rooms most efficiently, several filling areas may be grouped together. This approach has the disadvantage of requiring sterile, or clean, access corridors and
may complicate the product flow paths. Consider the generalized cases of Figures
6 through 9.

Figure 6 illustrates a process utilizing a single filling area. The functions of
equipment and container preparation, product preparation, product accumulation,
and personnel gowning all can be separated and simple nonintersecting flow paths
maintained. Figures 7 and 8 illustrate arrangements where filling areas are clus-
tered to utilize a common facility, in this case, gowning. Other functions, such as
product preparation and/or material preparation, must be dispersed in order to
maintain direct access to the gowning rooms. Figure 9 illustrates the cross-flow
problems associated with a multiple-use filling area or a common filling area with
partial segregation of operations.

Figures 7 through 9 are generalized and do not illustrate all multiple room
variations. The important point to note is that to achieve maximum control each

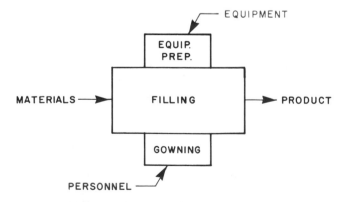

Figure 6 Single filling area.

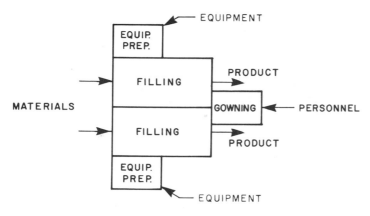

Figure 7 Two-room filling area.

filling line is a dedicated and fully supported operation. However, this approach is often not practical when the realities of product volume and construction and operating costs are considered. Multiple-use areas and banks of filling areas may be necessary, with administrative or procedural steps being taken to minimize or eliminate cross-flow or cross-contamination. The multiple-use room is an example where several pieces of equipment are located in the same room, although only one piece of equipment is used at a time. A bank of filling rooms with a common access corridor could be considered in many respects to be a variation of a multiple-use room. Although the multiple-use room can minimize facility costs, it increases environmental control problems.

By use of multifloor concepts, a third dimension can be added to production layouts. For filling operations where the product is difficult to pump, locating the product preparation area above the filling area presents obvious advantages. These should be weighed against the higher construction costs, lack of visual communication between rooms, and the physical problems such as leakage through floor or ceiling openings or access to services between the vertically stacked rooms.

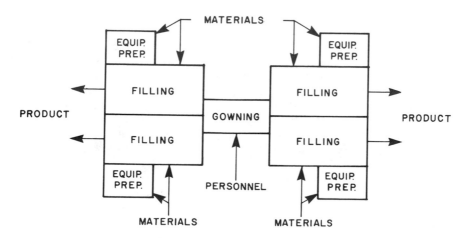

Figure 8 Four-room filling area.

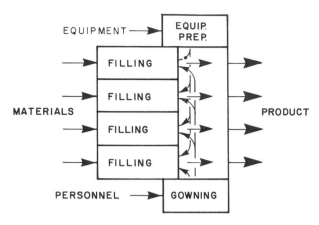

Figure 9 Multiple-use filling area.

B. Wall and Floor Treatment

The concern with filling areas, or more generally, controlled environment areas, involves many seemingly minor details. The proposed LVP–CGMP specifies particular design and construction features for controlled environment areas. These requirements include having smooth, cleanable walls, floors, ceilings, fixtures, and partitions. The basic cleanability requirement eliminates the "open" types of building construction where columns, wall studs, bracing, pipes, and so on, are exposed.

1. Walls

All inside walls must be finished; common methods of finish are block, plaster, or gypsum board. Concrete block walls are sturdy and easily constructed. The porosity of concrete block walls can be reduced by coating with a block filler prior to painting. But even filled concrete block walls have a surface texture that is not conducive to cleaning. Painted concrete block walls are particularly susceptible to peeling if they are subjected to moisture, as from leakage or rain on the back side. A final problem with block walls is the tendency to crack along joints due to the inevitable movements of building structures. Use of ceramic–faced block can overcome the surface finish problems of concrete block, but are still subject to cracking along joints and still present a cleaning problem at the joints.

Plaster walls are becoming increasingly rare due to their relatively high cost and the scarcity of skills required. A plaster wall requires a good substantial base such as a block or concrete wall or wire–reinforced gypsum board. The plaster wall is relatively sturdy against personnel wear and has moderate resistance to movement cracking. It is, however, quite vulnerable to nicks, chips, and so on, from equipment. Repairs are relatively easy, but finish options are few; painting is the usual finish.

Gypsum board is the modern version of plaster. For most industrial use, 5/8 in. thick paper–faced gypsum sheets are fastened to wood or metal studs. When the joints are taped and sealed, a smooth, continuous surface results. A properly constructed gypsum board drywall is very resistant to cracking. Finishing is normally limited to painting and gypsum board is very susceptible to equipment damage.

To overcome the surface weaknesses of most walls, various heavy coverings are available. These coverings are applied in sheets that must be glued or otherwise fastened to existing walls. Although these coverings are much more durable, the sealing of the joint between sheets is still a problem. For severe usage conditions, a metal-clad wall may be useful. Although the metal-clad wall is durable, any damage incurred will often produce permanent scars which are difficult to repair. Painted metal walls are often used in clean room applications. Stainless steel walls, although expensive, eliminate a maintenance painting. The disadvantages of metal-clad walls is that they are available in relatively small (3 or 4 ft wide) panels. Unless glued to the wall, the fasteners will present a cleaning problem, and the seams must be carefully sealed.

2. Floors

Selection of floor materials poses a particularly difficult problem since they must be durable, seamless, and easily cleaned and sanitized. To achieve good floor results, the application must be matched to the particular characteristics of the floor system.

The simple concrete slab is the ideal base for a good floor, but is not suitable alone. Plain concrete is relatively soft, thereby scratching or "dusting" easily, especially when subjected to heavy foot or machinery traffic. The surface of concrete is porous, and becomes more so as it is subjected to frequent cleaning with aggressive cleaning media. To minimize porosity, concrete can be finished to a very smooth surface. However, this tends to increase the problem of slippage when the floor is wet. Commercially available sealers also can be applied to concrete to reduce the dusting problem.

Hardeners may be added to concrete to increase the surface hardness by a factor of 3, greatly improving the floor's resistance to scratching and dusting and are available in colors to improve the appearance of the floor. These hardeners are spread by hand and worked into the concrete while still wet, so the colors may not always be true and uniform. Sealers can be used to reduce dusting further and generally are more effective on a hardened surface than on a plain concrete surface. The worker fatigue and slippage problems of the hardened concrete floor are no different than for a plain concrete floor. In terms of durability, the hardened concrete floor is excellent.

Cracks are a serious problem with concrete floors, whether hardened or not. A well-designed reinforced concrete slab is very strong, but due to any of a number of factors—poor concrete, poor installation, shrinkage, soil movement or settling—cracks often develop. Once cracked, a concrete floor can be repaired only if the floor movement stabilizes. Otherwise, the crack can only be filled with a resilient filler that will expand and contract as the floor moves.

Another general group of floor types consists of epoxy or urethane applied as a coating over a cured concrete surface. Application procedures vary with the particular product, but generally require a new or acid-cleaned surface, followed by one or more coats of finish. Advantages of these coatings include being able to apply them over existing concrete floors, the availability of colors and improved resistance to dusting and slippage, and the provision of a continuous seal. When compared to hardened concrete, these finishes are generally less resistant to scratching or cutting. In areas where there is primarily foot traffic, they may be ideal. Such coatings cannot "patch" cracks in the concrete base, but if the movement that caused the crack has stabilized, the coating can cover a fine crack or a patched crack. However, if the base moves, the crack will propagate through the surface.

A third general type of floor is composed of large sheets of vinyl or PVC laid on a concrete base floor and "welded" together with heat or sealed at the seams with cement. Vinyl and polyvinyl chloride (PVC) products vary as to porosity and must be checked for suitability before use. These floors are relatively easy to install, can be installed over existing floors, and can cover considerable cracks and movement. They are available in colors and a variety of slip-resistant finishes and are compatible with similar wall coverings. Vinyl and PVC surfaces are more susceptible than concrete to cutting by wheels and glass, but are often easily repaired by rewelding. Their resiliency make them more comfortable for standing workers.

The performance of any floor will be enhanced by the control of the traffic it sees. Keeping heavy equipment traffic off floors is desirable but often not practical. Selection of compatible materials for material-handling equipment wheels and for floors will reduce floor damage. All caster manufacturers offer a variety of composition materials.

3. Wall Junctions

To aid sanitation, all wall and ceiling junctures must be coved, or rounded. A 1 1/2 to 2 in. radius on the corners aids cleaning and strengthens the corners to help prevent cracking. Similarly, floors are normally coved up the wall about 4 in. to prevent damage to the wall by floor cleaning and to prevent cracks at the junction of floor and wall.

C. Miscellaneous Controlled Area Details

To obtain a pharmaceutically clean environment, attention must also be given to many other items which are necessary in a production area. Although minor, these details can create potential contamination entry points.

1. Door Hardware

Hospital-type hardware, which replaces the usual doorknobs with push plates or arm hooks, is preferred. If available hospital hardware does not fit the exact need, custom hardware may be fabricated easily due to its relatively simple design. The primary goal is to eliminate surfaces, such as doorknobs, where worker's hands may be contaminated. Difficult-to-clean ledges and crevices should also be avoided, as around hinges, door closers, and screw heads. Windows should be flush-mounted on the clean side to avoid ledges, or the ledges should be beveled to aid cleaning.

2. Lighting Fixtures

Lighting fixtures should be recessed flush with the ceiling. Since most lighting fixtures are not tightly sealed, the diffuser should be sealed integrally with the ceiling, and the lamps changed from outside the room. Often this is not possible and access must be from inside the clean room. Either recessed or surface-mounted fixtures can be used, but particular attention needs to be given to both the front and back of each fixture to ensure that potential contamination is sealed out and that internally generated contamination, as from a failed ballast, is sealed in. Special "wash down" fixtures are well sealed, but protrude obtrusively into the room and have clips and sealing lips which are difficult to sanitize.

3. Sprinkler Systems

By their very nature, sprinkler systems present a potential contamination problem in controlled areas. The most common sprinkler type is the "wet pipe" system, where a water-filled sprinkler system stands ready to supply water to an area when a heat-sensitive sprinkler head is activated. This water is stagnant, however, and often nonpotable. In the event of fire, this would be no particular problem since a complete cleanup and resanitization would most likely be required. However, in the event of a more minor malfunction, such as leaking sprinkler heads or accidental damage, this contaminated water could leak into the area so slowly that it is unnoticed. An alternative to the wet pipe system is the "dry pipe" system. The latter, normally used in freezing areas, uses compressed air in the sprinkler system. When a head activates, the resulting drop in pressure allows water to flow. Although this system keeps stagnant and nonpotable water from close proximity to the controlled environment, it is questionable whether or not the potential for contamination by the compressed air is any less. Other alternative systems using dry powders or gases can also be used, but are more complex, expensive, and have problems of their own. Normally, the risk of the wet pipe system is accepted as a necessary safeguard for life and property. The cleanability of the exposed sprinkler heads can be improved by use of semirecessed heads and protective caps, although these caps cannot be sealed.

4. Communication

Communication in a controlled area is usually via membrane plates mounted in windows, telephones, or intercoms. Membrane plates cannot be installed in existing tempered glass windows and, when installed, offer marginal performance and are a cleaning problem. On the other hand, telephones require use of hands, are difficult to clean, and may be damaged internally by sanitizing fluids or sprays. Special intercoms, sealed, cleanable, and requiring a minimum of hand contact are often the best means of communication.

5. Pass-Throughs

The transport of miscellaneous items (paper, writing instruments, tools, samples, etc.) in and out of a controlled area can create a significant contamination potential. For best control, anything going into a controlled area should pass through a sterilizer or, at a minimum, be surface-disinfected in a change room area. For outbound materials, an unprotected wall opening or a double door pass-through can be used. The double-door pass-through, when equipped with an interlock to prevent opening both doors simultaneously, maintains the positive pressure within the area and prevents blow back of contamination. For small openings, contamination is prevented by the outflow of air caused by the positive pressure in the controlled area. The permissible size of the opening is a function of the excess air supplied to the area.

6. Change Rooms

Personnel access to all controlled areas should be through change rooms. Change room concepts and layouts vary from single closet size rooms to expansive multiroom complexes. Although the cleanliness needs of the controlled area and of the entering personnel both affect the specific requirements for a change room, Figure 10 illustrates the basic elements of a typical change room. The finish details of a change room are comparable to the area served. Entrance to a change area is normally through vestibules whose doors are electrically interlocked so that both cannot be opened simultaneously, thus maintaining the necessary air pressure differential to prevent the entry of airborne contamination. The flow of personnel through the change area should be planned to encourage the following of prescribed

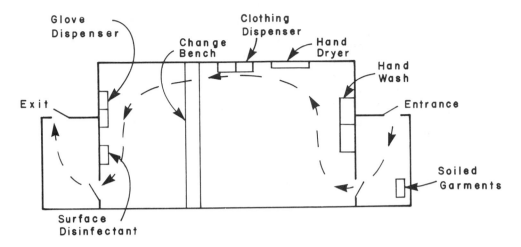

Figure 10 Typical change room.

cleanup and gowning procedures without congestion. Upon entry into the change
room, wash sinks are provided for scrubbing hands and forearms. Automatic or
foot-operated controls for water and soap eliminate hand contact with contaminated
surfaces. Next, hands are dried by hot air blowers. Although commercial hand
driers are often used, they may create undesired airflow patterns and may circulate
particulate laden air. Special filtered driers are available to minimize the creation
of particulate contamination. Further control may be achieved by using filtered and
heated compressed air for drying to reduce further particulate potential. After hands
are dry, garments are taken from dispensers and donned while moving across a
dressing bench. As a final gowning step, aseptic gloves are put on and sanitized.
Exit from the change room to the controlled area is, like entrance, through an interlocked vestibule. Depending on the degree of disrobing required, separate gowning
facilities may be provided for men and women. When leaving the controlled area,
depending on the practice in a particular company, garments may be discarded or
placed in a special locker for reuse. These lockers typically have ultraviolet lamps
and HEPA-filtered air supplies.

D. Warehousing

Once the basic production area has been defined, warehouses and service areas may
be addressed. Warehouses, whether centrally located or split according to function,
must be designed to do much more than merely provide storage. From the moment
goods are unloaded, they must be protected from contamination while being sampled
and quarantined until released for use. Inside docks are a common means of increasing environmental control and security, but do not provide more positive protection
from outdoor contamination when the outside doors are opened to admit trucks, an
especially important factor in windy areas.

Environmental air conditioning is normally not considered a problem in warehouse areas. Temperature control in summer months often consists of nothing more
than exhaust fans, and winter heating may be by ceiling-mounted unit heaters. For
general storage, these conditions may be adequate. However, if product require-

ments (e. g. , stability) dictate closer temperature control, better environmental control may be necessary.

Layout of a warehouse requires attention similar to that required for a production area. A first consideration is to prevent contamination while unloading materials. Near the point of unloading must be a receiving area equipped to sample the incoming materials under whatever protection is necessary to prevent sample contamination or exposure of personnel to hazardous materials. A well-designed exhaust hood is normally adequate. Security measures in the form of clearly designated quarantine areas are necessary to provide separation of materials in accord with their receipt status. Materials do not always flow smoothly through receiving procedures. Therefore, the warehouse must be adequate in size and must be flexible enough to hold materials in an indefinite status if necessary. Basic factors must be known or assumptions must be made concerning material-handling equipment early in the layout of a warehouse. The size and type of forklift and the unit load characteristics will have direct bearing on aisle widths and on type, capacity, and style of storage racking. The opposite approach, first to determine the warehouse size, then choose the best forklift and racking, will usually result in a less than optimum utilization of space. This approach may be required, however, if an existing facility is being remodeled.

Thought must also be given to the transfer of materials into a production area. If the environmental conditions of the warehouse and production areas differ greatly, or if it is undesirable to carry the receiving packing materials (e.g. , wooden pallets) into the production area, some type of cleaning and/or transfer area may be required. This area would be contiguous to both areas and might serve as a staging area for materials required for production. Here bulk quantities may be vacuumed, unpacked, washed, or transferred to another transport means such as a metal or plastic pallet or cart. In some cases, the materials may be delivered to a transfer area by one set of material-handling equipment and be picked up by a separate set, dedicated for exclusive use in a cleaner, more controlled environment.

E. Mechanical Services

One of the most tedious and complex problems in plant design, yet one of the most important, is that of providing mechanical services. Mechanical services are a variety of production support functions which are normally supplied to production areas from a remote location through a type of fixed and permanent distribution system. These services include the common public utilities such as electrical power, water, gas, and sewage as well as plant-generated utilities such as steam, compressed air, air conditioning, oxygen, nitrogen, and vacuum. Providing these services involves unique problems in a parenterals plant. First, the wide variety of services needed requires a large amount of floor space and creates a complex coordination problem in the service areas. Second, there is an urgent need to keep the service systems and distribution networks remote from the production areas in order to reduce cleaning problems and congestion. Finally, parenteral service systems require very careful design to ensure controllability and reliability, additional control and monitoring instrumentation, and adequate accessibility. The task of defining a mechanical service system progresses step by step from the general question of mechanical equipment location, to the more specific definition of utility requirements, to the very specific details of system components and specifications.

1. Utility Equipment Location

Public utilities require space for metering. In addition to metering, electrical power systems require space for switchgear and transformers. Water systems usually require treatment to ensure consistent quality. Plant-generated utilities typically require steam boilers, air compressors, and distillation equipment. Many of those utilities lend themselves to handling in a central location, the typical "boiler room" approach. Grouping mechanical equipment in a centralized utility area helps ensure that all equipment is properly monitored and maintained. Although a central location minimizes distribution problems and minimizes service distribution distances, it is often impractical unless a multifloor layout is used. If mechanical equipment, especially air compressors and water treatment equipment, is dispersed through a production area, there is more difficulty in properly monitoring the equipment during use.

Rooftop equipment location makes use of otherwise unusable space, but leads to other problems. The roof is a harsh operating environment and will shorten equipment life and increase equipment maintenance. Proper equipment maintenance is difficult in foul weather, especially winter. Heavy equipment may damage the roof structure, particularly if the equipment vibrates. Finally, overhead equipment location requires numerous penetrations through the roof which, coupled with equipment vibration, will invariably lead to leakage.

A mezzanine equipment platform eliminates the problems of operation in a harsh environment and roof loading, but still poses an overhead leak potential, although leakage due to the weather is minimized. Another possible equipment location for multifloor facilities is a lower level or basement. The lower level provides a protected operating environment, usually has easy access for service, and leakage will flow away from the production area. The basement location may require that some space be provided on the lower production levels in order to extend service distribution lines to the upper levels. Care must also be taken to ensure that the basement area can be kept clean and dry enough to prevent contamination of the utilities and that sufficient access is available for moving large equipment in and out.

2. Definition of Utility Requirements

If a facility is being designed for true general-purpose use, all or most of the service systems may have to be convenient to all production areas. This approach can be extremely expensive and can lead to systems difficult to control because of large amounts of unused and static service lines. Ideally, exact production and equipment needs should be known so that the necessary systems can be tailored to only those needs. A potential problem with the latter system is that future additions or changes may be quite costly and may even require significant system redesign. Although general-purpose systems may be desirable, the reality of cost and the capriciousness of the future require that service system design be based on a reasonable assessment of actual needs. Therefore, a general and ordered approach to the design problem should be followed:

1. Determine product requirements. In a parenteral facility, a piping system must not merely deliver a product to a point of use, but must do so without contaminating the product and must be controllable, a controlled system being one that responds in a positive, predictable manner to corrective actions. For example, if a piping system has been designed to supply water at all points of use at a specified temperature, the system should include a means of varying the temperature if that temperature is found to be out of specification. To maintain product quality, the distribution system must be as inert as possible with respect to the product handled as well as to any substance that may be used to clean the system. Product condition is important. Water, for example, can present different corrosion potential depending on whether it is raw city water, deionized, distilled, hot, or cold.

2. Evaluate point-of-use requirements. How much is needed and where? Minimal usage of a compressed gas at isolated locations may indicate that supply should be from portable cylinders, while high-volume use in concentrated areas may indicate the practicality of a bulk storage and distribution system.

3. Determine maintenance procedures. A water system for Water for Injection (WFI) must withstand rather severe cleaning and must be capable of steam sterilization. A piping system for nitrogen, on the other hand, may only need to be free of oils and particulate matter. Consider, especially, routine and frequent maintenance functions that are related to the product requirements in step 1. For example, if a system requires periodic flushing or cleaning, it is necessary that the system be constructed so that it is drainable, with all piping sloped toward a drain point. If sterilization is required, a source of clean steam must be nearby and provisions must be made for condensate draining and air venting.

3. System Component Details

The need for absolute control of utility systems in a parenterals facility requires that attention be given to details of system design which might otherwise be considered unimportant. This attention to detail is necessary to ensure compatibility of all system components and to ensure that each design criteria and each component is in concert with the overall system specification.

To completely design, specify, and install a utility system, specifically a piped system, requires attention to details such as material and alloy selection, surface finish, sizing, joining technique, types of valving, cleanability, insulation, and so on. A thorough treatment of these items is beyond the scope of this text, but some details—selection of type of distribution system, materials, surface finish, joining technique, valving, and utility service connection arrangement—can significantly affect the maintenance of a pharmaceutical environment and should be considered further.

Selection of Type of Distribution System. Utilities are distributed from supply to points of use via a network of main and branch supply lines arranged to provide the required utilities in the most efficient manner (i.e., with minimum loss at least cost). Figure 11 illustrates a simple branch line distribution system such as could be used for electrical power, water supply, gas supply, ventilation air supply

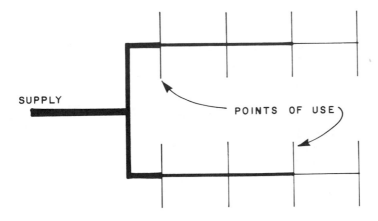

Figure 11 Branch line distribution system.

and so on. The identifying characteristic of this system is the stepwise reduction in size as the system splits into smaller branches. This distribution system is well suited for electrical systems because of the ease with which each branch may be protected against overload. The simple system is also most frequently used for general-purpose utilities such as domestic water supply. The branch line system in reverse becomes a collection system, as for sewage.

In addition to the ease of providing overload protection, the branch line distribution system is usually least expensive since material is minimized by the decreasing branch sizes. If, however, a significant increase in utility need occurs at a terminal point, the branch line system may not be able to supply that need and major modifications may be necessary. Another disadvantage of this system is that each branch must be sized for its maximum anticipated needs. Thus, if the utility need is not constant, there may be areas of the system where the flow rate is very low or even static, an undesirable condition for critical systems such as water for injection. The branch line system is also vulnerable to interruption since a failure in a main supply line will interrupt flow to all of the following branches.

The disadvantages of the branch line distribution system can often be overcome by use of a loop distribution system, as in Figure 12. In contrast to the branch line system, the entire supply line of the loop system is of constant size and forms a closed loop. Changes in utility need can be easily accommodated, provided that the basic system capacity is not exceeded, and failures can be easily isolated. Variable point-of-use requirements can be more easily accommodated by the loop because of the possibility for flow from either direction. For increased reliability or for increasing system capability, a second feed can be added to the loop, usually opposite the first feed. Although the flow in a loop system is static only if all usage is curtailed, flow rates are variable. For systems where a minimum constant flow rate is necessary, as in a water for injection system, a circulating pump may be incorporated to prevent stagnation.

Material. The selection of material for a piping system depends on the product to be handled, the product purity desired, material cost, and installation cost. A design engineer can often provide a comparison of two or more alternate materials, leaving final selection to the user based on product purity requirements. For example, consider the materials commonly used for pharmaceutical utility systems:

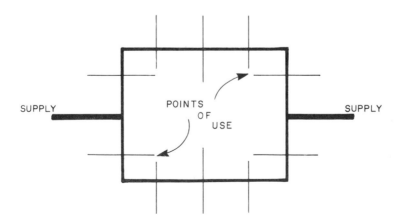

Figure 12 Loop distribution system.

Carbon Steel. Carbon steel pipe, manufactured according to ASTM Standard A53 or A106, is commonly available in various schedules or wall thicknesses. The standard schedule is No. 40. Carbon pipe of appropriate grade and schedule may be used for almost any inert or mildly aggressive material up to pressures of 17,200 kPa. Common uses include water, compressed air, oil, nitrogen, steam, and steam condensate. Carbon steel pipe rusts quite readily, so it is unacceptable for use where rust would create a problem, as in compressed air systems supplying air for controlled environment use.

Copper. Copper is commonly used for water and compressed air piping because of ease of installation. Copper pipe is available according to standard pipe dimensional specifications or as tubing. Type K tubing has greater wall thickness than type L, therefore being suitable for higher pressures. Either type K or type L tubing is available in annealed form, making it more flexible. Copper has a smooth surface finish compared to that of carbon steel and is relatively resistant to corrosion. Copper loses strength rapidly at higher temperatures and is not recommended for steam use.

Type 304 Stainless Steel. Type 304 stainless steel is probably the most common alloy of a group of steels known as austenitic stainless steels. These alloys are generally characterized as containing approximately 18% chromium and 8% nickel, being nonmagnetic and nonhardenable. Type 304 is resistant to attack by nitric acid but is attacked by sulfuric or hydrochloric acids. Type 304 is a good general-purpose alloy for pharmaceutical applications where pitting corrosion is not a problem.

Type 316 Stainless Steel. Type 316 stainless steel is similar to Type 304 except that Type 316 has 2 to 4% higher nickel content, 2% less chromium, and has 2 to 3% molybdenum. The molybdenum gives Type 316 improved resistance to pitting corrosion as compared to Type 304 and slightly improved general corrosion resistance. Type 316 is usually specified for product contact surfaces, especially if heating is involved due to the superior pitting corrosion resistance.

Both Type 304 and Type 316 stainless steel are susceptible to integranular corrosion adjacent to welded areas. When austenitic stainless steels are heated to 425 to 870°C and cooled slowly, as adjacent to a weld, the carbon tends to form chromium carbides which precipitate at the grain boundaries, resulting in reduced resistance to intergranular corrosion. Alloys 304L and 316L were developed to avoid this problem by reducing the alloy carbon content to below 0.03%, compared to 0.08 and 0.10% for Type 304 and Type 316, respectively. The low-carbon alloys of either 304 or 316 should be used when the piping system requires welding and when annealing after welding is impractical.

Surface Finish. Surface finish is very important for pharmaceutical applications. For less corrosion resistant materials such as carbon steel or copper, surface finish specifications are unimportant because these materials are not used for product contact surfaces or for corrosive applications. For stainless steels, improved surface finishes provide a more sanitary surface and improve corrosion resistance. Surface finish specifications often refer to 3-A Sanitary Standards. These standards were formulated by the cooperative efforts of three industry and regulatory groups of the dairy industry [2]. The standards have since become commonly accepted throughout the dairy, food, and pharmaceutical industries as valid for equipment that must be sanitized. The writers of the 3-A standards recognized that a polished surface is easier to sanitize than a rough surface and helps expose or remove impurities that may have been embedded in the metal during forming.

According to these standards, a product contact surface should be polished to a No. 4 finish, a finish obtained by polishing with a 150 grit sanding belt. The removal of surface impurities by polishing also enhances corrosion resistance by removing possible sites for pitting corrosion. Pitting can occur when a small electrolytic cell is formed at the site of an inclusion. In addition to mechanical polishing, electropolishing has been used to improve further the surface finish of stainless steels [3]. Electropolishing is a process of metal removal by electrolytic action. Because the mechanism of electropolishing is the same as pitting corrosion, a secondary benefit of electropolishing is that it emphasizes any imperfections in the surface being polished. The electropolished surface exhibits somewhat better corrosion resistance than mechanically polished surfaces. There is some evidence to indicate that, under certain conditions, electropolishing may actually eliminate the necessity for the No. 4 polish [4].

Joining Techniques. Piping systems can be joined by threading, welding, or clamping. Threaded connections are common for noncritical applications where iron pipe might be used. Threading is easily done on thicker materials and a large selection of threaded fittings are available. High-quality welding produces the smoothest internal surface in a piping system. Welding requires more skill than threading, makes maintenance or modification more difficult, and may induce corrosion due to carbide precipitation. For sanitary piping requiring frequent disassembly, a clamped and gasketed flange is commonly used. Each pipe end has a tapered flange with a gasket-retaining groove. Two pipe ends are held together with a gasket between, as shown in Figure 13. Although this sanitary clamp fitting provides a rather smooth internal surface, it is prone to leakage and must be disassembled for complete sanitization.

Valving. The selection of valves for a pharmaceutical application requires as much consideration as any other element of utility system design. Although the basic function of a valve, to block flow in a pipeline, is simple, the actual selection and application of valves can become a complex problem. Common valve types include gate, globe, ball, diaphragm, plug, and compression valves. Gate and globe valves are most common for general use but are seldom used in pharmaceutical

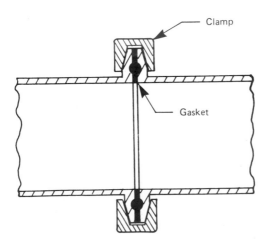

Figure 13 Sanitary clamp fitting.

applications because of stagnant areas inherent in their design. Ball, diaphragm, and plug valves are available with connections, materials, and finishes acceptable for pharmaceutical use, but none can be fully categorized as acceptable for sanitary or pharmaceutical use. If properly selected and installed, these valve types are acceptable. As a general rule, valve material, finish, and joining technique must be compatible with the parent piping system. Beyond that, each valve has particular advantages and disadvantages which can be maximized or minimized by careful selection and installation.

A typical ball valve as illustrated in Figure 14 has a ported ball that is rotated 90° to regulate flow. If the valve port is smaller than the pipeline, it may prevent complete draining of the pipe if installed in a horizontal position. Some ball valves use a seal ring on either side of the ball to prevent leakage but in turn create a nondrainable stagnant area around the ball. Depending on the criticality of the application, the core of fluid trapped within the ball when the valve is closed may be an unacceptable feature. Ball valves are particularly well suited for simple on-off control, but their use for throttling is limited by their nonlinear flow characteristics.

A diaphragm valve, as in Figure 15, controls flow by compressing a diaphragm against a wire placed across the direction of flow. Although diaphragm valves are often described as meeting 3-A sanitary standards, they are acceptable for sanitary or pharmaceutical use only if installed at an angle so as to prevent entrapment of fluid behind the wier. The selection of diaphragm material must consider the product characteristics to avoid premature cracking, erosion, or leaching of harmful compounds by the product. A particular application must also consider the potential for product stagnation at the joint between the diaphragm and valve body, an area very difficult to flush by product flow. Diaphragm valves are slower to operate than ball valves and can be damaged by overtightening. Diaphragm erosion may also occur, especially at low valve opening settings.

A plug valve is similar in concept to a ball valve except that a tapered plug is used to control flow rather than a ball. The taper makes possible a close fit between plug and body without the seal rings necessary in a ball valve. The plug valve is also well suited for use in three-port designs for diverting flow. The main ad-

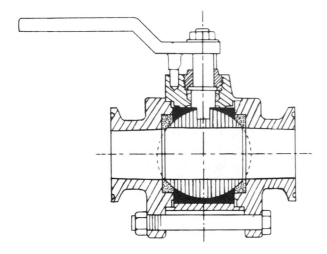

Figure 14 Typical ball valve. (Courtesy of Pittsburgh Brass Manufacturing Co., Irwin, Pennsylvania.)

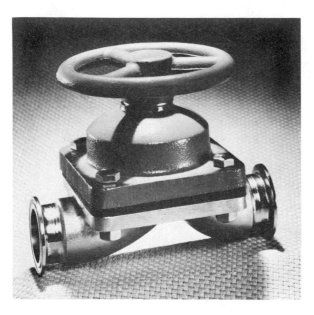

Figure 15 Typical diaphragm valve. (Courtesy of Ladish Company, Kenosha, Wisconsin.)

vantage of the plug valve is ease of disassembly. Its disadvantage is its tendency to leak. Its best use is for relatively low pressure applications where frequent disassembly for cleaning is necessary. Compression valves, as illustrated by Figure 16, control flow very simply by compressing a plug against a round seal surface. Compression valves are available in many configurations for a variety of uses and are readily adaptable to powered actuation. Compression valves have good throttling characteristics and when specifically designed for such, have excellent throttling characteristics.

   Utility Service Connection Arrangement. The arrangement of services within the production area and the connection of services to the points of use and equipment can have a significant impact on the plant environment. Utilities must be carefully connected to avoid stagnant areas and to avoid difficult-to-clean areas just as would be done for the utility distribution system. To minimize contamination potential, typical utility arrangements and typical service connections should be defined during planning.

   Utilities can be arranged so that the service connections enter a room vertically upward, horizontally, and vertically downward, with various advantages and disadvantages. Vertical upward service connections, with connections under machinery, create a very neat appearance, allow full unobstructed machine access, and require only short connection lengths. However, these service connections create obstacles to cleaning and for service systems that must be drainable, are unacceptable unless distribution piping is located below the floor with access from a lower level. All equipment locations must be determined when utilities are installed and relocation of equipment may require floor excavation.

   Horizontal service connections are often used in single-level facilities to avoid floor excavation during equipment relocation or utility maintenance. Maintenance access to the utility distribution system is usually better because the

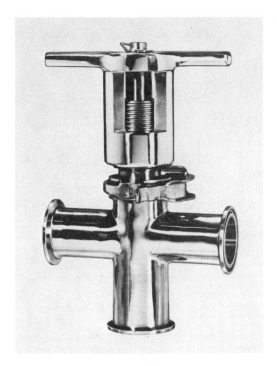

Figure 16 Typical compression valve. (Courtesy of Ladish Company, Kenosha, Wisconsin.)

distribution feedlines are located in a wall where access is provided from a less critical environmental area. Service connections above the floor can be easily drained if necessary. Horizontal service connections do limit machine access, create some congestion, and may necessarily be longer than vertical service connections.

Service connections extending vertically downward allow full machine access and contribute to an uncluttered floor. The connection lines are drainable and easily relocated if necessary. Maintenance access may be difficult if the distribution lines lie between the ceiling and an upper floor. Vertical downward services create a visually cluttered appearance and may restrict access to the working surface of equipment. This type of connection may also be undesirable if laminar flow coverage of the equipment is necessary.

F. Heating, Ventilation, and Air Conditioning

One of the most critical plant service systems is heating, ventilation and air conditioning (HVAC). HVAC design is a complex and tedious task that requires a well-trained and experienced engineer. Operating personnel involved in the design or modification of a pharmaceutical facility must have a basic understanding of HVAC in order to give direction to the HVAC designer and to provide necessary base information. Of the many systems for heating, ventilating, and air conditioning buildings, the environmental control requirements of a parenteral facility dictate the use of a forced-air system. By means of such a system, an area can be heated, ventilated, or cooled while maintaining a defined environmental cleanliness level. To define an air handling system, one must consider the general arrangement, the method of air distribution, the filtration requirements and method, the control method, and the heating/cooling method.

1. Standards

There are three important references to consider when designing an air handling system for pharmaceutical use, varying from the more general to the more specific. First is the ASHRAE Handbook, published by the American Society of Heating, Refrigeration and Air-Conditioning Engineers [5]. The ASHRAE Handbook is a four-volume encyclopedia of data and "common practices" covering all aspects of system design and installation. ASHRAE standards are not binding on anyone, but are the guidelines of the industry. Next is Federal Standard Number 209 B, Federal Standard Clean Room and Work Station Requirements, Controlled Environment [6]. The objective of 209 B is "to prescribe air cleanliness classes and certain other environmental air conditions required for achieving and maintaining the levels of environmental cleanliness specified in the product specifications." This is the industry's standard definition of cleanliness classes and of terms applicable to controlled environments and contains suggested means of achieving the specified cleanliness levels. Also included are means of monitoring and testing cleanliness levels. Standard 209 B is a standard specification used by federal agencies in the procurement of controlled environment facilities, but like ASHRAE, is not binding on anyone except when referred to as, for example, ". . . shall meet the requirements of Federal Standard 209 B." The last and most specific requirement for pharmaceutical air handling systems is the proposed CGMPs for LVPs published June 1, 1976 [1]. Paragraph 212.221, in total, specifies: "Air in controlled environment areas shall have:

(a) A per-cubic-foot particle count of not more than 100,000 in a size range of 0.5 micron and larger when measured with automatic counters, or 700 particles in a size range of 5.0 microns or larger when measured by a manual microscopic method.
(b) A temperature of 72°F ± 5° or 22°C ± 3°.
(c) A maximum relative humidity of 50 percent and a minimum of 30 percent.
(d) A positive pressure differential of at least 0.05 inch of water with all doors closed in relation to less clean adjacent areas.
(e) At least 20 air changes per hour."

2. General Considerations

Figure 17 illustrates the basic elements of a forced-air HVAC system. Outside air, air returned from the conditioned space or a mixture of the two is filtered upon entry into the air handling unit. Two purposes are served by air filters in the general system: First, the air is cleaned for the end use. Second, the air is cleansed of particles that may clog or damage the mechanical elements of the air system. The level of filtration for a given application will depend on the relative importance of these two purposes. If the cleanliness of the final air stream needs to be no better than the ambient air, then the air filters may be the panel type of 20% or less efficiency (filter types and efficiencies are discussed on p. 390). If, however, the final air quality must be cleaner, as in a library, filters of approximately 80% efficiency may be used. Applications requiring cleaning efficiencies of up to approximately 40% usually have a single set of filters. Systems requiring

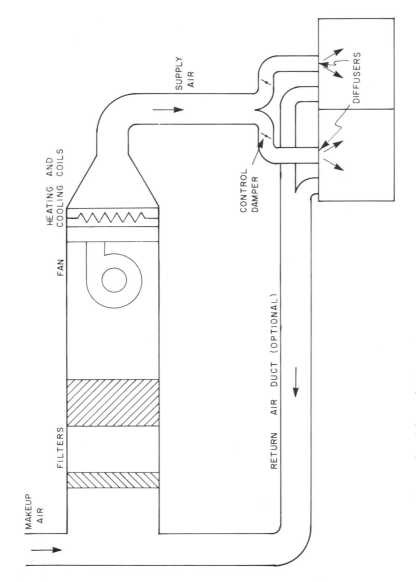

Figure 17 Generalized forced–air system.

higher efficiencies often have two sets of filters, where the less expensive, low-efficiency filter is used to increase the life of the more efficient filter.

After being filtered, the air is heated or cooled as necessary and moved into a distribution system by a fan. The air is introduced into the conditioned space through diffusers at ceiling level. These diffusers are designed to distribute the air uniformly throughout the work space.

Most air handling systems recirculate conditioned air from the work space. Figure 17 shows a return duct system which returns air from the ceiling level of the work space. If the work space has open space above the ceiling, that space can often be used as a return system in lieu of ductwork.

The generalized air handling system is a very flexible system but it is usually to heat, cool, and provide fresh air (ventilate). Humidity control and air cleaning are often considered secondary functions.

3. Clean Room Application

Air handling systems for clean air applications, as illustrated by Figure 18, are very refined versions of the generalized air handling system. A clean air system must satisfy the CGMP requirements discussed on page 386. The generalized system can satisfy only the temperature requirement (b) and the air change requirement (e). Additions to the system are necessary to satisfy the cleanliness requirement (a), the humidity requirement (c), and the pressure differential requirement (d).

Cleanliness levels of Class 100,000 or better, as defined by Federal Standard 209 B, require the use of high-efficiency particulate air (HEPA) filters. It is customary, although not absolutely necessary, for a nonlaminar flow room to install the HEPA filter at the point where the supply air duct enters the room. This location prevents the inadvertent introduction of contamination into the ductwork during filter changes and, most important, facilitates close monitoring of the filter for failure. Because HEPA filters are expensive, delicate, difficult to install, and have a limited dust holding capacity, medium- to high-efficiency filters are necessary as prefilters. Federal Standard 209 B suggests two prefilters in clean air systems. The initial prefilter, located at the entry to the air handling unit, should be of 20 to 30% efficiency. The intermediate prefilter of 80 to 90% efficiency can be located after the air handling unit, as shown, or may be located immediately after the initial prefilter. This staging of filters reduces the chance of damage to the very fine final filter by a coarse particle and prolongs the life of the more expensive and usually harder to change final filters.

The CGMP humidity specification requires moisture removal in humid weather and moisture addition in dry weather. Moisture addition is usually accomplished by steam injection in the distribution duct system. Moisture removal is accomplished through use of a cooling coil in the air handling unit and a heating coil following the air handling unit—called a reheat coil. A typical set of operating parameters for a system meeting CGMP requirements might first cool the air to 7°C. This cooling will remove excess moisture by condensation and produce air at 100% relative humidity unless the incoming air is very dry, as in winter. The air is then reheated to approximately 13°C to lower the relative humidity level to 40% before introducing air into the room. By varying the temperatures to which air is cooled and heated it is possible to control the amount of moisture and thus the relative humidity of the air as well as the final air temperature. These temperatures are not fixed by specifying only the final room air temperature and relative humidity, but also require that the room heat and moisture loads be known or assumed since the room environmental conditions are determined after mixing of supply air with the room air.

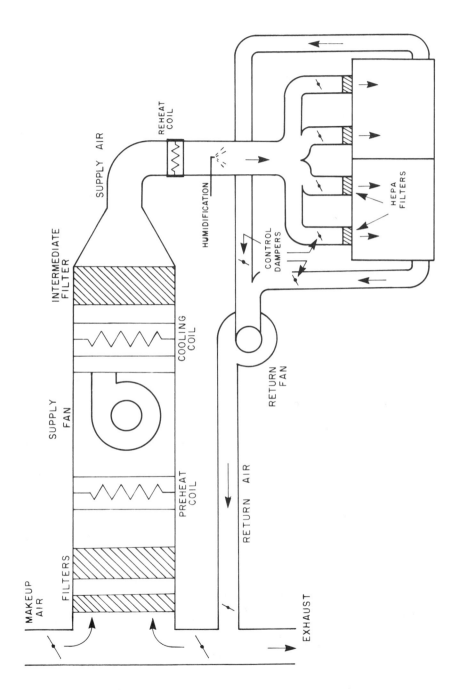

Figure 18 Typical air handling system for pharmaceutical use.

To prevent infiltration of contamination into a clean environment, a net positive outflow of air is necessary. This positive outflow is the difference between the volume of conditioned air supplied and the volume of air returned by the return fan. Because of the impracticality of measuring and monitoring air leakage through the various openings from a controlled environment area, it is common practice to measure and monitor the air pressure differential caused by the excess air supply. CGMP requires that this pressure differential be maintained at or above 0.05 in. of water [see requirement (d) on page 386]. The volume difference between supply and return necessary to produce the necessary pressure is not fixed but is determined by the air escape area. Wider openings or more frequent opening of entry doors will require a greater excess supply. Clean air systems usually have return fans to help maintain pressure differentials, but systems without return fans can produce the positive pressure differential by using dampers in the return air ductwork. These dampers are adjusted to restrict the return airflow, causing outward leakage. Creation of positive air pressure by using return dampers is less efficient than by modulating supply and return fan volume. The most important use of dampers is in the supply duct system. Most air handling systems supply more than a single room. Dampers are used in the supply ducts for accurate balance of the airflow to the various rooms so that each room at the same cleanliness level has the same positive air pressure.

For economical operation, the conditioned return air is recirculated. Outside or makeup air is added to compensate for building losses, exhausts, and to provide fresh air. Minimum makeup rates on the order of 10% are usual. When the return air is noxious or excessively heated, makeup air rates of up to 100% may be necessary. Local building codes may require certain makeup rates or ASHRAE standards may be used for good system design.

Turbulent airflow is to be avoided in a clean room. Turbulent airflow enhances temperature and fresh air distribution but also circulates particulate contamination. Therefore, ceiling diffusers are usually not used in a clean air system and return air is taken from near floor level. Stagnation may be avoided in clean rooms by splitting the supply duct so that air is introduced at several points of the ceiling. Similarly, dispersion of several return air connection points throughout the work area will avoid stagnant conditions and reduce particulate circulation.

4. Air Filtration

Effective air filtration is absolutely essential to those pharmaceutical operations that must be conducted in a controlled environment. While physical cleaning and sanitization can remove surface contaminants from people, equipment, tools, containers, and so on, only air filtration can prevent contamination of all of these by airborne contaminants. While air filter selection for most applications takes into consideration the factors of initial cost, filter efficiency, power costs, maintenance labor costs, maintenance requirements, filter life, system resistance, amortization, and return on investment, the filtration system for a pharmaceutically controlled environment is selected to provide the cleanest environment possible, with the factors listed above being of secondary concern.

There are many types of filters available for air filtration and there are an equally large number of manufacturers and techniques. Except for Federal Standard 209 B, which pertains to clean rooms, there are no widely accepted performance or design standards for air filtration, making the definition of a typical system difficult. Air handling or air conditioning systems typically employ one or two sets of filters to reach the desired level of air cleanliness. Air handling systems for

pharmaceutical use, as in Figure 18, usually employ three sets of filters with increasing efficiencies as outlined in Federal Standard 209 B.

To understand air filtration more fully, it is necessary to understand the characteristics of atmospheric dust, the mechanisms of filtration, the types of filters,
and the associated testing and rating systems:

Characteristics of Atmospheric Dust. Atmospheric dust is acknowledged to
vary in particle size and constituents. Table 2 illustrates the relationship between
weight analysis and particle count analysis of atmospheric dust. Although these
values are representative only, they serve to illustrate two important points about
air filtration. First, because of the wide range of particle sizes found, it is difficult and usually impractical to attempt to remove all particles with a single grade
of filter. Second, because of the inverse relationship of particle weight and volume,
it is impossible to meaningfully rate high-efficiency (HEPA) filters according to the
standards used for low- to medium-efficiency filters. Two filters which vary considerably in volume removal might differ imperceptibly in their removal efficiency
on a particle count basis. Similarly, filters with very different removal efficiencies
by count might differ only slightly on a weight removal basis.

Mechanisms of Filtration [8]. A screen may be thought of as a filter, capable
of retaining particles larger than the opening size. Because of its two-dimensional
configuration, the screen would become plugged quickly. For practical use, filters
are a three-dimensional array of fibers, often coated with an adhesive to hold them
in place and to retain intercepted particles. Rather than screening, particles are
removed by (1) direct interception, (2) settling, (3) inertial effect, (4) diffusion,
and (5) electrostatic effect.

Direct interception occurs most frequently with particles too large to diffuse
due to Brownian motion but too small to settle appreciably. Direct interception is
simply a collision of the particle with a filter fiber.

Filtration by settling occurs only with relatively large particles which are
heavy enough to fall from the streamline and settle on the surface of a fiber.

As air flows through a filter it must continually change directions. The inertia
of larger particles will prevent them from changing direction and will cause them
to strike filter fibers.

Table 2 Size Distribution of a Typical Atmospheric Dust Sample

Particle size range (μm)	Proportionate particle count	Percent by particle count	Percent by volume or weight
10–30	1,000	0.005	28
5–10	35,000	0.175	52
3–5	50,000	0.25	11
1–3	214,000	1.07	6
0.5–1	1,352,000	6.78	2
0–0.5	18,280,000	91.72	1

Source: Data from Ref. 7.

Diffusion is the predominant removal mechanism for smaller particles which diffuse in a manner similar to molecular diffusion and are subject to turbulence within the filter. Due to these effects, the smaller particles tend to remain in the filter a long time, increasing the opportunity for collection.

Electrostatic charges which may occur in certain types of filters may attract and hold particles from the airstream. In the case of electrostatic air filters, high-voltage plates or wires give an electrostatic charge to the particles, which are then attracted to collection plates of opposite polarity.

Types of Filters. The performance standards for clean rooms as defined by Federal Standard 209 B require the use of high-efficiency particulate air (HEPA) filters such as illustrated by Figure 19. HEPA filters are typically box shaped with a thin glass fiber filter medium folded accordian style to provide a very large surface area. Approximately 23 m^2 of filter medium is folded into a filter measuring 61 cm X 61 cm X 30.5 cm deep. Flow resistance of HEPA filters usually ranges from 25 mm water gauge initially to 75 mm when loaded (recommended filter replacement). HEPA filters are rated according to their ability to remove 0.3 μm particles from the airstream. The standard efficiency of a HEPA filter is 99.97%, but ultra HEPA filters of up to 99.99% efficiency are available. Many HEPA filter options are available. Some (extracted from Ref. 9) are:

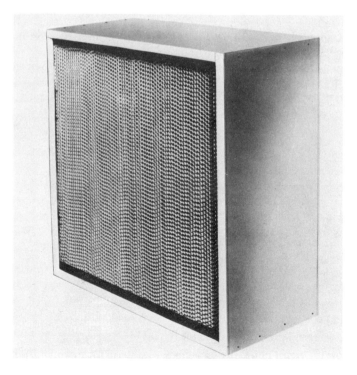

Figure 19 Typical HEPA filter. (Courtesy American Air Filter, Louisville, Kentucky.)

Frame material:
Particle board, standard or fire resistant
Plywood, standard or fire resistant
Cadmium-plated steel
Stainless steel
Aluminum

Separator material:
Aluminum
Kraft paper
Asbestos

Bond (media to sides):
Polyurethane foam
RTV silicone
Neoprene rubber
Glass mat packing

Gasket material:
Neoprene
Fiber
Silicone

Test standard:
99.97% DOP
99.99% DOP
99.999% DOP
Full scanning

The standards and options above are by no means rigid or all-inclusive. HEPA filters are individually tested and are commonly built to customers' specifications. HEPA filters are usually changed when their airflow resistance reaches 75 mm water gauge. The filters can withstand higher flow resistance, but as airflow resistance increases, airflow volume will decrease. The number of hours required for a HEPA filter to reach maximum loading depends on the efficiency of prefiltration.

Intermediate prefilters are usually of the extended surface pocket type illustrated in Figure 20. These filters typically use a fine glass fiber medium whose efficiency depends on the density of fibers. Federal Standard 209 B recommends an efficiency of 80 to 90% for intermediate prefilters. This efficiency is determined not by a DOP test but by a dust spot (discoloration) test, as will be discussed on page 395. The two rating systems cannot be directly compared. For filters of 90% efficiency, airflow resistance will vary from approximately 12 cm to 25 cm water gage and will have a gross media area of about 20% of a HEPA filter having comparable flow capacity. Prefilter specifications are more standardized than for HEPA filters and customized designs are usually not available. This type of filter is also disposable.

Initial prefilters may be lower-efficiency pocket-type filters similar to the intermediate prefilters or may be of the disposable panel filter type illustrated in Figure 21. Federal Standard 209 B suggests an efficiency of 20 to 30% for initial prefilters, according to the same rating system as for intermediate prefilters. Panel filters are often rated according to their weight removal ability, a test different than that used for either HEPA or pocket filters. Panel filters are disposable and have a typical airflow resistance of less than 12 cm water gauge.

The final decision regarding prefilter selection is an economic decision considering initial cost, power cost, maintenance labor cost, filter life, system resistance, and other factors. In some cases, the initial prefilter might be omitted. The HEPA filter will adequately clean the air, although its useful life will be directly affected by the efficiency of prefiltration. Because of the complexity of the

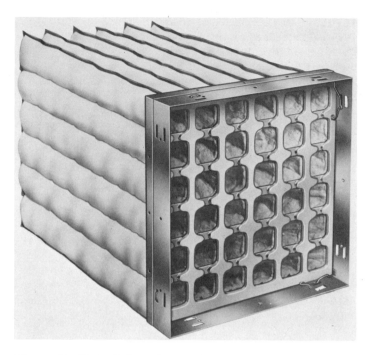

Figure 20 Extended surface pocket-type filter. (Courtesy American Air Filter, Louisville, Kentucky.)

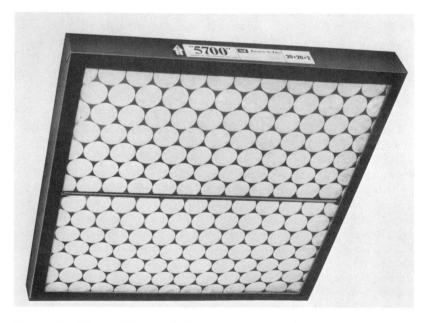

Figure 21 Disposable panel filter. (Courtesy American Air Filter, Louisville, Kentucky.)

filter selection process, filter manufacturers have developed computer programs
to analyze the specific needs of an installation and recommend the optimum filters.

Filter Testing and Rating. The various types of air filters are used for different purposes: for example, panel filters to remove large quantities (weights) of
large particles while HEPA filters remove large numbers (little weight) of small
particles. Further, different users attach different values to various filter quali-
ties. Accordingly, many different agencies have developed terminology, standards,
and test procedures for filter evaluation. Standard 52-76 [10], developed by the
American Society of Heating, Refrigeration and Air-Conditioning Engineers
(ASHRAE), is a National Voluntary Consensus Standard developed to evaluate and
rate air filters uniformly. ASHRAE Standard 52-76 is intended for testing all filters
except those with air cleaning efficiencies greater than 98%. Standard 52-76 references Military Standard 282, DOP Smoke Penetration Method, for particle removal
performance testing. Various other procedures and methods also exist for testing
HEPA filters.

Three performance characteristics are of interest in describing filter performance: particle removal ability, airflow resistance, and operating life. A filter's particle removal ability is described by atmospheric Dust Spot Efficiency
(efficiency) and Synthetic Dust Weight Arrestance (arrestance). Both efficiency and
arrestance are reported when describing a filter's performance, except that efficiency is normally not reported if it is less than 20%. Airflow resistance data include an airflow resistance curve, the initial resistance to airflow, and the rated
final resistance as recommended by the manufacturer. Operating life is determined
by the rated final resistance of the filter.

Atmospheric Dust Spot Efficiency, commonly called efficiency, is a measure
of a filter's ability to remove atmospheric dust. Two airstreams, one from upstream of the filter being tested and one from downstream of the filter, are filtered
through "targets" of Hollingsworth and Voss H-93 glass paper. The upstream sample is cycled on and off to maintain approximately equal opacities on the two targets.
Efficiency is determined by

$$E = 100 \times \left(1 - \frac{Q_1 O_2}{Q_2 O_1} \right)$$

where

Q_1 = total quantity of air drawn through upstream target

Q_2 = total quantity of air drawn through downstream target

O_1 = opacity of dust spot on upstream target

O_2 = opacity of dust spot on downstream target

Synthetic Dust Weight Arrestance, commonly called arrestance, is a measure
of a filter's ability to remove a standard prepared synthetic dust. The ASHRAE
synthetic test dust is 72% by weight standardized air cleaner test dust fine, 23%
Molocco black and 5% No. 7 cotton linters ground in a Wiley Mill to pass a 4 mm
screen. In the arrestance test, a measured quantity W_1 of synthetic dust is fed to
the test filter. The air passing through the filter is then filtered through a final
filter of no less than 95% efficiency, 98% arrestance. The amount of dust collected
on the final filter is weighed W_2. Arrestance is

$$A = 100 \times \left(1 - \frac{W_2}{W_1}\right)$$

Airflow resistance is expressed as a pressure differential, in pascals, between the air pressure upstream of the filter and the downstream air filter. This resistance is a function of both airflow rate and filter loading. An airflow resistance curve is determined by measuring the resistance at a minimum of four airflow rates of 50, 75, 100, and 125% of the manufacturer's airflow rating. Airflow resistance must be carefully considered in the design of an air filtering system and must be monitored during operation. Airflow resistance caused by dirty filters may reduce airflow volume, thereby reducing the air change rate in critical areas, possibly causing a loss in relative air pressure. If filters are not changed when they reach the maximum resistance as specified by the manufacturer, they may begin to lose their physical integrity or rupture, thereby releasing some of the dust they have accumulated. The initial resistance to airflow and the rated final resistance are used to compare filters. The initial resistance to airflow is the resistance of a clean filter operating at its rated airflow rate. The rated final resistance is the maximum allowable resistance specified by the manufacturer for the rated airflow rate.

The arrestance and rated final resistance are often used to determine dust holding capacity, a fourth comparative characteristic. Dust holding capacity is the product of the weight of dust fed to the filter during the Synthetic Dust Weight Arrestance test times the average arrestance until either (1) the filter reaches its rated final resistance or (2) two consecutive arrestance values are less than 85% of the maximum arrestance. The dust holding capacity is a more complete indication of filter life than the rated final resistance.

HEPA filters, designed to collect a specified percentage of particles in a specified size range, require different and more closely controlled test methods. No industry consensus standard exists for testing and rating HEPA filters, but Military Standard 282 is cited by ASHRAE Standard 52-76 as a uniform HEPA test procedure. HEPA testing, whether according to Mil Std 282 or according to other procedures, involves generation of an aerosol of uniform particle sizes and measurement of the number of particles passing through the filter. Dioctyl phthalate (DOP), when heated in an airstream, generates a smoke containing a large quantity of particles of $0.3 \mu m$ size. This smoke is mixed with the airstream of the filter to be tested. The upstream smoke concentration is sampled to determine initial loading and the downstream air is sampled for filter leakage. This sampling is done by removing a portion of the airstream with an isokinetic probe and passing that sample through a penetrometer. Isokinetic sampling is a technique of removing the sample stream at the same velocity as the parent airstream. If the sample stream velocity is too high, the probe will draw in more air, and thus more particles with a higher proportion of small particles than otherwise would be found in the space occupied by the probe. Similarly, a low sample velocity will cause an erroneous low result. Two methods of filter scanning are used, depending on the criticality of the installation. First, the downstream air may be allowed to mix and is then sampled so as to indicate an average value for the entire filter. This method is quick, but will not indicate a possibly serious leak. A second more rigorous procedure is to scan the filter face with the sample probe. Often a test pattern of one sample for each 150 mm $\times$ 150 mm square of filter face is used unless a high test reading is observed, when a small test pattern is used to pinpoint a leak. Testing of a HEPA filter also requires sampling along all seals and gaskets intended to prevent air from bypassing the filter. Minor leaks in a HEPA filter can be repaired using RTV (room-temperature vulcanizing) silicone rubber. The percentage of area that can be covered by RTV before complete replacement is necessary depends on the filter usage. As before, filter resistance is important. If the repair causes the filter resistance to increase beyond the manufacturer's maximum specification or beyond the capability of the air supply fan to maintain an adequate airflow, it should be replaced. If a HEPA filter is used to supply a laminar flow installation, the disruption of the laminar flow stream by the patch must also be considered. Further, whether the patch is actually sealing the hole or simply spreading the leaking contaminants must be evaluated.

G. Laminar Flow

Laminar flow, as it pertains to environmental control, is an extension of HVAC systems, utilizing control of airflow direction and velocity as a technique to improve environmental cleanliness. Laminar airflow was described on page 363 as an environmental control zone but is a fundamentally different barrier to contamination than physical barriers such as walls or air filters. HEPA filters, when properly installed, tested, and maintained, provide a supply of very clean air to the work area, creating a conventional clean room. However, introduction of personnel, equipment, and materials into the work area provides sources of particulate matter which may contaminate the product. Very small particles are not heavy enough to settle due only to the force of gravity, but instead are carried and directed by air currents. If generated upstream of the product or if caught in turbulent air, particles may be driven into the product. Federal Standard 209 B defines laminar flow as "airflow in which the entire body of air within a confined area essentially moves with uniform velocity along parallel flow lines." An average air velocity of 90 ft min^{-1} (27.5 m min^{-1}) has been accepted as the standard for laminar flow applications. A variation of 20% across the laminar flow area is acceptable. This airflow velocity satisfactorily sweeps the area yet does not create unacceptable turbulence. In the event that a contaminant particle is introduced into the laminar flow environmental zone, whether by having been carried in or having been generated there, the unidirectional laminar flow air movement will carry it away quickly, minimizing the time of the particle in the protected zone.

The advantages of laminar flow can only be realized by its careful application. The nature of the task or product to be protected and the potential source of contamination must be considered. An entire room may be swept by laminar flow or only localized areas may be protected. The direction of flow may be horizontal or vertical. Figure 22 illustrates a vertical laminar flow room. Note the raised floor for air return and the ceiling plenum for air distribution. Multiple blowers are usually required to handle the large volumes of air required. Unitized laminar flow systems are also available in vertical or horizontal configurations, as illustrated in Figures 23 and 24. Portable units are useful in areas where they must be moved for cleaning or maintaining the protected equipment.

Although it might seem ideal to have an entire room protected by laminar flow, there are disadvantages. A laminar flow room is relatively expensive to construct and operate. To illustrate, consider a room measuring 6 m X 6 m X 3 m (20 ft X 20 ft X 10 ft). To provide vertical laminar flow would require 36 m^2 (400 ft^2) of filter surface and sould require an air flow rate of 990 m^3 min^{-1} (36,000 ft^3 min^{-1}). Horizontal laminar flow would require 18 m^2 of filter surface (200 ft^2) and an airflow of 495 m^3 min^{-1} (18,000 ft^3 min^{-1}). A conventional clean room of the same size supplied with the minimum 20 air changes per hour would require only about 0.5 m^2

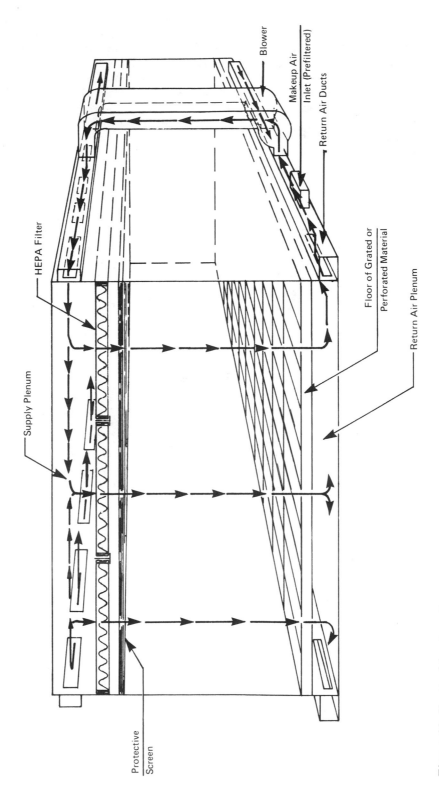

Figure 22 Vertical laminar flow room.

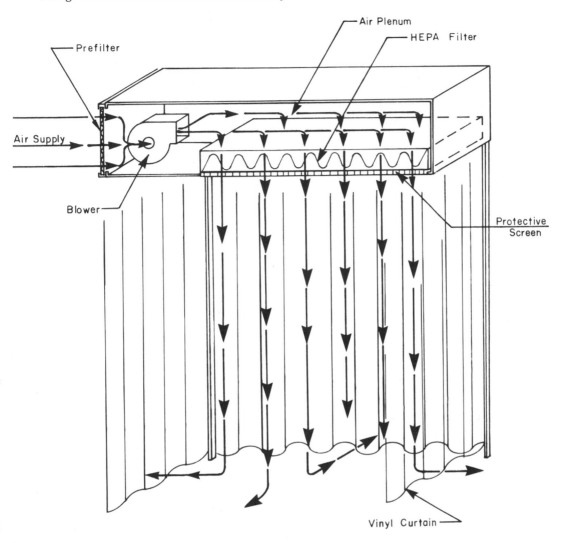

Figure 23 Portable downflow laminar flow unit.

(6 ft^2) of filter surface and only 36.7 m^3 min^{-1} (1333 ft^3 min^{-1}) of supply air. Operationally, a horizontal laminar flow room provides laminar flow conditions only at the first workstation, after which point turbulence may be created or particulate matter introduced. Vertical downflow rooms are flexible in work surface layout, but are usually inefficiently utilized due to the relatively small area which actually requires laminar flow protection. Pharmaceutical production areas are usually constructed as conventional clean rooms (Class 10,000 to 100,000) with portable or ceiling-mounted laminar flow units located immediately above those areas where product or product contact surfaces are exposed. Table 3 summarizes the characteristics and anticipated performance of the various types of laminar and nonlaminar flow installations.

Table 3 Typical Performance of Various Clean Room Installations

Type of Facility	Cleanliness class		
	100	10,000	100,000
Laminar airflow Vertical flow room Vertical flow curtain unit Vertical flow bench	Entire work area usually meets requirements at normal working height locations	Entire area normally meets requirements	Entire area meets requirements
Crossflow room Tunnel room Wall-to-floor room Crossflow bench	First work locations normally meet requirements	Entire work area normally meets requirements if particle generation, work locations, and personnel are reasonably controlled	Entire area normally meets requirements
Nonlaminar airflow Conventional clean room	Will <u>not</u> meet requirements under operation conditions	In some cases, can be upgraded to meet requirements by placing laminar airflow devices (benches, modular units, tunnel rooms, or downflow curtain units) within the room and continuously filtering the recirculated air; personnel and operation restrictions and janitorial maintenance are also required	Will usually meet requirements with strict observation of rules governing personnel, operations, garmenting, and janitorial procedures

Source: Ref. 6.

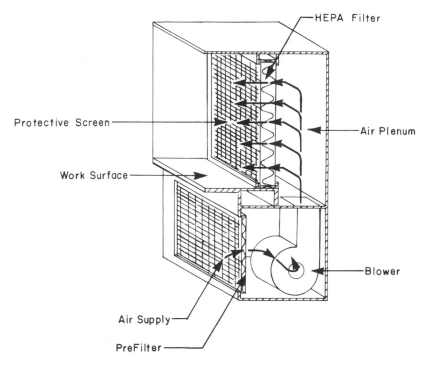

Figure 24 Horizontal laminar flow bench.

H. Steam

In an industrial plant, steam is important as an energy transfer medium. It may be used for space heating, water heating, process heating, or to drive engines or turbines. In a pharmaceutical plant, steam further serves as a means of sterilization. Many additives used with industrial steam systems to enhance operation and prevent corrosion are unacceptable in a pharmaceutical application.

1. Generation and Distribution

The most common steam generation system consists of a gas- or oil-fired boiler producing saturated steam at medium pressure [up to approximately 960 kPa (125 psi)]. To prevent scaling and corrosion in the boiler, various additives usually are added to the boiler feedwater. These additives may be carried over, either intentionally or unintentionally, into the steam distribution system. If the additive is volatile at the steam temperature, the carryover will be gaseous. Nonvolatile additives can be carried over as liquid if the boiler is overdriven or if a sudden steam demand causes a temporary drop in system pressure. Steam condensed by heat loss or process use is called condensate and is returned to the boiler for reuse. In the usual industrial plant steam is distributed and returned in piping systems of "black iron" pipe of strength suitable for the pressures involved. When condensate combines with the carbon dioxide carried over with the steam, corrosive carbonic acid is formed. If this corrosion is unchecked, return piping may fail within a year. The usual method of controlling such corrosion is to introduce a volatile additive in the boiler which will carry over with the steam and inhibit condensate corrosion.

Industrial systems use filming amines to coat the surface of return piping to reduce corrosion, but they are strictly unacceptable where steam contacts food or drug products or product contact surfaces.

Steam at higher temperatures and pressures carries more energy, thus is more efficient than low-pressure steam. Pressures of 10,000 to 20,000 kPa or more (1450 to 2900 psi) and at superheated temperatures (heated above saturated conditions) greatly increase steam system efficiencies, but also increase system cost. Such systems are usually found in power plants, generating stations, and turbine application. In an industrial plant, particularly a pharmaceutical plant, the temperatures required are usually in the range 100 to 150°C. System flexibility is important and plant maintenance personnel, who may not be highly trained in steam system work or who are equipped for only light-duty piping work, must be able to handle the system. The basic purpose of the system is to recover (use) the latent heat of vaporization when steam condenses. In the boiler, energy is added—approximately 2000 Jg (868 B lb^{-1})—to the steam and at the point of use this same energy is removed. The process is efficient except for various heat losses:

a. Piping heat loss: Even though insulated, heat loss through piping is inevitable and substantial. This loss creates condensate which must be trapped (drained away) and returned to the boiler or it will create "wet" steam, which reduces process efficiency. Uninsulated piping loses heat through conduction and radiation. Well-insulated piping minimizes radiant loss due to the lower outside surface temperature and reduces conduction loss by wrapping the pipe with materials having a lower heat conductance. Heat losses also occur at valves and fittings due to their odd geometries.
b. Friction losses: All piping causes loss due to the friction of flowing fluid, and all fittings and valves introduce their own loss, which may be expressed as equivalent lengths of pipe. These losses are all proportional to velocity. Thus, in a static or pseudostatic system where flow rates are low, no friction loss occurs, but in a high-flow-rate system, friction losses are significant and will cause fluctuating pressure dependent on system loading. Therefore, if pressure control is important, system velocities must be minimized.
c. Makeup water: Water and steam lost through leaks, process use, or flushing must be replaced, creating an additional heat requirement on the system.

2. Sterilization Process

When used for sterilization, steam must be at saturated conditions and be as free from impurities as possible. Thus a superheated steam boiler is not suitable for use to produce steam for direct steam sterilization. The problem of superheat may occur with a saturated steam boiler if the pressures are high enough. Consider, for example, saturated steam being generated at 960 kPa absolute (equivalent to approximately 125 psi) flowing through a distribution system and expanding to a lower pressure in a steam sterilizer. This expansion process is illustrated graphically in Figure 25. This figure is a plot of steam conditions known as a Mollier chart. Key features of the Mollier chart are:

a. The ordinate is enthalpy, a measure of the steam's energy.
b. The abscissa, entropy, is a thermodynamic property defined as the amount of heat taken in by a process divided by the absolute temperature at which the heat is taken in. This property is not used directly in interpretation of this steam process but is merely a convenient means of graphically expressing steam characteristics.

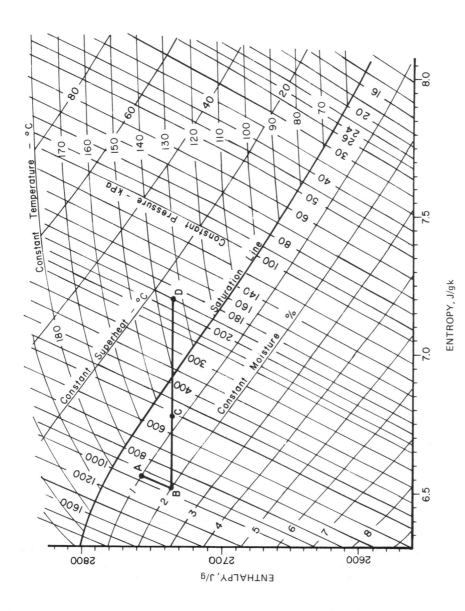

Figure 25.   Steam expansion process.   (Data from Ref. 11.)

c. The saturation line is a locus of points where water vapor and liquid exist in equilibrium (100°C at 101 kPa is such a point).

d. The lines at about 60° from horizontal are lines of constant absolute pressure.

e. The lines paralleling the saturation line on the lower side represent constant moisture percentage conditions, while the lines above the saturation line are degrees of superheat. Superheat is the temperature above theoretical saturation temperature for a given pressure.

To start the process, assume that due to carryover of moisture during boiling, the steam is not pure vapor, but contains 1% moisture. At point A (pressure = 960 kPa, moisture = 1%), the enthalpy = 2756 Jg^{-1}. As the steam flows through the distribution system at constant pressure, it loses energy, reducing its enthalpy to, perhaps, 2736 Jg^{-1}. Since the pressure remains constant, point B indicates a higher moisture content of 2%. In most steam systems, the distribution system pressure is reduced at the point of use by a pressure reducing valve. The path from point B to point C illustrates steam flow through a pressure reducing valve. Although no energy is added (or lost) by the valve, the steam conditions are much nearer saturation conditions. Further pressure reduction to point D, representing conditions inside a typical sterilizer, show a superheated steam condition. This superheated condition occurs due to a pressure reduction and the concurrent reduction in the amount of energy required to maintain saturated conditions. Note that temperature was not used to describe this process since temperature will vary depending on several variables. The only reliable means of determining theoretical steam temperature is by consulting steam tables. For actual temperatures, measurements are usually necessary since the losses are difficult to calculate accurately. In the event that a comparison of theoretical saturation temperature (found from steam tables, knowing pressure) with actual measured temperature indicate that superheated steam exists, only two alternatives are practical. First, the pressure of the boiler may be reduced. Reference to Figure 25 shows how this action would reduce the energy available for creating a superheat condition. If the system pressure cannot be changed, a de-superheater may be necessary at the point of use. A de-superheater injects water, which is evaporated by the "excess" energy, thereby reducing the energy available for superheat. In actual practice, superheat is a problem only where the system heat losses are low compared to the total energy transferred—as in a well-insulated high-flow system.

3. Clean Steam

Most pharmaceutical facilities that require steam for general plant use choose a dual system. Plant steam is provided by a conventional low- or medium-pressure boiler with maximum return of condensate and an industrial water treatment program as recommended by a reputable boiler water treatment specialist. "Clean" steam is produced for critical product contact use through use of steam-to-water heat exchangers. Termed re-boilers, these heat exchangers usually generate steam from distilled water and are constructed of stainless steel to withstand the relatively corrosive distilled water. Because of the potential for contamination, clean steam condensate is normally not recovered for reuse. For plants not having a utility steam system for heating a re-boiler, a conventional water still can be modified to provide clean steam. Both re-boilers and stills can be fed with other than distilled water, but must be used more carefully since any contaminants, including pyrogens, can be carried over in water droplets if the unit design capacity is exceeded.

I. Compressed Air

Compressed air, like steam, is an energy transfer medium. The principal use of compressed air in many plants is to actuate air cylinders or drive air motors. Within a parenterals plant, additional important uses include cleaning, drying, or vessel pressurization. Direct and indirect product contact is common, thus requiring utmost care in assuring the quality of the compressed air.

A basic compressed air system is composed of a compressor, a distribution system, and points of use. For pharmaceutical use, a much more refined system is required, including filtration and drying equipment, as in the general compressed air system of Figure 26. Compressed air systems can be centralized or dedicated. In a central system, a single compressor installation supplies air to the entire facility. With dedicated systems, several compressors feed separate areas of the facility. The advantages of the central system are obvious:

a. A single installation is easier to control.
b. The total initial and operating costs are likely to be lower.
c. A better grade of filtration and drying equipment can probably be justified.
d. A single distribution system is easier to maintain.
e. Greater total reliability results from fewer total components.
f. A central system may be able to use compressors more efficiently at or near their rated capacities due to the "averaging" of plant load.

But there are many instances where the advantages of the dedicated separate systems are significant:

a. If compressed air needs are widely separated, the cost of the distribution system may be significant and favor the use of separate systems.
b. Separate systems may be more flexible, making scheduling of maintenance, for example, easier when fewer activities must be coordinated. There is often a reluctance to place total plant dependence on a single system, where the failure of one element may affect all plant operations.
c. All air uses may not require the same quality of air. If a large portion of the compressed air requirements are for general utility use, it may be more practical to split the system than to operate a relatively expensive and complex system designed to produce clean air when it is not needed.

1. Clean Air Requirements

The proposed Current Good Manufacturing Practices for Large Volume Parenterals require (Sec. 212.223, June 1, 1976) that compressed air used in controlled environment areas meet the requirements for particle count and size of a class 100,000 room, be supplied by an oil-free compressor, and be dehumidified. Strict interpretation of these guidelines dictates the use of oil-free compressors and compressed air dryers to obtain air of the required cleanliness, the usual practice. Many feel that air meeting the required cleanliness levels can be obtained by a combination of coalescing, drying, and filtration, as illustrated by the compressed air purification system of Figure 27. At least two circumstances exist where such a system may be required in addition to oil-free compressors:

a. If an existing compressed air system is being upgraded, it may be impossible to remove all the accumulated contamination and oil residue from the distribu-

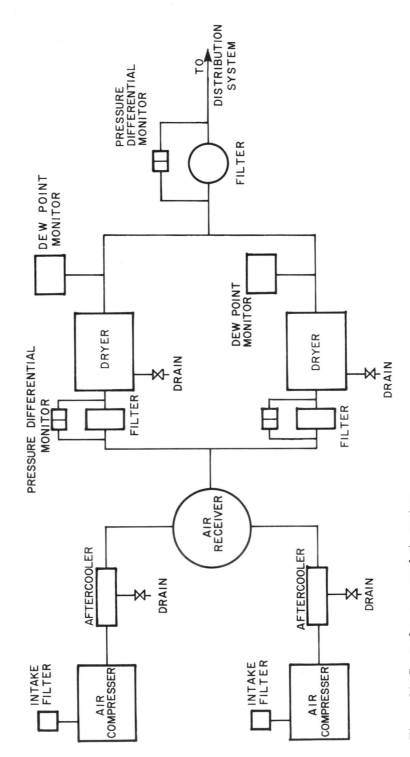

Figure 26 General compressed air system.

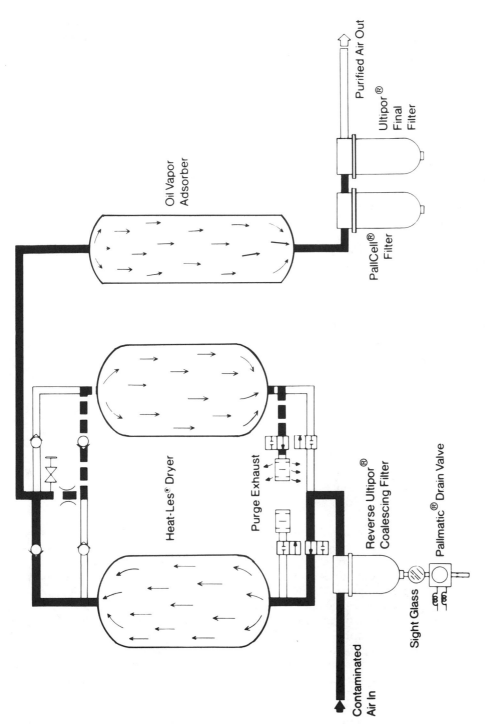

Figure 27 Compressed air purification system. (Courtesy Pall Corporation, Glen Cove, New York.)

tion system. If the distribution system must be reused, a combination oil removal and particulate matter filtration system would be required.
b. An oil-free compressor may not produce oil-free air if the intake air is sufficiently contaminated, as might be the case if the compressor intake was located
near a boiler stack.

2. Equipment Selection

In either a centralized or dedicated system, the actual compressor equipment
can be composed of a minimum number of large units or a series of smaller modular units. The easiest compressor selection process involves planning for maximum plant usage plus 50 to 100%. A single compressor may be sized to handle
the total plant load, while a second duplicate compressor will act as a standby or
provide capacity for expansion. This system is simple but creates problems in
normal use. First, compressed air loads are seldom constant. Thus the single
compressor will often operate at part load, an inefficient procedure for some compressor types. Second, as compressed air usage grows, the second (standby) compressor will be required to run constantly but inefficiently to provide only a small
quantity of air. At this point the backup protection of the second compressor is
lost. In the modular compressor approach, a smaller compressor size is selected
to nearly equal the minimum plant usage. The range to maximum usage is then
covered by multiple compressors of the same type and size, plus one or more extra
units for backup and expansion. To illustrate, assume that anticipated air usage is
100 to 400 m^3 hr^{-1}. The large compressor installation would require two compressors of 400 to 500 m^3 hr^{-1} capacity each. The modular concept would require five
compressors of 100 m^3 hr^{-1} each. Although the trend in recent years has been to
the large central compressor concept, the arguments for the modular concept are
becoming more important:

a. Energy consumption and electrical demand changes favor the modular compressors. Only the motors actually required are in use at a given time.
b. The modular concept lends itself to recovery of waste heat. The heat of compression, absorbed by either water cooling or air cooling, can be used more
readily since the smaller compressors can be more easily located near a use
point and are less likely to be cycling on and off.
c. The modular installation requires less idle investment for backup protection.

Oil-free compressors are of three types: reciprocating piston, rotary screw,
and centrifugal. No compressor is truly oil-free since the crankcase must be lubricated. The term "oil-free" applies to the components in contact with the compressed air. Each type of oil-free compressor has its own advantages and disadvantages for a particular application.

Reciprocating piston compressors are the more common compressor type.
Although some manufacturers have designed reciprocating piston compressors specifically for oil-free service, most oil-free reciprocals are a modified lubricated
type. For oil-free applications, the connecting rod is lengthened to prevent oil
carryover from the crankcase into the cylinder, and the steel piston rings, which
require lubrication, are replaced by rings of Teflon or a Teflon compound. The reciprocating piston compressor, as a general rule, requires more maintenance and
is less reliable when used for oil-free service than when used as lubricated units.
Reciprocating piston compressors are generally used for small to medium volume
requirements (up to approximately 850 m^3 hr^{-1}). A single-stage reciprocating
piston oil-free compressor can be used up to approximately 700 kPa pressure. For

higher volumes, compressors can be infinitely paralleled. For higher-pressure requirements, two-stage compressors (two cylinders in series) are used up to 1000
kPa. Multistaging beyond two stages is generally not done for general plant use.

Rotary screw compressors tend to be more compact than piston-type nonlubricated compressors and tend to require less maintenance due to their simpler construction and closer tolerances. Most rotary screw compressors require oil mist
lubrication, but several "nonoil" types are available, using water or silicone mist
as a lubricant. One that is widely used in the pharmaceutical industry relies on
fine machine tolerances to prevent metal-to-metal contact of the compressing elements while holding leakage, a problem in nonlubricated compressors, to a minimum. Although more compact than piston compressors, rotary screw compressors
are less efficient, especially at part load. This problem is most significant if the
compressed air system has only one compressor, sized for peak loads. Although
rotary screw compressors are usually more noisy than reciprocating types, they
can usually be silenced easily because of their compactness. Because of the in-
efficiency of the rotary screw compressor, it has not found wide acceptance as an
oil-free unit except in the medium to large capacities (over 750 m^3 hr^{-1}), although
the use of water or silicone as a lubricant may make smaller units more practical.
Like reciprocating piston compressors, rotary screw compressors can be staged
for higher pressures. A single-stage oil-free rotary screw compressor can be used
at pressures of 350 kPa, while two-stage units operate in the 1000 kPa range. When
paralleled for additional capacity, rotary screw compressors may be affected by
surges from other compressors, especially reciprocating piston compressors. Additional care in the sizing of piping and compressed air storage tanks should be exercised.

Centrifugal compressors are not widely used to provide utility air. Their
most frequent application is to meet large constant-volume requirements since they
must be designed for a specific capacity. Operation at reduced capacity can cause
stalling or surging of the compressor.

3. Heat and Moisture Control

Pharmaceutical compressed air must be cooled to remove the heat of compression. This aftercooling is usually accomplished with a shell-and-tube heat exchanger using ordinary potable water, cooling tower water, or plant chilled water.
Aftercooling causes condensation and leaves the air at saturated condition. Any further cooling in the plant distribution system or at the point of use would cause more
condensation, creating a potential for both system corrosion and bacterial growth.

To reduce the moisture content below the capability of an aftercooler, a dryer
is used. Most common is the refrigerated dryer, available for either 2°C (35°F) or
10°C (50°F) dew point. Dryer ratings are confusing since the dew point (that point
at which moisture begins to condense in air) changes with pressure. To select a
dryer properly, one must know the system working pressure and the anticipated
temperatures of the distribution system and points of use. Figure 28 shows the relationship of atmospheric dew point and pressure dew point for a pressure of 690
kPa. A dew point of 10°C at 690 kPa will give a dew point of -17°C at atmospheric
conditions. The dryer specifications required depend on the lowest temperature
expected at any point in the distribution system.

Desiccant drying using absorption or adsorption can be used to reduce the dew
point and will, in fact, reduce the dew point much below that of the refrigerated
dryers. Adsorption systems using silicagel (S_1O_2) or activated alumina (Al_2O_3) are
the most common industrial desiccant systems. Desiccant dryers can be made

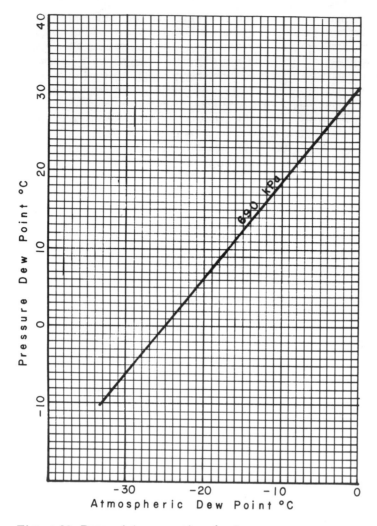

Figure 28 Dew point conversion chart.

regenerative, making them quite economical to use. Their use has not been wide-spread in the pharmaceutical industry, due to the potential for particulate carry-over.

4. Filtration

Particulate filtration of compressed air is necessary if it is to be used in controlled environment areas. Compressor intake filtration is normally intended to remove contaminants likely to cause equipment damage. Special filters comparable in efficiency to HEPA filters can be installed on a compressor intake, but are of questionable value since the air may be recontaminated by particles generated by corrosion or abrasion within the compressor. Filters causing a significant pressure drop will also significantly affect compressor performance when used on the intake.

After cooling and drying, the compressed air can be filtered before being introduced to the distribution system. Here a depth-type filter can be used to produce air quality consistent with end-use requirements. Bacteria retentive filters can also be used, but must be protected by suitable prefilters to prevent filter damage by larger particles. The need for a bacteria-retentive filter after compression is questionable since filtration prior to distribution would not protect from bacterial growth within the distribution system. Second, the heat generated during compression and the dry conditions caused by the air dryer create an atmosphere that should not support bacterial growth.

Point-of-use compressed air filtration is of two basic types. First, there is the relatively gross filtration done to protect air-powered equipment. With a pharmaceutical grade system having good filtration after drying, such filtration is unnecessary, but is often done as a matter of good practice. The second type of point-of-use filtration for pharmaceutical use is the bacteria-retentive filter, which must be used where the air will enter controlled areas or be used for product contact.

5. System Control

Control of a compressed air system is quite simple and straightforward. For small compressors, a pressure switch is used to start the compressor when system pressure falls to a level just above the highest point of use pressure requirement and stops the compressor when system pressure reaches the maximum operating pressure of the compressor or maximum desired system pressure. For multiple-compressor systems, the "start" pressure points can be "staged" automatically to bring more compressors on line if necessary.

For larger compressors and in systems where large pressure fluctuations are undesirable several types of modulating controls are available. For piston compressors, one or more intake valves can be held closed to reduce compressor capacity or allow it to idle. For rotary screw compressors modulating controls can restrict the inlet or bypass air for part load operation.

Compressed air filters, like environmental air filters, must be monitored to ensure that they are not overloaded with accumulated particulate matter. For small systems where the filter elements are relatively inexpensive, the filters are often changed on a fixed schedule designed to ensure replacement before failure under all operating conditions. For larger systems, pressure differential monitoring is used to determine filter condition. Because compressed air systems typically have a widely fluctuating flow rate, it is necessary to monitor both air flow rate and pressure differential to assess filter condition accurately.

Refrigerated air dryers have a fixed cooling capacity and a fixed minimum discharge temperature. Failure of the refrigeration system or exceeding the maximum flow rate will result in an increase in discharge temperature, which in turn will result in less moisture being removed by condensation, indicating that corrective action is required. For additional monitoring assurance or for desiccant drying systems a dew point measuring system can be used. A measured flow of air is directed across a mirror cooled to the desired dew point temperature. Condensation, indicating a dew point equal to or above the mirror temperature, is detected by an optical system. The dew point monitor can then activate an alarm, automatically shut down the compressed air system, or switch to backup equipment.

J. Compressed Gases

Compressed gases found in a pharmaceutical plant may include nitrogen, oxygen, liquid propane, ethylene oxide, and various specialty gases. For limited usage, these can be supplied from pressurized cylinders located near the point of use. The use of portable cylinders is relatively expensive, requires more quality control testing, requires more material handling, and requires provisions for fire prevention or operator safety at each point where a portable cylinder is located.

1. Nitrogen

Nitrogen is often used in sufficient quantities in a pharmaceutical plant to justify a central nitrogen storage system such as that illustrated in Figure 29. Nitrogen is delivered and stored as a liquid at a temperature of approximately -195°C and a pressure of approximately 200 kPa. As needed, liquid nitrogen is vaporized in an air-to-liquid heat exchanger and fed to the distribution system. An economizer can be utilized to use the gas which might otherwise escape to the atmosphere through a pressure relief valve. Being inert, nitrogen can be distributed through ordinary black iron pipe. Threaded fittings create no serious quality problem, but can lead to indirect problems such as leakage or contamination due to excessive use of thread sealant. Therefore, a welded system is best. Once the system is well cleaned, bacterial or particulate contamination are minimal problems due to the low temperatures involved and the inertness of the gas. Point-of-use filtration for produce contact uses is, however, advisable common practice.

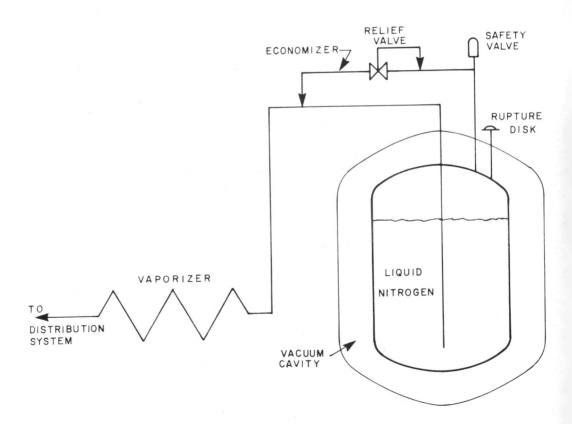

Figure 29 Nitrogen storage system.

2. Oxygen

Oxygen is required if large amounts of glasswork, ampul sealing, for example, are done. Storage and distribution are similar to that for nitrogen, except that oxygen requires a more nonreactive piping system than nitrogen. 304 stainless steel is commonly used. If used for combustion, point-of-use filtration of oxygen is normally not necessary.

3. Propane

Liquid propane gas is often used as a fuel gas when natural gas is unavailable. Although propane has a higher heating value than natural gas (approximately 94×10^6 Jm^{-3} versus 37×10^6 Jm^{-3}) both burn with approximately equal flame temperature. The two gases cannot be used interchangeably without modifications to burners to account for the different heating values. When available, natural gas is usually less expensive. Black iron pipe with threaded connections is commonly used, but leak-free joints are essential.

4. Specialty Gases

Various specialty gases may be required for both process and analytical use. Detailed handling requirements for each are too complex to pursue here. Compressed gas suppliers can provide valuable assistance in solving usage problems and willingly provide data on gas characteristics and industry standards for the handling and use of various gases. Generally, compressed gases must be considered hazardous for one or more of the following reasons:

a. Pressure: Gases may be stored in portable cylinders at very high pressures. If released in an uncontrolled manner, as when cylinder or valve is damaged, the escaping gas can propel the storage cylinder at dangerous velocities.
b. Fire or explosion: Many specialty gases are highly flammable or are strong oxidizers. At the pressures and concentrations associated with portable cylinders, many materials will burn.
c. Toxicity: As with flammability, toxicity is more serious at higher concentrations.
d. Suffocation: Many gases, although nontoxic or inert, can cause suffocation due to oxygen starvation.

K. Water Treatment

Water treatment is one of the most important and complex problems in a pharmaceutical facility. Although a simple chemical mixture, water is never found in a pure state. Instead, it is found with a variety of contaminants depending on the source of the water. Well water, river water, and rain will obviously contain different contaminants. Well water quality varies according to location, and since most systems use more than one well, the water quality will depend on the wells in use. Obviously, river water quality will vary due to a multitude of factors associated with the fact that it is surface water. Water treatment, then, although it must be designed for a particular input quality, must be sufficiently flexible to adapt to the infeed variation.

1. Basic Pretreatment

Water treatment for pharmaceutical use is a two-part operation: treatment to meet public health standards and treatment for process use. Treatment to meet public health standards is normally done by a municipal treatment facility and often consists only of chlorination. In some areas, simple sand bed filtration or settling is also done to clarify the water. If done, softening is usually a convenience for the community rather than a health requirement.

To produce water of controlled and repeatable quality according to fixed standards, some combination of filtration, softening, deionization, or distillation is necessary. The capabilities of each process vary according to the input water quality and equipment design. Design of an efficient treatment process requires the experience and knowledge of a water treatment specialist. Some of the techniques used in water treatment are:

Filtration. Filtration removes suspended solids. Filtration efficiency can be improved by addition of chemicals such as alum or ferrous sulfate to produce coagulation. Removal of particles is accomplished by filtration through screens, fabric, or sand beds.

Softening. Hardness is defined as the presence of scale-forming impurities such as calcium, magnesium, or silica. The compounds formed have decreasing solubility with increasing temperatures, and thus tend to deposit in piping and equipment where the water temperature increases. Water can be softened chemically by adding lime (calcium hydroxide) to react with the soluble calcium and magnesium bicarbonates to form insoluble carbonates, which precipitate. Scale-forming calcium sulfate can be removed by use of sodium carbonate, which reacts to form insoluble calcium carbonate and sodium sulfate, which is soluble and non-scale forming.

Hardness may also be removed by cation exchange using a zeolite process. Zeolite materials have the property of exchanging sodium ions for calcium and magnesium ions. Before the zeolite bed is exhausted of sodium ions, it must be regenerated by a strong sodium chloride brine. Before returning the softener to use, the spent brine is flushed with filtered water.

Softening by lime treatment is a time-dependent function and affected by the degree of mixing and separation efficiency. Neither lime treatment nor zeolite softening effectively remove silica, although the lime process, if done as a hot process (95 to 120°C), will remove some silica.

Deionization. Demineralization by deionization utilizes synthetic organic resins to remove undesirable cations or anions by replacing them with hydrogen or hydroxyl ions. The treatment may be done by using separate cation and anion beds or by using a mixed bed. The cation bed is regenerated using an acid rinse while the anion bed is regenerated by a caustic soda rinse. Although more effective than separate beds, the mixed bed arrangement is more difficult to regenerate.

2. Distillation

Distillation is the traditional method of producing Water for Injection. In its basic simplicity, distillation involves evaporating the feedwater and subsequent condensation by cooling. Impurities are left behind in the evaporator. Distillation for pharmaceutical purposes requires a high degree of refinement to prevent recontamination by carryover, material degradation, or bacterial growth in isolated areas of the system.

The most common distillation method uses an evaporator pot and condensing heat exchanger and is an energy-intensive process, requiring approximately 2250 Jg^{-1} of water for evaporation and an equal amount of energy for condensation.

Multiple-effect stills use two or more evaporators in series, utilizing the condensing steam to evaporate water in a following stage. Figure 30 illustrates the components of a conventional still in a multiple-effect configuration. The conventional still is easiest to understand and is mechanically simple, thus usually involving the least operator attention and maintenance. If desired, the still can be modified to produce "clean steam" for process use as well as distilled water. Conventional stills are more expensive to operate unless configured as multiple-effect systems, in which case the initial cost is increased. The evaporator still can be powered by steam or electricity, whichever is least expensive. High-capacity units often require high ceiling clearances. Output pressures are limited, so the distillate must usually be pumped to storage. The output rate of a conventional still can be varied simply by varying the input energy.

Vapor compression stills use an evaporator pot only to begin the distillation cycle. Once steam is formed, it is compressed by a centrifugal compressor to a higher temperature and used to evaporate the feedwater. As the feedwater is evaporated, the pressurized steam is condensed. The energy in the distillate is then used to preheat the feedwater. A simple vapor compression cycle is illustrated in Figure 31. Vapor compression systems are, as a rule, more energy efficient and compact, but most of the energy required is electrical. Thus, in areas where electricity costs are high, the energy efficiency may be offset or negated. The complexity of the system requires more operator attention and maintenance and increases the potential for contamination due to mechanical failure.

Either conventional distillation or vapor compression can produce high-quality distilled water. Selection of a distillation system must consider all the advantages of each in a particular application.

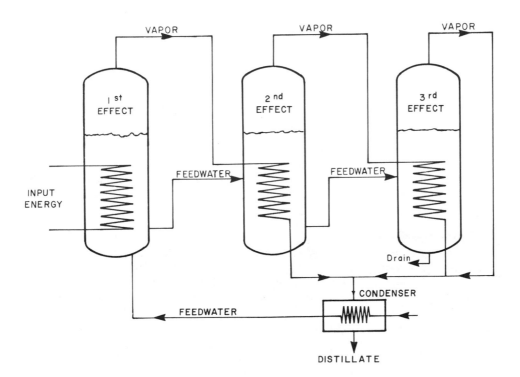

Figure 30 Multiple-effect evaporator.

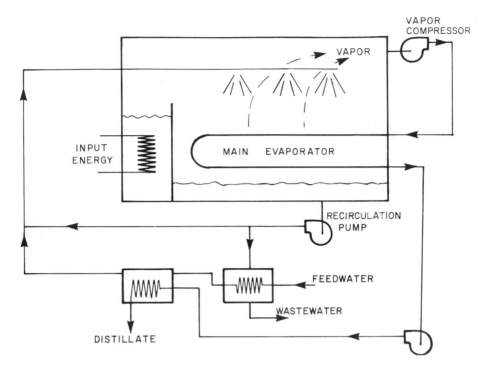

Figure 31 Simple vapor compression cycle.

L. Water for Injection

1. Definition and Requirements

Water for Injection (WFI) is an ingredient common to almost all pharmaceutical plants, certainly to all parenteral plants. The United States Pharmacopeia [12] defines several types of Water for Injection, depending on its use. For purposes here, the general definition is appropriate:

> . . . water purified by distillation or by reverse osmosis, and it meets the purity requirements under Purified Water. It need not be sterile but, in order to meet a test for freedom from pyrogens, it must be produced, stored and distributed in such a way that microorganisms, if present, do not produce pyrogens.

To maintain and assure WFI quality, all elements related to the pretreatment, generation, or distribution of WFI must be evaluated and integrated as a system, from pretreatment to point of use. A key shaping element in the philosophy of WFI systems at this time is the current requirement of the CGMP for large volume parenterals that WFI must be held at a temperature of 80°C or above or be discarded after 24 hr. For small WFI users, it may be practical to generate WFI for each day's needs and discard or recycle any unused portion at the end of the day. Such a system, although relatively inexpensive on a first-cost basis, can create operational scheduling problems, especially if needs cannot be accurately forecast, and requires a large amount of labor for periodic sanitization.

Water for Injection systems include (1) distillation equipment, (2) storage tanks, (3) distribution loop, (4) points of use, and (5) control components. Each element presents unique design problems that must be addressed in concert with particular system specifications.

2. Distillation

Distillation equipment was discussed on pages 414–416. In addition to pure equipment design considerations, system-related requirements must be considered when distillation equipment is selected. These considerations may include the relative positions of the storage tanks (which may affect the means of transfer from still to storage), the intermittent flow rates, and the temperature requirements. Conventional stills characteristically have limited capability for pressuring the distillate. If the storage tanks are located above or remote from the stills, a pump installation must be included in the still arrangement. Vapor compression stills, because of their internal pumps, can usually provide the pressure necessary to transfer the distillate to storage. If water usage rates fluctuate widely or are intermittent, consideration of the startup and operating characteristics of the two basic still types may be necessary. Conventional stills can be started easily and quickly and can be controlled quite simply by throttling the input energy. Vapor compression stills require a more complex startup procedure and operate efficiently only at a specific flow rate. Conventional stills provide distillate at condensing temperature (100°C), while vapor compression stills will normally provide distillate at approximately 10°C above feedwater temperature since the hot distillate is used to preheat the feedwater. Either type of still can be modified to provide distillate at any temperature desired but will require additional initial and operating costs.

3. Storage

WFI is normally stored in stainless steel tanks. Sizing of the storage is a function of daily usage, testing/hold time, makeup (distillation rate), and storage concept. Two concepts are possible: batch storage and dynamic storage. In batch storage a specific quantity of WFI (batch) is generated and stored as a segregated entity while quality assurance testing is performed. Only after all test results are verified as being acceptable is the batch released for use. Batch storage has the obvious advantage of providing maximum product/batch accountability and ensures that all water is tested and released prior to use. In contrast, dynamic storage is a procedure where the storage vessel is primarily a surge tank. As the level of WFI falls, more WFI is produced and filled into storage, mixing with the WFI already there. The dynamic system is less costly, less complex, and easier to operate than a batch system but obviously does not allow batch-wise accountability of the WFI. WFI used for product formulation usually requires batch-wise accountability, but less critical uses such as equipment rinsing may allow use of dynamic systems.

To maintain the required storage temperature, WFI storage tanks are normally provided with steam-heated jackets around the lower portion(s) of the tanks, as in Figure 32. Although total heat loss can be calculated rather accurately to determine the heating requirement, the placement of the heating jacket to prevent temperature stratification is somewhat empirical. Disadvantages of the jacketed tank include the potential for increased corrosion in the area of the heating jacket due to the higher temperatures and higher tank fabrication costs. An alternative externally heated WFI storage tank uses an external heat exchanger and circulating pump (Fig. 33). WFI is constantly circulated through the external heat exchanger and returned to storage. Since a separate heat exchanger, pump, and added piping is needed, total

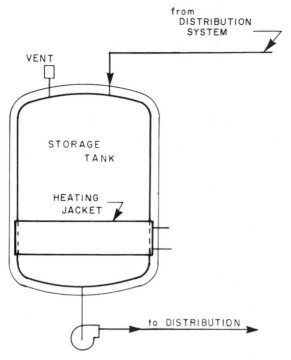

Figure 32 Steam jacketed WFI storage tank.

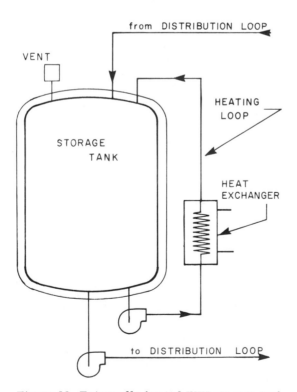

Figure 33 Externally heated WFI storage tank.

initial cost for this heating method is probably higher than for the jacketed tank. Although the circulating pump will minimize temperature stratification, the external pump and heat exchanger introduce additional complexity to the system, thus decreasing reliability and increasing contamination potential. At this time, there are no known data to conclusively compare the expected life of a jacketed tank versus a nonjacketed tank, so life-cycle cost comparisons of the two systems are not possible.

The tank physical construction requires careful attention. The high-temperature distilled water service requires the use of 316 series stainless steel to minimize the potential for pit corrosion, as discussed on pages 381-382. The welding requires the use of a low carbon grade (316L) to prevent carbide precipitation in the weld zones.

Mechanical polishing of the tank interior is necessary to produce a cleanable surface, although the degree of finish is highly debated. The 3-A sanitary standards suggest the use of a No. 4 polish (approximately 150 grit), but others [4] contend that electropolishing produces a more cleanable and inert surface, even compared to a No. 3 (approximately 120 grit) mechanically polished finish. An advantage of electropolishing, apart from the question of surface quality, is the fact that visibility of surface imperfections is magnified by the process so that inspection and repair are easier.

Tanks rated for atmospheric pressure use are suitable for WFI storage, but present several deficiencies. First, the tanks must be sterilized periodically. While sterilization can be accomplished at atmospheric pressures, it is a much longer process than pressure sterilization. To obtain lethality equivalent to a 15 min sterilization at 121°C (approximately 100 kPa) would require 1888 min at atmospheric pressure [13]. Second, a venting arrangement is needed to relieve pressure as a tank fills and empties. A non-pressure-rated tank may rupture if any significant pressure differential is created across the vent during filling. Tremendous vacuum pressures are created when the steam inside a tank is cooled, and if not adequately relieved, may collapse the tank on cooling. A storage tank rated for full vacuum and at least 1 atm pressure (100 kPa) at 121°C greatly facilitates sterilization.

4. Distribution

The state of the art for WFI distribution is the WFI loop distribution system illustrated in Figure 34. The distribution system must provide an adequate supply of WFI to each point of use while preventing stagnation and maintaining WFI temperature. The loop system utilizes a constant circulation of water to satisfy these requirements. Points A to G represent point-of-use control valves, all of which must be located within a distance equal to six times the diameter of the piping (dead legs) to avoid stagnation.

The loop system may be arranged as either a series system, a parallel system, or a hybrid system. Points A, B, E, F, and G represent a series arrangement, where WFI circulates past each point in turn and is returned to the storage tnak. The series arrangement is preferred because it offers positive assurance of flow but may require excessive piping if the points of use are widespread and may be impractical for areas of limited access.

The pairs of points E, F and C, D represent a parallel arrangement where the circulating flow is split into separate streams. The parallel arrangement may be desirable for complex systems and for cooling, as will be explained later. A hybrid system contains elements of both series and parallel arrangements. Both hybrid

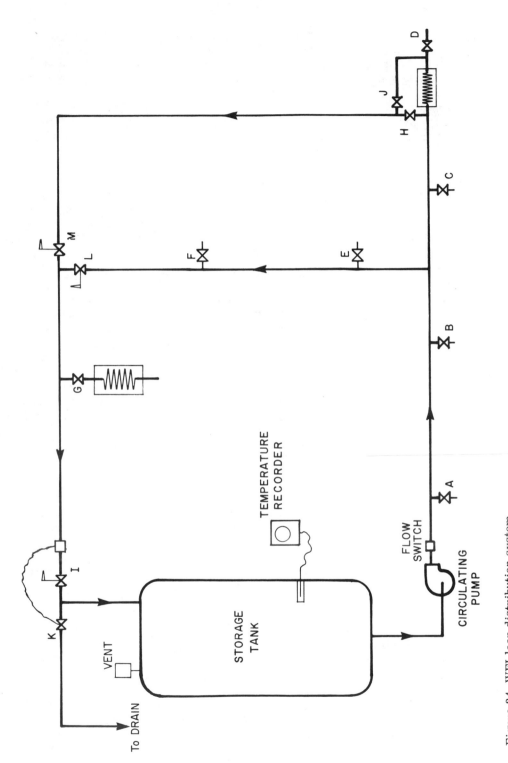

Figure 34 WFI loop distribution system.

and parallel arrangements must have pressure control to assure adequate flow through all branches.

The most significant operating disadvantage of the loop distribution system is that many points of use do not require or cannot use water at a temperature of 80°C or higher. For these uses, a cooling arrangement is necessary. Point G in Figure 34 illustrates a series cooling arrangement which is satisfactory for points of use requiring a constant flow of cooled water. This arrangement is not suitable for intermittent uses because the heat exchanger becomes a stagnant area. For intermittent uses, a cooling arrangement illustrated by point D can be used. In the cooling mode, valve J is closed and valve H is open. The heat exchanger is in use and in series with the use point as at point G. When cooling is not required, valve H closes and valve J opens, putting the heat exchanger flow in series in the circulating system until cooling is again required. As with all WFI piping, the connections for the heat exchanger must be made within six pipe diameters to prevent stagnation.

5. Control Components

Control and monitoring instrumentation must be provided to ensure that temperature is maintained at all points and that flow is continuous. Operationally, the system must maintain minimum pressure at all times and the equipment must be protected. To ensure that temperature requirements have been met, a continuous recorder/controller is needed for each storage tank. Measurement of water temperature just before return to the storage tank may indicate a need to hold the storage tank temperature somewhat above 80°C to compensate for heat loss through the circulating loop. As a further precaution, a temperature sensor may be installed near the point where the return loop enters the tank. In the event that cool water is detected, for example, because of heat exchanger flushing, the sensor will cause valve K to open, diverting the cool water to drain.

System flow must be monitored to ensure constant flow and to detect possible pump failure. Flow detection can be indirect by measuring pressure or temperature or it can be direct, as by a flow switch following the circulating pump, as illustrated in Figure 34.

To maintain system pressure, it is necessary to install pressure control valves at strategic points. For a series system, a pressure control valve located near the end of the loop, as at point I, is adequate. This valve will restrict flow until a preset minimum pressure is reached. Parallel or hybrid systems require a pressure control valve at the end of each branch, as illustrated by points L and M.

Air must be supplied to or vented from the storage tank as the water level fluctuates and during sterilization. This venting must be bidirectional and must prevent airborne bacterial contamination. Figure 35 illustrates two general venting schemes that have been successful. The first scheme uses a bacteria-retentive filter as a vent. The filter housing and piping to and from the filter are constantly heated to prevent condensation, which would wet the filter and increase pressure drop, perhaps causing sufficient pressure to damage the tank. A second scheme involves the use of an overpressure of compressed air or nitrogen supplied through a bacteria-retentive filter. Using the same philosophy as for HEPA-controlled environments, the constant pressure prevents the entry of contamination. To relieve the pressure that would be created during tank filling, a pressure relief valve is needed. The first scheme is easiest, but it is totally dependent on the heating of the vent and there is a possibility that the alternating flow direction will cause premature filter failure. The second scheme avoids the condensation concern but requires additional relief valves, which are difficult to calibrate for low-pressure applications.

To protect the storage tank in the event of control malfunction, rupture disks are commonly used. Rupture disks are thin diaphragms held between two flanges

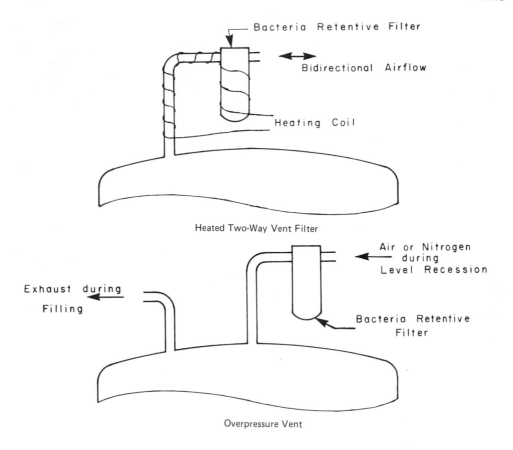

Heated Two-Way Vent Filter

Overpressure Vent

Figure 35 Tank venting arrangements.

and connected directly to the tanks. Any pressure or vacuum outside design limits
will cause the diaphragm to flex against knife edges, causing it to rupture and vent
the excessive pressure or vacuum. Although effective, rupture disks require constant monitoring to detect failure.

M. Waste Disposal, Sanitation, and Equipment Cleaning

1. Waste Disposal

Waste disposal is as important a consideration in the building of a pharmaceutical facility as is the control of raw materials, water, or air. Waste disposal is
not merely the trash left over at the end of a production day, but is the separation of
undesirable contaminants from the production stream. This separation can begin as
early as the receipt of incoming raw materials, with the separation of packaging
from the raw materials, or with the separation of out-of-specification raw materials from acceptable raw materials. The waste may be in the form of liquid,
solid, or airborne. Contamination by waste materials could be direct, via cross-
contamination where the waste becomes mixed with the "good" material or the
waste could be the carrier for another contaminant, such as becteria-laden sewage.

The accumulation and disposal of process wastes is an extension of the manufacturing process. Throughout the manufacturing process wastes are generated:

spillage, packaging materials or containers, defective product, and so on. Estimates should be made of the waste quantities and characteristics at various points in the manufacturing process and means of collection provided. The wastes must be effectively separated from the process stream to provide positive assurance that the product will not be contaminated. Examples of such disposal means are clearly marked and covered waste containers, dust collection equipment, vacuum collectors, or even separate sewage systems. Wastes, like product, must be controlled throughout the process. To illustrate the need to identify and separate waste streams, consider the liquid waste discharge from a pharmaceutical facility. This waste may include waste from rest rooms, lavatories, kitchens, rinse water from process areas, tank drainage from compounding areas, or laboratory wastes. The rest room, lavatory, and kitchen waste, known as domestic sanitary sewage, is compatible with and usually can be discharged directly to a sanitary sewage system. All other wastes are generally classified as industrial wastes or process wastes and may require, individually or as a group, some pretreatment prior to discharge. The subject of pretreatment is beyond the scope of this discussion because the reasons for and methods of pretreatment are usually very specific to the particular waste.

To facilitate the separation and possible pretreatment of toxic, noxious, or hazardous liquid waste streams, most production facilities have multiple sewage systems. Domestic wastes are collected and discharged directly. Process wastes are evaluated as to possible pretreatment or special handling needs and sewage collection systems are designed accordingly. If all process wastes are similar in nature, a single process sewage system may be adequate. If, however, several unique types of process waste are identified, it may be necessary to have multiple process sewage systems. Each of the process systems that requires pretreatment must carry the waste directly to a pretreatment basin or holding tank prior to discharge to the sanitary sewage system with the domestic waste.

The previous paragraphs deal with the need to separate liquid waste streams for the protection of the municipal sewage treatment system and facility. Internally, the separation of process waste from domestic waste is necessary to help maintain the necessary controlled environment conditions. If all liquid wastes were discharged via a single system, any blockage or overflow condition in that system could cause a backflow of domestic waste into a production area, introducing an unacceptable and indeterminate bacterial contamination. To preclude the possibility of this condition, pharmaceutical facilities must have separate domestic and process waste systems which do not connect within the plant. These systems must also be equipped to prevent backflow of waste into the facility. Backflow may be prevented by check valves placed outside the facility, or the sewage systems may be designed to discharge into a manhole or collection basin which is outside and below the level of the facility floor. Any excess flow or backflow would then occur outside the facility.

Control of the waste disposal problem then involves a three-element system: solid waste disposal, liquid waste disposal, and airborne waste (dust) collection. For each ingredient or item of waste, thought must be given to: what is to be collected, what quantities are expected, and how the waste must be moved through and out of the area to prevent accumulation and possible contamination. Finally, how must the material be disposed of? Wastes that are common and nonhazardous can usually be disposed of through such means as depositing in landfills, municipal sewage systems, or incineration.

2. Sanitation

Effective sanitation of both physical facility and equipment is essential to the maintenance of a clean production environment. Sanitation includes the accumulation and disposal of process wastes, facility cleaning, and equipment cleaning. Well-defined procedures are necessary, but effective sanitation is enhanced by facility design details, such as those discussed on pages 372–376, which reduce bacterial growth areas and improve surface cleanability. Beyond design details, broader consideration must be given for the space and utility needs of sanitation.

Sanitation equipment must be controlled like all other equipment entering controlled environments. It must be cleaned, sanitized, and sterilized if for aseptic use. After use, the equipment must be removed from the controlled area for storage and cleaning prior to reuse. The equipment required will depend on individual needs but may include buckets, mops, sponges, sprayguns, brushes, and vacuum hoses. Areas must be provided adjacent to the controlled-environment areas where sanitation equipment can be cleaned and stored without subjecting it to potential contamination.

Utility needs for controlled-area sanitation are unique. Both sewage drains and nonaseptic water supplies are contamination potentials to be avoided. Use of Water for Injection eliminates the potential water contamination. After cleaning, the wastewater may be picked up by mops, which may redistribute contamination rather than remove it. One alternative approach is to spray the cleaning solution onto the surfaces and remove it by a central vacuum collection system. The vacuum connections are sanitized as part of the area sanitation activity to prevent contamination of the controlled environment. Although this method is effective, the vacuum piping must be planned and installed in the walls of the facility during construction.

Equipment cleaning, like facility cleaning, requires consideration during planning stages. It lends itself to a central operation, at least for closely allied production areas, but cannot be located so that travel through noncontrolled areas is required. Equipment cleaning involves cleaning of compounding equipment: tanks, mixers, pumps, filling equipment and all associated hoses, pipes, transfer vessels, filters, etc. The cleaning may involve disassembly, removal of product residue, reassembly, integrity testing, sterilization, and storage. The area should be separate from but adjacent to the controlled production area and will probably function at irregular hours. An adequate supply of water, including WFI, steam, compressed air, and nitrogen, is typically required. If equipment is to be used aseptically, provision must be made for sterilization prior to use.

REFERENCES

1. Current Good Manufacturing Practices in Manufacture, Processing, Packing or Holding of Large Volume Parenterals, Fed. Regist., 41(106) (Tuesday, June 1, 1976).
2. Nissen, R. L., Bull. Parenter. Drug Assoc., 32:44–49 (1978).
3. Grimes, T. L., Griffin, J. C., Fonner, D. E., and Rathbun, L. R., Bull. Parenter. Drug Assoc., 29:64–73 (1975).
4. Valley, J. A., and Rathbun, L. R., Bull. Parenter. Drug Assoc., 31(2):94–102 (1977).
5. ASHRAE Handbook, 1981 Fundamentals, American Society of Heating, Refrigeration and Air-Conditioning Engineers, New York, 1981.
6. Federal Standard Number 209 B: Federal Standard Clean Room and Work Station Requirements, Controlled Environment, Apr. 24, 1973.
7. An Evaluation of Atmospheric Dust, American Air Filter Company, Inc., 1958.
8. Austin, P., Design and Operation of Clean Rooms, Business News Publishing Company, Detroit, 1970, pp. 82–103.

9. Brochure AF-1-1956, American Air Filter Company, Inc.
10. Standard 52-76: Method of Testing Air Cleaning Devices Used in General Ventilation for Removing Particulate Matter, American Society of Heating, Refrigeration and Air-Conditioning Engineers, Inc., New York, 1976.
11. Keenan, J. H., Keyes, F. G., Hill, P. G., and Moore, J. G., eds., Steam Tables, Thermodynamic Properties of Water Including Vapor, Liquid and Solid Phases, International Edition, Wiley, New York, 1969.
12. The United States Pharmacopeia XX, The United States Pharmacopeial Convention, Inc., Rockville, Md., 1980, p. 1040.
13. Pflug, I. J., in Industrial Sterilization (G. B. Phillips and W. S. Miller, eds.), Duke University Press, Durham, N.C., 1972, pp. 239-282.

10

Personnel: The Key Factor in Clean Room Operations

CECELIA J. LUNA

E. R. Squibb & Sons, Inc.
New Brunswick, New Jersey

The problem of contamination dates as far back in time as man's presence on earth. However, it has been only recently that the problem has taken on significance to a wide variety of industries, including the pharmaceutical industry. More specifically, the parenteral products operation is affected by contaminants from a variety of sources, the most important of which is personnel. Contamination control principles apply particularly to that area in a pharmaceutical company where the manufacture of sterile injectable drug products is performed, since these products require a special environment, special equipment, and most of all, special people. The importance of the role that personnel play in the production of a high quality drug product is illustrated by the following comments.

> . . . people are the largest single source of contamination. [1]

> Personnel contribute markedly to product contamination by releasing inert and viable material in a continuous shower of material. Personnel are disintegrating. [2]

This chapter discusses personnel-related sources of contamination in the clean room and the measures taken to overcome this problem. Other sources of contamination are discussed only briefly since they are covered elsewhere in this book.

I. CONTAMINATION

Personnel working in a clean room contribute both viable (microbial) and nonviable (particulate) contaminants to the surrounding environment. The following lists a few of the categories into which these contaminants may be classified:

1. Skin flakes and scales
2. Fragments of human hair
3. Droplets of moisture from breathing and coughing
4. Cosmetics, including hair spray and heavy use of aerosol deodorants

5. Lint and starch particles from washable fabrics
6. Fibers and frayed particles of wool, cashmere, or similar loose-weave fabrics

A. Microbial Contamination

The surface of the skin releases squamous cells which serve as a source of both microbial and particulate contamination to the clean room environment. The microbial contaminants that are shed are associated with the skin scales and are indigenous to the particular person. These organisms are referred to as <u>resident organisms</u>. However, not all skin scales or particles carry microorganisms. For those particles bearing bacterial contaminants, a mean of four viable organisms per particle has been determined, with large particles carrying more organisms than smaller ones.

Microorganisms can also be transferred to and from objects which the operator has touched or handled. These are called <u>transient organisms</u> since they are carried from one location to another by all personnel touching these surfaces. These organisms may come into direct contact with equipment and/or components utilized in the operation. They must be eliminated or destroyed if product integrity is to be maintained.

B. Particulate Contamination

People are continuously shedding skin cells. Each adult loses approximately 6 to 14g of dead skin material each day. Each person loses a complete layer of skin

Table 1 Personnel as Sources of Bacterial Aerosols

Conditions	Number of particles generated per minute	Mean settling rate of particles
Surgical Teams:		
Good practices	5,000	0.6 fpm
Average practices	10,000	1.0 fpm
Poor practices	50,000	2.4 fpm
Average per person laboratory personnel:		
Great activity	15,000	>2.4 fpm
Moderate activity	8,000	2.4 fpm
Slight activity	4,000	1.4 fpm
Simulated sneezes:		
12 HAT-CHOO per minute	84	0.2*fpm
*Excluding drops too large to be airborne		

Source: Ref. 4. Reprinted with permission, Institute of Environmental Sciences, Mount Prospect, Illinois; originally published by the American Association for Contamination Control.

about every 4 days, which is equivalent to a minimum shed rate of 10^7 particles per day [3]. Ordinary walking movements emit approximately 10^4 particles per minute. Even while standing perfectly still a person releases particles from the surface of the skin. The average adult has approximately 40 ft^2 of body surface area; however, it cannot be assumed that everyone will shed the same number of particles under the same conditions. Table 1 illustrates that personnel exhibiting good aseptic technique emit a significantly fewer number of particles than those demonstrating poor technique. The rate of dispersion is expressed as the number of particles shed per minute. Following this train of thought, it would seem that bacteria are being shed as a steady, continuous stream of particles; however, this is not true. Instead, "bursts" of particles are generated from the body in relation to the person's movement. Thus it is the average of all the individual dispersion rates which gives the appearance of particles being shed at a constant, steady rate.

Airborne particles released from the skin surface are assumed to be spherical in shape in order to calculate their settling rates in the clean room. The behavior of naked particles is similar to that of spheres 8 μm in diameter, but particles carrying bacterial cells react as if they were spheres about 14 μm in size. The settling velocity of the latter size particles has been calculated to be 30 centimeters per minute. In a conventional clean room, these particles remain suspended in air for long periods of time and can cause serious problems for the operation.

II. PERSONNEL CHARACTERISTICS

The level of contamination in a clean room is influenced by the characteristics of the people working in the area. Such factors as number of bacteria present on the skin and within the body, types of bacteria and their location on specific areas of the body, and the rate of dispersion affect the overall bacterial and particulate counts.

A. Bacterial Load

Studies have shown that many factors influence the total bacterial count on the skin surface at any given time. The bacterial load supported by each individual is directly related to personal hygiene habits. Furthermore, the amount of microbial contamination increases as the number of people increases within a confined area, being concurrent with the period during which the individuals are unable to practice their normal hygiene habits. One study demonstrated that bacteria are not evenly distributed over the surface of the body. This is due, in part, to the formation of microcolonies of bacteria on the surface of the skin. Bacterial cells normally do not exist as single units on the skin surface, but rather exist as clumps of cells which vary in size from as few as 10^2 to as many as 10^5 cells.

B. Types of Microorganisms

Microorganisms causing contamination of a drug product can be divided into two major groups according to their structure: bacteria and fungi. Viruses are sometimes added to this classification; however, they are not capable of proliferating outside a living cell. Bacteria are further subdivided into two classes: gram-negative organisms and gram-positive organisms. The former are usually bacilli and are rarely derived from human sources; the latter are usually cocci, are frequently found in the air, and are usually derived from a human source.

Many studies have been done to determine more specifically the types of bacteria emitted by personnel working in the clean room. The most common inhabitants of the skin were found to be micrococcaceae, corynebacteria, streptococci, spore-forming bacilli, yeasts, and organisms from the Propionibacterium acnes group. Staphylococci, streptococci, tubercle bacilli, and viruses such as influenza were emitted from the respiratory tract. From the gastrointestinal tract, such organisms as gram-negative bacilli, spore-forming Clostridia, viruses, and yeasts were isolated.

One of the studies performed attempted to determine quantitatively and qualitatively the predominant types of microbial contaminants in both conventional and laminar flow clean rooms. As would be expected, the data showed that reducing the level of particulate contamination also reduced the levels of airborne and surface microbial contamination. This was especially evident in the horizontal laminar flow clean room. The types of organisms isolated from the air and surfaces included Staphylococcus spp., Micrococcus spp., and the Corynebacterium-Brevibacterium group, the types normally found on human skin, hair, and in the respiratory tract.

C. Body Areas Shedding Organisms

The surface area of the body is divided as follows: legs, 18% each; trunk, 37%; arms, 9% each; head, 9%; axilla and perineum, less than 2% of the total area. Body flora may vary from person to person, but specific organisms tend to be found in specific areas of the human body. The kinds of organisms dispersed into the environment depends to a large extent upon two factors: (1) the types of organisms present on the individual and (2) the activity of the individual—not only the degree of activity, but also that part of the body which is engaged in the particular activity. Table 2 indicates the numbers of aerobic and anaerobic bacteria isolated from different regions of the body as reported in one study.

Viable contaminants are emitted from the skin, nose and ear, mouth, respiratory tract, and intestinal tract. In diseases of the skin, such as eczema and psoriasis, investigators isolated increased levels of Staphylococcus aureus and Streptococcus pyogenes from the skin of the test subjects. Shedding the aforementioned organisms is especially critical if the person carrying these pathogens is part of the clean room staff.

In the nose and ear, pathogenic cocci have been found in 75% of the subjects examined, as well as diplococci and hemophilus. Microorganisms indigenous to the oral cavity included Streptococcus salivarius, lactobacilli, and Candida albicans, a pathogenic organism. Saliva contains approximately 100 million organisms per milliliter. Generally, the intestinal tract contains anaerobic, nonsporulating rods (putrefactive bacteria) and gram-positive lactobacilli. Some aerobic organisms are present, but in smaller numbers. They include coliforms, Proteus, enterococci, and staphylococci.

Large numbers of microorganisms are also emitted by a person exhibiting heavy oral and nasal discharge due to bacterial infection. In this instance, coughing, sneezing, and nose blowing dramatically increase the number of organisms emitted from the nasopharynx and respiratory tract. Placing this infected, sneezing person in a clean room can greatly increase the level of contamination, thereby increasing the possibility of product contamination. The horizontal laminar flow clean room poses more of a threat in this situation than does the vertical laminar flow room. A sneeze is emitted at a velocity greater than the room air velocity of 100 ft min^{-1} and particles are carried downstream. The organisms are disseminated a specific distance from the source, depending upon the initial velocity with which

Table 2 Geometric Mean Count per Square Centimeter of Skin Surface in
Eleven Normal Healthy Males and Eleven Normal Healthy Females

	Aerobic flora		Anaerobic flora	
Site	Males	Females	Males	Females
Forehead	2075	1225	8000	13500
Sternum	2125	165	50000	3500
Subclavicular area	350	130	18500	2275
Center back	450	155	67500	7500
Shoulder	128	48	1025	1075
Deltoid area	118	65	57	127
Forearm	250	35	9	13
Palm	98	155	33	85
Lower axilla	500	92	14	12
Lumbar area	300	33	178	142
Periumbilical area	850	175	55	80
Thigh upper front	325	140	9	35
Thigh lower front	350	67	14	16
Thigh back	325	82	4	5
Shin	190	77	7	8
Calf	173	20	2	5
Dorsum of foot	80	122	3	10
Sole	22750	675	10	4

Source: Ref. 5. Based on data summarized in D. A. Somerville and C. T.
Murphy, J. Invest. Dermatol., 60:232 (1973); 1973 The Williams & Wilkins Co.,
Baltimore, Maryland.

they were discharged and the size of the droplets. Thus these particles may affect
both the contamination level and the operation in another part of the room. However, in a vertical laminar flow room, only the area directly in front of the person
will be affected by the sneeze. Placing a barrier between the person and the work
area will eliminate this problem.

D. Male Versus Female Shed Rates

Upon further examination of the characteristics of people working in the clean room,
another variable becomes apparent: the difference in the bacterial dispersion rate
between males and females. The mean dispersion for males was determined to be
2506 organisms per contact plate, while that for females was 692. These results
indicated that males dispersed, on the average, between 2.5 and 5 times as many
bacterially contaminated particles as did females. Table 3 represents the differences in dispersion for various locations on the body surface. Generally speaking,
movement of both male and female subjects increased the number of bacteria shed
from the skin surface.

Because of the presence of S. aureus on the skin and the problems that can
result from its dissemination in the clean environment, studies have been done to
determine the dispersion rate of this organism. In one study, 13% of the men tested
shed S. aureus, while only 1% of the women shed the organism. Further studies

Table 3 Total Counts of Organisms at Various Sites on the Body Surface of Males and Females

Method of sampling (area sampled)	Site	Mean count* for		Statistical significance (t test)
		Males (n = 38)	Females (n = 34)	
Scrub count (4 cm^2)	Thigh	10,470	1,230	P < 0.1%
	Abdomen	2,344	646	P < 1%
	Shin	2,455	692	P < 1%
	Arm	549	389	NS
	Chest	3,890	741	P < 1%
	Back	468	309	NS
Contact plate (25 cm^2)	Hair	324	81	P < 0.1%
	Thigh	873	220	P < 0.1%
	Shin	549	234	P < 5%
	Arm	178	109	NS
	Chest	263	126	P < 5%
	Abdomen	162	107	NS
	Back	55	48	NS
Alginate swab (not defined)	Axilla	147,900	53,700	NS
	Nose	19,500	30,200	NS
	Perineum	275,400	186,200	NS

NS = not significant (P > 5%).
*Arithmetic values given. Analysis performed on log values.
Source: Ref. 6.

with the male subject showed that the number of this organism dispersed increased by a factor of 3 above the waist and 6 below the waist as the subjects began to move. However, some studies have been performed which indicate no significant difference between the dispersion rate of S. aureus from male and female subjects.

E. The Carrier Concept

Each person carries specific types of organisms on the surface of the skin. However, changes may occur which support the growth and colonization of organisms other than the person's normal body flora. Such a person is referred to as a carrier. McDade defined the term carrier as "an individual in or on whom pathogens reside and multiply, without producing demonstrable disease or ill effect on him" [7]. Two types of carriers exist: (1) temporary carrier, on which the pathogenic organism is carried by the person for a relatively short period of time; and (2) permanent carrier, on which the pathogen is conveyed on the person for a very long period of time. Studies have shown that carriage of a particular pathogen does not always result in dispersal of the organism; some people have more of a tendency to shed pathogenic organisms than do others. These individuals are referred to as shedders or disseminators and can contribute significantly to the microbiological contamination within the clean room.

The pathogen of most concern to hospitals and industrial clean rooms alike is S. aureus. This organism may be carried in the nose or throat, on the skin, or in the hair. Even though people may be identified as carriers of this organism, relatively few have been found to be disseminators. Studies have shown that the ability to disperse S. aureus is a property of the patient rather than the organism. Usually, the organism is dispersed into the air attached to skin scales from the body surface.

III. SELECTION OF CLEAN ROOM PERSONNEL

Selection of clean room personnel may be the most important step in the contamination control program. Because the clean room operation is so critical, only those individuals who meet special requirements should be permitted to work in this environment. The choice is based upon four factors: (1) physical requirements, (2) skill trait, (3) job performance, and (4) psychological characteristics. The following discussion describes the characteristics that clean room personnel should possess, as well as the procedures and regulations to which the employees must adhere while working in the area.

A. Characteristics of Clean Room Employees

All clean room employees should be neat and clean. Their personal hygiene habits must ensure an acceptable level of cleanliness for clean room operations. Since hair is a source of contamination, it should be kept clean and remain covered while working in the area. Personnel who have dandruff or any other condition causing flaking of the scalp should be precluded from working in the clean environment. Male employees with beards or mustaches must cover facial as well as head hair.

The general condition of health for clean room personnel must be satisfactory. Each potential clean room employee should be given a physical examination to determine factors such as the degree of dryness and particle shedding rate of the skin, the presence of asthma, emphysema, or other allergies causing mouth breathing, coughing or sneezing, and the existence of eczema or similar conditions. The medical examination may also include a microbiological examination—throat swabs and stool specimens. A coughing/sneezing test, using an agar plate, can be used to determine the types of oral flora which the employee disseminates. A contact plate test identifies the various kinds of skin flora which are present. Employees should also be given an eye examination to determine whether their level of visual acuity is acceptable for the job requirements.

Personnel with skin and/or upper respiratory diseases should be excluded from the clean room operations. Persons with allergies to synthetic fabrics or solvents used in the operation should also be eliminated from this critical area. Persons suffering from eczema or other scaly conditions, hives, or similar problems should not be permitted to work in the clean room because of the excessive skin shedding caused by these conditions. If personnel are sick or have a cold, they should report to their supervisor immediately, and be assigned to another work location or sent home until completely recovered from the illness. People considered heavy smokers are likely to demonstrate periods of excessive coughing, which emits large numbers of bacteria from the oral cavity, and they may wish to enter and exit the clean room more frequently than a nonsmoker.

Personnel hygiene control and discipline are extremely important for the successful operation of any clean room. Persons assigned to this area must receive periodic reinstruction on good personal hygiene habits and the effect of these habits on the work performed in this special environment.

The skills and aptitudes that a clean room employee should possess include the following: (1) a minimum of two years of high school education, (2) above-average intelligence, (3) good manual dexterity, (4) good work habits, and (5) an understanding of the operation being performed. Management must be certain that employees have the ability required to perform the job and that their work habits are acceptable for clean room operations. If not, those habits must be changed to comply with the practices required for the area. An understanding of the overall clean room operation provides employees with a better perspective of their own jobs and the importance of their roles in the operation being performed.

To determine the success with which a person can be expected to perform a specified task, an aptitude test may be given to determine the employee's ability. Also, the employee's past work performance record should be considered. Employees must be thoroughly instructed in all aspects of the job required. As they assume their newly assigned responsibilities, employees should be closely observed to be certain that they are performing the job in the proper manner. Studies have shown that aptitudes and skills actually <u>do</u> change when the work is performed within a clean environment. The same job <u>inside</u> the clean room is more difficult to accomplish because of the many restrictions placed on each person. An employee's manual dexterity often improves as the shift progresses. However, at the same time this person's mental alertness may decline and he may become less attentive to the performance of the job, thereby enhancing the possibility for error. As the end of the shift approaches, the operator may begin to slacken the pace, and again the chance for error increases. Management must be aware of this situation and plan ways to minimize its occurrence.

Employees should not be selected for clean room operations on the basis of seniority alone. Sometimes senior employees find it difficult to adjust to a new area and the restrictions placed on them working in that area. Also, they may have difficulty in changing their work habits to comply with required procedures.

Satisfactory physical job performance is essential, but it is not enough. Employees must also be concerned about the cleanliness with which they are performing the assigned tasks. They must be aware of contamination control principles and the consequences that may befall the operation by violation of these procedures.

Not every employee is suited to working in the clean room. Everyone does not have the mental makeup required to adjust to the stringent regulations governing an operation in an area that is enclosed and restrictive. Others cannot adjust to wearing a uniform, hood, mask, booties, and gloves. Sometimes showing an employee the new work area and the uniform that will be required can be helpful in selecting the appropriate type of person. The maintenance of proper personnel behavior is absolutely essential to ensure maximum efficiency. Violations of procedure by personnel can increase the contamination load in the area, thereby decreasing the overall effectiveness of the facility.

Psychologists have tested qualified clean room operators and have found that they score high in emotionally stable characteristics, average in active and sociable characteristics, and low in impulsive, dominant, and reflective characteristics [8]. Clean room personnel should have an even disposition. Persons who are nervous or highly emotional should not be placed in the clean area. Nervousness produces excess movement, which in turn disseminates more particles from the body. Emotional individuals also have a tendency to perspire more easily. Persons who suffer from claustrophobia should not be assigned to clean room operations. Also, employees who are unable to follow clean room rules and regulations should be excluded from working there. This area more than any other in a pharmaceutical company requires the enforcement of and strict adherence to regulations.

Since personnel problems in adapting to a clean room are sometimes psychological in origin, there must be some "reward" for those employees who are selected for the operation. Management can provide monetary compensation, longer break periods, or other incentives. These individuals are special and therefore must be treated in a special way.

Additional traits that clean room employees should possess include: (1) a high level of motivation, (2) pride in a job well done, (3) a better than average attitude about the job, (4) a willingness to assume personal inconveniences, (5) an interest in maintaining cleanliness, (6) conscientiousness, (7) dedication to quality, (8) orderliness, (9) reliability, (10) mental alertness, (11) a sense of responsibility, (12) carefulness, (13) a positive attitude toward repetitive operations, (14) attentiveness to details, (15) punctuality, (16) good listening ability, (17) truthfulness, and (18) a sense of duty. Pride is a key word for working in a clean room. This concept, together with a sense of togetherness, must be instilled in all clean room employees to ensure an effective operation.

IV. PERSONNEL FACTORS REQUIRED TO CONTROL CONTAMINATION

Parenteral products require manufacture in a clean room for the following reasons [9]:

1. To maintain sterility for the aseptic manufacturing and filling processes
2. To prevent pyrogenicity of terminally sterilized products
3. To prevent particulate contamination of the product

To fulfill these requirements, several elements must be controlled.

Factors such as bacterial and particulate shedding, personal hygiene, personnel activity, traffic flow, and clean room garments play a significant role in the level of contamination, and therefore must be controlled to protect the integrity and purity of the finished drug product. To a lesser degree, facility design, the air handling system, and maintenance and cleaning procedures also affect clean room operations. The latter factors will be discussed only as they relate to the problem of personnel contamination.

Many studies have been done to determine the effect of bathing on the mechanism of bacterial dispersion. From the data, investigators concluded that showering or washing increases the number of particles dispersed from the body, even though many thousands of organisms are removed in the process, and reaches its peak between 30 and 45 min after showering. The presence of bacterial microcolonies on the skin surface explains this observation. The mechanical process of washing removed many of the bacterial cells in the colonies and at the same time spread the remainder over the surface of the body. Thus more skin scales become contaminated by bacterial cells after bathing. Also, during the washing process sebum is removed from the skin surface. This temporarily causes the skin scales to become dry, curl up, and peel off the body surface. Therefore, initial dispersion rates after showering show a marked increase, despite the reduction in the total bacterial count on the skin surface. Within 2 hr after bathing, the surface of the skin resumes its original pattern of microcolonies. In general, the data indicate that the largest concentration of bacteria was found near the perineum and on the face. Investigators speculated that bacterial dispersion from the perineum occurred as a result of friction between areas of the body carrying large numbers of organisms. Applying 70% ethyl alcohol or lanolin to the medial thigh and perineum of the naked subject greatly reduced the number of bacteria shed.

During the summer months, contamination in the clean room increases. Part of this increase is caused by personnel becoming suntanned. Suntanning dries out the skin and causes it to flake and peel more easily. Although the use of creams that are absorbed into the skin can help to control the degree of shedding, in cases where an employee exhibits an excessive amount of peeling, the person should be placed in another work location outside the clean room for as long as the condition persists.

Employees assigned to a clean room operation must practice good personal hygiene at all times. All personnel must bathe or shower routinely and wash their hair. Using antibacterial soaps can reduce the number of microorganisms present on the skin; however, studies have shown that these agents can cause tissue damage and/or photosensitization to the user. Soaps containing hexachlorophene are especially effective in reducing bacterial counts on the body surface, but have been found to cause brain damage in newborn babies in the hospital. Because of this recent finding, governmental control over the dispensing of material containing hexachlorophene has been instituted. Preferably, the employee should not bathe immediately before beginning work since this will temporarily increase the number of particles and skin scales shed from the body. Fingernails should be given special attention since they harbor a variety of microorganisms underneath them. Clean clothing must be worn each day upon entrance into the clean area. Shoes should also be kept as clean as possible.

Additional studies have been done to determine the effect of clothing on the dissemination of bacteria from the skin surface. The data confirmed the assumption that friction between the clothing and skin increased the rate of bacterial dissemination. Up to 10 mg of skin particles may be deposited in a person's clothing during a 2 hr period. Furthermore, the dispersion of certain organisms increased as the test subjects wore the clothing for longer periods of time. A study performed by the Illinois Institute of Technology showed that the level of particulate contamination increased by a factor of 1.5 when personnel wearing dust-preventive clothing, booties, caps, and gloves entered the clean room [10]. As they began utilizing the equipment in the area and moving around the room, the level increased to six times that of the baseline value obtained during static conditions. Thus investigators concluded that personnel movement increased the degree of friction between the clothing and skin, thereby increasing the number of particles emitted from the skin surface. The studies also showed that certain materials effected an 80% reduction in the bacterial dissemination rate, while others completely eliminated the dispersion of microorganisms into the environment [11]. However, with the latter there was too much discomfort to the subject when this type of impermeable material was worn for long periods of time.

Investigators also discovered that wearing stockings increased dissemination from a woman's legs. The friction created between the stockings and legs released bacterial particles and skin scales. An average skin scale measures 20 to 30 μm in diameter, but the pore diameter of a nylon stocking measures several hundred micrometers. Thus the particles shed from the legs pass through the pores of the stocking. This phenomenon has been referred to as the "cheese-grater" effect.

The clean room garment is sometimes considered the first line of defense in controlling the problems caused by human contamination. The type of uniform selected for use is dependent upon the type of contamination to be controlled. Currently in the pharmaceutical industry, two types of material are being used for clean room garments: continuous synthetic filament Dacron and Tyvek. Dacron is the trade name for a polyester textile fiber and Tyvek for 100% high density polyethylene fibers. The latter is marketed in several different grades. Tyvek is considered to be more effective than woven uniforms in preventing contamination of the clean room with particles shed from the skin surface and in reducing airborne contamination levels associated with personnel movement. However, users must select the appropriate garment based upon the requirements of the operation. When barrier effects from both airborne and human particulates is a major concern, Tyvek appears to be the garment of choice. If particulates generated from the garment itself are a greater concern, the uniform made of Dacron polyester may be more suitable.

Regardless of the type of garment selected, the clean room uniform must meet two criteria: (1) it must be comfortable to the wearer, and (2) it must be functionally designed to contain contaminating particles and bacteria shed from the skin and clothing of personnel, thereby preventing contact with the drug product and/or its components. The uniform must fit snugly at the neck, wrists, and ankles to enhance its efficiency in containing particulates. It should also release as few fibers as possible from its external surface. Clean room garments must be properly laundered and, if appropriate, sterilized prior to use. To maintain their effectiveness, they should be worn only one time prior to relaundry. By wearing a special type of uniform, employees are constantly made aware of the environment in which they are working, and the importance of cleanliness in the performance of their jobs.

The level of airborne contamination in a clean room is also related to the number of personnel present, their activity, and the traffic flow within the area. Figure 1 demonstrates the direct relationship between the airborne contamination level and clean room population [12]. As the graph indicates, increasing the number of

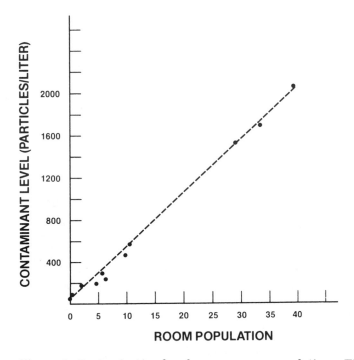

Figure 1 Contamination level versus room population. This plot shows increased contamination with an increase in personnel. (From Ref. 12.)

people in the clean room causes an increase in the level of contamination in the area.
Table 4 presents Austin's Contamination Control Index, an average of particle emission rates based upon the activity of personnel in the clean room [13]. As employees begin working and moving about the area, the number of particles emitted increases, due partially to friction between the clean room garment and the operator's skin. The more rapid the movement, the greater the number of organisms shed. By relating personnel activity to particle emission patterns, the contamination level in a clean room can be predicted [14]. Thus the contamination load for any clean room can be projected prior to its construction. This can be a valuable tool in the design and work layout of the area and in the selection of the appropriate air handling system. Moreover, the Contamination Control Index can be used to facilitate the operation of an existing clean room.

Figure 2 shows the contamination levels that occur during the course of the day's activity in the clean room. On the graph, the value of 10 represents the maximum contamination level at which the room should operate. This number varies, depending upon the class of clean room. For a Class 10,000 clean room, the value of 10 represents 10,000 particles 0.5 μm and larger; for a Class 100, the value of 10 represents 100 particles 0.5 μm and larger. The graph shows that the greater the activity of the people working in the area, the larger the number of particles emitted, and therefore the higher the contamination level in the room. Thus the purity and integrity of the injectable product may be jeopardized by the interrelationship of these factors.

The following will be helpful in minimizing the aforementioned problems caused by personnel:

Table 4 Contamination Indices

Position	Activity	Particles emitted per minute 0.3 micron
1	Standing or sitting—no movement	100,000
2	Sitting—light head, hand and forearm movement	500,000
3	Sitting—average body and arm movement, toe tapping	1,000,000
4	Changing position—sitting to standing	2,500,000
5	Slow walking—2.0 mph	5,000,000
	Average walking—3.57 mph	7,500,000
	Fast walking—15 mph	10,000,000
6	Climbing stairs—15 tmu	10,000,000
7	Calisthenics	15,000,000 to 30,000,000

Source: Ref. 13. Reprinted with permission, Institute of Environmental Sciences, Mount Prospect, Illinois; originally published by the American Association for Contamination Control.

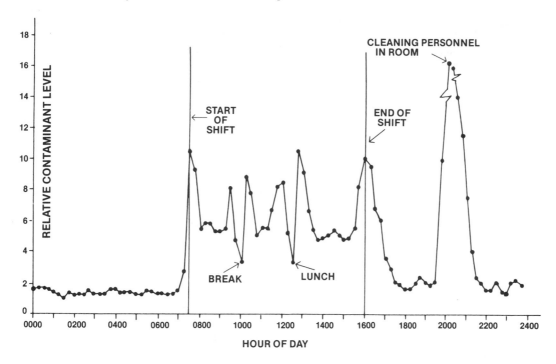

Figure 2 Typical clean room contaminant levels. (From Ref. 15. Reprinted with permission, Institute of Environmental Sciences, Mount Prospect, Illinois; the American Association for Contamination Control.)

1. Limit the number of personnel working in the clean room.
2. Instruct personnel to move slowly and calmly to avoid turbulence.
3. Do not allow personnel to wander from their immediate work area.
4. Do not allow personnel to congregate in the vicinity of the work area.
5. Personnel must be aware of the direction of the airflow, and must not interrupt it by placing any part of their body between the source of the airflow and the work area.

Since airflow patterns affect the dispersion rate of particles, the direction of the clean air can be used to facilitate contamination control procedures. The use of laminar airflow, high efficiency particulate air (HEPA) filters, a specified number of air changes per hour, and thorough cleaning procedures are utilized to achieve the desired class of clean room. To minimize human contamination of the drug product, the work area is placed as close as possible to the source of the clean air. However, a laminar airflow system cannot serve as a substitute for aseptic procedures. The best clean room facility can very easily be negated by personnel performing improper and unacceptable practices.

V. PERSONNEL PRACTICES AND PROCEDURES

The degree of cleanliness required in the clean room dictates the practices and procedures of personnel—their activity as it relates to the job and how much control management must exercise to achieve the level of cleanliness required by the product. All aspects of the clean room operation must be detailed in a written document, but especially those procedures relating to personnel and their activity. A compilation of acceptable clean room practices is presented below [16, 17]. The list is not intended to be all-inclusive since each facility and each operation are different, but rather is designed to indicate those practices which may be applied to any pharmaceutical clean room operation.

A. Practices Related to Gowning

1. All personnel entering the clean room must be familiar with the established gowning procedure. Approved procedures for entering and leaving the clean room must be followed.
2. Hands and fingernails must be scrubbed thoroughly with the disinfectant soap provided before entering the clean room.
3. Hands should be dried with the hot air dryer. The use of paper or fabric towels in the clean area is forbidden.
4. Skin lotions or lanolin base soaps should be provided for employees to tighten the skin and guard against epidermal scale.
5. Eyeglasses must be washed and dried with lint-free tissue prior to entering the clean room.
6. Special procedures must be observed in utilizing air locks and air showers when present.
7. Shoes must be covered with nonshedding booties or changed to approved clean room footwear. If special footwear is provided, it should not be worn outside the clean room.
8. Approved clean room garments must be worn.
9. The hood must be tucked completely inside the uniform, and the uniform zippered securely to the neck.
10. If any part of the clean room uniform becomes damaged, torn, or soiled during routine operations, the employee must return to the gowning area and replace the damaged part.
11. Normally, no clean room garment may be used a second time without being rewashed and resterilized. A clean garment should be used with each entry into the clean room.
12. All hair is to be completely covered at all times.
13. Personnel should avoid reaching under the hood or other parts of the garment with gloved hands.
14. Coveralls are not to be unzipped in the clean room.
15. No skin area is to be exposed between the gloved hand and coveralls.
16. If they become contaminated, gloves must be rinsed in the disinfectant solution provided.
17. Cosmetics are not to be worn or applied in the clean room. This includes: rouge, lipstick, facial powder, eye shadow and eyebrow pencil, mascara, eyeliner, false eyelashes, fingernail polish, hair spray, and the heavy use of an aerosol deodorant.
18. No jewelry (i.e., large rings, necklaces, earrings, lockets, watches, bracelets) is to be worn in the clean room.
19. Valuable items such as wallets may be carried into the clean room in the company-supplied uniform pockets, provided that they are not removed inside the clean room.

20. Personal items such as keys, coins, cigarettes, matches, pencils, handkerchiefs, watches, tissues, and combs should not be carried into the clean room.
21. Used clean room garments are placed in a receptacle outside the clean area.
22. In powder filling operations, used garments must be kept separate from other garments to prevent contamination with the product.

B. General Clean Room Procedures

1. Before entering any clean environment, personnel should understand the responsibilities of their position and know aseptic techniques.
2. Traffic into and within the clean room should be restricted to authorized personnel. Personnel should not walk around the room unnecessarily.
3. Movement in the clean room should be slow and rhythmic.
4. Once inside the clean room, personnel should remain until the break or lunch period.
5. Nervous relief-type mannerisms such as head scratching or rubbing hands, face, or parts of the body must be consciously avoided.
6. Loud, unnecessary talk through the mask should be avoided. Laughing, whistling, singing, and shouting increase the number of bacteria emitted from the mouth.
7. Horseplay is strictly forbidden in the clean room.
8. Soiled or dirty work clothes must not be worn in the clean room.
9. No eating of food, chewing of gum or tobacco, or smoking is permitted in the clean area.
10. No pencils or erasers should be used in the clean room. Ball point pens, magic markers, or felt tip pens are suggested.
11. Paper in any form (except that produced expressly for clean room operations, and meeting Class 100 conditions as specified in Federal Standard 209B) is not allowed in the clean facility. When it is necessary that paper forms be used, the form should be shielded with a clean plastic covering that has a window exposing the area on which the operator is to write.
12. No one who is physically ill, especially with a stomach or respiratory disorder, may enter the clean room.
13. All verbal communication with people outside the clean area should be accomplished through the use of an intercom or telephone.
14. Paper, pens, keys, and so on, must not be passed from the nonclean to the clean area, or vice versa.
15. Air locks are used as a barrier to the ingress of unclean air from the critical area, and as a passageway for equipment to be brought into and removed from the clean facility.
16. The air lock is not to be occupied by personnel or equipment from the clean and nonclean areas simultaneously.
17. All vials, bottles, and ampuls must be handled in covered trays.
18. Product containers should not be exposed unnecessarily to the clean room environment.
19. Trays containing product containers should be opened only under a laminar airflow device.
20. Personnel should not reach over or lean over open vials on the line.
21. Personnel should keep their hands away from vial openings. Vials should be handled from the bottom.
22. Glassware and stoppers generate particulates and must be handled with care.
23. Components that have fallen onto the floor must not be picked up and used.

24. Personnel must report any irregularities or adverse changes in environmental conditions (temperature or humidity) to the supervisor.
25. When personnel are in doubt as to the appropriate action, the supervisor should be contacted.

C. Safety Procedures

1. Personnel should be taught the proper procedures to follow for power failures— how to protect the product and exit the clean area. Emergency lights and generators should be provided.
2. Emergency fire exits should be provided if the normal exits are inadequate or are likely to be inaccessible.
3. Fire extinguishers should be provided and all personnel should be instructed in their use.
4. Emergency fire drills should be held regularly.
5. Emergency teams, such as first aid, should be trained and readily available during all working hours.

VI. TRAINING PROGRAM FOR CLEAN ROOM EMPLOYEES

Training in good manufacturing practices is one of the more important factors that influence the quality of the finished drug product. The best design, layout, and materials are worthless unless the people working in the clean room understand the operation and its significance. The federal Current Good Manufacturing Practices (CGMPs) regulations [18] state the following:

> Each person engaged in the manufacture, processing, packing, or holding of a drug product shall have education, training, and experience, or any combination thereof, to enable that person to perform the assigned functions. Training shall be in the particular operations that the employee performs and in current good manufacturing practices . . . as they relate to the employee's functions.

Thus the governmental regulations are actually fulfilled by clean room personnel. Management establishes the rules and regulations, operating conditions, and processes and procedures for the clean room. However, each operator performing a specific job function on a daily basis serves as the fulfillment of compliance with CGMPs.

One of the major problems with training personnel to work in the clean room is the communication of technical information to persons with a nontechnical background. There are various methods by which this can be accomplished. The following discusses one specific procedure for the development of a training program that will provide knowledge of the federal regulations and teach employees those functions required for the performance of particular jobs.

A. Development of the Training Program

All training programs, regardless of their content, should have three common objectives:

1. Training material must relate CGMPs to the individual's own job and how it fits into the total compliance aspect.
2. The program must be individualized to increase its effectiveness.
3. CGMP material must be easily revised to keep current with operational changes.

Satisfying these objectives is important for the success of the training program. Employees must see how the federal regulations pertain to their particular job functions. This should give them an understanding of the importance of their jobs, and serve as an incentive to perform to the best of their ability. Current material and individualized programs geared to a particular group must not be overlooked in program development. The training program would be of no value if the information presented were outdated. When operational changes are made, the new procedures must be incorporated into the program. Without this, the training program loses its credibility. Furthermore, if the program can easily be corrected and edited, it can be used to present information that is specific for one job or even one person. Since each person comes to a job with a different background and different experience, the program must be tailored to each person's strengths and weaknesses. The word processor can help to fulfill these two objectives. The word processor provides greater efficiency in utilizing classroom time to explain contamination control principles and their relationship to the specific job. Complete training manuals or parts of manuals can be corrected and duplicated very easily and with a time-saving factor of 90% compared to the conventional method of making corrections using an electric typewriter. Furthermore, material can be inserted into or deleted from the text by a few simple manipulations on the machine. Respacing of added letters or written text occurs automatically. The word processor has many other advantages. Further details of its operation can be found in the literature [19].

Based upon the objectives cited above, there are four fundamental steps to follow in developing a training program: (1) select the appropriate medium, (2) develop a training syllabus, (3) select a person to perform the training function, and (4) select the appropriate techniques and methods [20]. Generally speaking, there are four media which are commonly used in the design and implementation of a training program: (1) slide/lecture presentations, (2) slide/tape programs, (3) videotapes and films, and (4) workbook programs. An important consideration is that the media used be interesting and easy to understand. Cost and the ease of program revision are also determining factors. The training syllabus outlines the contents of the program. The underlying theme of each program is the basic concept of CGMPs and how they relate to the employee's job. Employees should understand their roles in the overall operation, and why jobs are performed in certain ways. They should also understand the consequences of not following procedures as specified. The course content is determined by the needs of the company and its operation.

After the development of the outline for the training program, it must be presented to top-level management for their approval. Without the support of this group, the training program would have only a limited degree of success. Intermediate management levels become involved after the completion of the first draft. Their comments are used to make improvements and changes in the program's content.

Any training program should begin with supervisory training. The completed program should contain an introductory segment which is shown just to supervisors. It should cover such topics as the attitude of the supervisors toward production personnel. It must also encourage the supervisors to ask for help with any problems they cannot resolve. First-line supervisors should be instructed to praise good work performance. On the other hand, they must discover why some employees perform poorly. In many cases, a company's violation of the CGMPs result from inadequate training. This situation is caused by management personnel who fail to familiarize themselves with the requirements of the CGMPs and neglect to provide operating personnel with the appropriate training.

Selecting the appropriate person to perform the training function is a major decision in the development of any training program. At one time the line supervisor was solely responsible for the training of new employees. The advantages of this type of arrangement are numerous: (1) existing rapport between the supervisor and employees; (2) employees identify the supervisor with the concept of CGMPs and the importance of quality in the performance of the job; and (3) employees recognize the basic responsibility of the supervisor to train them. However, within the last several years a change has taken place and a new concept has been introduced—the development of a training specialist. This person is responsible for conducting both CGMP and job function training programs. The new position brings with it distinct advantages: (1) uniform instruction for all personnel, (2) more extensive knowledge and understanding of the CGMPs, (3) better communication skills, and (4) feedback occurring through one person who can then modify the training program to achieve more significant results. Training specialists must possess very distinct characteristics. They must be part actor, part teacher, and part comedian. They ought to be enthusiastic about the program and present the material in an interesting fashion. They must believe that the training program is beneficial to both the employees and the operating department. This feeling has to be conveyed in order for them to develop credibility with the management of the operating department and those employees they train. Because training specialists are dedicated to the parenteral area, they can learn more details of the operation. This, too, will strengthen their credibility and enhance the job performance of the sterile products operators.

There are a number of training methods that can be utilized to instruct personnel: (1) formal classroom training, (2) on-the-job training, (3) training manuals, (4) audiovisual programs, (5) training by outside consultants, (6) vendor presentations or seminars, (7) discussion groups, (8) closed-circuit television programs, (9) teaching machine courses, and (10) train-the-trainer technique. In most cases, a company will use a combination of the methods to perform the required training. However, the method(s) selected must first and foremost satisfy the needs of the organization. The material must be presented in a simple form and in language that the trainees can understand. The trainer must explain how to apply the principles and concepts being discussed. Theories do not mean anything if they have no practical application for the employees.

When the program is first administered, members of top-level management should be present to demonstrate their support and commitment to the training effort. Often the comment is made: "Boy, I sure wish my boss was here to hear you say that! He's the one who really needs this program." Management attendance shows their regard for the importance of the program and its significance to the operation. Their participation also confers credibility on the training program. The practices and procedures illustrated in the training program must be reinforced by all levels of management, but in particular by the first-line supervisors. The trainer has the responsibility to present the concepts and ideas. Supervision demonstrates the importance of these concepts and ideas through their practical application to the performance of the job. In this way, work habits can be changed and employee performance improved.

B. Three-Step Training Program

There are many different programs that a company may develop to utilize in training their clean room employees. One popular and widely used approach in the pharmaceutical industry is a three-step program which includes the following: (1) class-
room/orientation training, (2) technical training, and (3) on-the-job training [21,22].

1. Classroom/Orientation Training

The first phase of the training program is an introduction to the clean room
environment. The trainer should discuss the requirements for parenteral products—
purity of all components and the absence of toxic substances and microbial contamination. Parenterals must be sterile and free from pyrogens. They are injectable
products, and as such, they bypass the body's natural defense mechanism—the skin
and mucous membranes. The presence of microorganisms can cause an adverse
reaction and even death in the patient since the body has no way to defend itself
against the invading organisms. Thus the trainee begins to see the need for a clean
room to manufacture this type of product.

Training programs are designed with regard to the particular operation which
they will service. In a parenteral operation, one important consideration is the
concept of contamination—what it is, where it comes from, and how it can harm the
drug product. Trainees should be given a thorough explanation of contamination in
terms they can understand and with examples to which they can relate. This instruction should depend on the employees' backgrounds and previous training. In
each case, the problem to the patient must be emphasized. At this point, the trainer may present a visual demonstration of microbial and particulate contamination.
Rubbing the skin or clothing will emit particles that can be seen by the naked eye in
a beam of light in a darkened room, such as from a projector. Trainees must also
realize that there are many particles which are <u>invisible</u> to the naked eye. The
trainer should relate the size of these invisible particles to particle sizes of objects
with which the trainees are familiar, and explain the unit of measurement for these
particles. Drawings or diagrams and photographic slides of different types of contaminants may be helpful. The use of petri plates and particle counters will also
demonstrate invisible contaminants. The trainer must explain that particles serve
as a means of locomotion. The trainer should also discuss pyrogens—what they
are, where they originate, and what harm they cause to the product and patient.

Personnel contributions to the level of contamination in the clean room can be
illustrated by Austin's Contamination Control Index (see p. 438). These values
represent individual emission patterns which are influenced by personnel activity.
The trainer must emphasize to all employees the importance of good personal hygiene and work habits. This is followed by an introduction to clean room regulations
and procedures. One of the first procedures discussed is gowning and entry into the
clean room. Equally important is an explanation of the reasons for these strict
rules. Improper behavior increases the level of contamination in the area, which
in turn can jeopardize the purity and integrity of the drug product. The orientation
to clean room operations also should include training in aseptic techniques. The
bacteriological information that is presented should be sufficient to enable operators
to understand the aseptic procedures required to perform their jobs.

The program must also include a discussion of clean room design: the concept of laminar airflow, HEPA filters, and the classes of clean rooms as specified
in Federal Standard 209B. The trainer must explain that Class 100 conditions are

required for the aseptic processing of all parenteral products. The trainer should also explain the sterilization processes and their importance to the operation. In an area outside the clean room, exercises may be conducted to demonstrate these methods. In each case, sublethal conditions are also employed to show what happens when failures occur in the sterilization procedures. In the last several years, the concept of validation has become important to the parenteral operation. The trainer should define this term and explain its significance to the clean room operation. Finally, the trainer should briefly describe the overall clean room operation to the employees, giving them an understanding of each job and why it is performed in a specific manner.

During the formal classroom period of instruction, trainers should vary their methods of presenting the required information to maintain interest in the program. Trainees are more likely to retain this information if it is presented in a manner that holds their attention. Furthermore, the specific information being presented usually lends itself to a particular form, thereby enhancing the trainer's delivery of the material. Trainers may use one or more of the following methods during this phase of the program: (1) lecture method, (2) questioning method (factual or recall), and (3) demonstration (problems and application).

"The importance of this phase of training cannot be overstressed, since it forms the basis of the worker's future attitude toward a job where such personal interest is demanded, and such inconvenience is assumed" [23].

2. Technical Training

The technical training involves teaching employees the specific knowledge and skills required for performance of the job. The job function should be presented in exactly the manner in which it must be performed. The first step in preparing an effective program for job function training is the performance of a comprehensive task analysis. Each job function in the clean room should be carefully evaluated and a detailed description written of the steps that operators follow in fulfilling their responsibilities. With a complex job function, the information gathered can be quite extensive. Some companies use this information to write a training manual thoroughly describing each aspect of the job. This manual is used as a guideline to instruct employees in the technical responsibilities of their assigned jobs. The procedures discussed are directly related to the product and the operation, and have been tailored to the company's needs. The use of an audiovisual program describing the particular job is sometimes helpful. Trainers must also stress the importance of each employee's job function, indicating how carelessness and violations in procedure can jeopardize the product and, more importantly, the patient. With this thought in mind, trainees can better understand the reasons behind the established job procedures. Showing employees the operation can be helpful at the conclusion of the verbal discription.

Studies have indicated that personnel performance is at its best where regulations are explicit and the employees know exactly what is expected of them. If instructions are vague, employees are likely to make mistakes that are costly to both the operation and the product. In industry today, a group of individuals is responsible for the manufacture of a sterile product. Each person is involved in only one part of the total operation. This situation is not conducive to the employee's understanding of the overall task. However, each worker must thoroughly understand the job that he is required to do if his performance is to meet satisfactory standards. Therefore, management must compensate for the enigma that is built into the system.

3. On-the-Job Training

When employees have satisfactorily completed the first two phases of train-ing, they are ready to work alongside a skilled clean room operator. Giving em-ployees an opportunity to do the job will indicate their ability and understanding of what has been taught. Hands-on experience is invaluable in learning a new job. The trainer must carefully observe the progress of new employees as they put into practice what they have learned. A trainer should be available in the work area to answer questions and correct violations in procedure or aseptic technique. When employees can perform the assigned task satisfactorily, they should be allowed to work on their own. However, their work should continue to be checked at frequent intervals. Gradually, the frequent observations can be eliminated and normal su-pervision of the employee assumed.

On-the-job training is probably the most beneficial form of training if it has been properly reinforced with previous information regarding the operation. Em-ployees need both practical experience and an understanding of the overall operation to appreciate fully their own roles. This is why the orientation and technical train-ing are so important, since they lay the groundwork for the last phase of the train-ing program.

However, the trainer's responsibility does not end at the conclusion of the formal training program. Sometime after the completion of the program, the train-er should follow-up on the employees' performances to be certain that they continue to adhere to all established procedures. Retraining should be scheduled at specif-ically defined intervals or when deemed necessary by the trainer and management from the operating department.

4. Documentation

An essential factor in any training program is documentation. Each company must establish its own procedure based on compliance with the federal regulations and the available resources. Paperwork containing pertinent information regarding the training administered—when, by whom, and the type of training—together with the employee's signature is all that is required. Some companies are able to utilize the computer to store the necessary training information. This system provides rapid recall of specific information, saves time in obtaining the data, and is capable of supplying a printed copy of the desired material. Storage of information in this manner also saves space. Whatever method of documentation is utilized, it must satisfy governmental regulations by furnishing the required information while satis-fying the particular needs of the organization.

5. Evaluation

At the completion of the training program, management must be able to evalu-ate the program in terms of its benefit to the operation. Evaluation is necessary to improve the cost-effectiveness of the training function and to meet the educational needs of the organization and the employees. The ability of trainees to perform their jobs and the effectiveness of the program in helping them achieve these results are both important.

At the completion of the training program, the trainer should not only see an improvement in employee performance, but be able to measure this improvement with the proper evaluation technique. The method of evaluation selected should an-swer the following questions:

a. Is the problem amenable to a training solution?

b. Which training method is most appropriate for the material and the target population?

c. Was the course material learned? Did the training result in the desired immediate demonstration of behavior change?

d. Did the immediate learning or behavior change translate into the desired on-the-
   job performance?

e. What changes could be made to improve the training program?

f. Are there particular types of trainees for whom the training is more (or less)
   effective?

g. What are the implications of the induced behavior change relative to meeting
   long-range organizational objectives?

These questions imply that evaluation can be directed at two basic components of
training effectiveness: (1) to what degree does in-class learning occur as a result
of training?, and (2) to what degree does this learning translate into on-the-job behavior change? These two elements represent the problems of external and internal
validity.

    Internal validity is defined as the degree to which changes in the dependent
variable (performance) can be directly attributed to the independent variable (training program). In other words, participation in the training program is singularly
responsible for both learning and noted improvements in employee performance
measured by the evaluation technique. Any extraneous factors that could be used to
explain the results of training will jeopardize the internal validity of the training
and its evaluation. These factors can be classified into two major categories:
history and maturation. The term history is used to relate an improvement in employee performance produced by a change in the work environment (i.e., new equipment, new supervisor). Maturation expresses a condition in which an improvement
in employee performance occurs simply because employees have become more familiar with the job and what is expected of them. There is absolutely no training
involved. Performance improves simply because employees become more profi-
cient in the execution of their jobs.

    External validity represents the accuracy with which one can predict employ-
ees' on-the-job performance based upon their performance in the training program.
To measure the external validity of a program, objective criteria and the effect of
training on both organizational and on-the-job performance must be utilized. Of the
two, however, internal validity presents more of a problem in the selection and
implementation of a suitable evaluation method.

    Thus the evaluation procedure has many pitfalls and problems which must be
resolved in order for it to measure program effectiveness accurately. The following suggestions may be helpful for making evaluation easier and more useful:

a. Describe all crucial elements in the training activity, not just program contents.

b. Choose an evaluation design that is appropriate for the situation.

c. Seek out naturally occurring opportunities for evaluation.

    There are four basic evaluation designs: (1) the before-and-after or AB de-
sign, (2) the control group design, (3) the reversal or ABA design, and (4) the multiple baseline design. Only one evaluation technique will be discussed in this chapter: the multiple baseline design [24]. Practical application has shown this design
to be adaptable to almost all training evaluation research. Furthermore, this method of evaluation is capable of demonstrating a functional relationship between improvements in employee performance and training program participation.

Multiple baseline design was established with the following two criteria as its focal point: (1) collection of two or more sets of baseline data, and (2) presentation of the training program to different groups of people at different times. There are three major types of multiple baseline designs: (1) multiple baseline across behavior or performance variables, (2) multiple baseline across subjects or groups, and (3) multiple baseline across settings or locations.

In a study utilizing the multiple baseline across behaviors or performance variables, baseline values for preselected evaluation indices must first be established. The baseline data must stabilize prior to startup of the training program. Next, a training program centered on one of the variables is administered. After the completion of this program, data are collected on all the variables. Then a second training program is presented, with emphasis on the second variable. The collection of data on all variables continues at the conclusion of the training program. The number of intervention phases should equal the number of variables or indices being examined. If possible, the data gathered throughout the study should be plotted on a graph. In this way, a visual inspection is all that is required to determine whether the training program has a positive impact on the variables being studied. If the training program is successful, the graph of each variable will rise above the baseline level after completion of the training for that particular variable. From the graph, the trainer can calculate the percentage of improvement posttraining. The cost of the entire training program can also be calculated. A comparison between these two figures represents the cost-effectiveness of the training program. Based upon this information, management will decide whether to implement the same program with other groups of employees.

Multiple baseline across subjects or groups is used to evaluate the effect of an intervention on one performance variable in two or more classifications or groups of employees. For example, this design may be utilized to determine the effect of a training program on one performance variable for employees in different geographic locations. The design has proven to be more valuable when using three different groups of subjects and when the groups are independent of each other. To implement this program, only one specific performance variable is selected. Next, three groups of employees are chosen. A baseline for the particular variable in question must be established using data from all three groups. As before, the data are plotted on a graph. One group of employees is trained at a time, while data are collected from all three groups. Each subsequent group is trained at specified intervals after the completion of the training for the first group. Based upon the data obtained, a conclusion is reached regarding the effect of the program on the variable being studied.

A practical example of a multiple baseline design across subjects or groups will demonstrate its usefulness as a method for evaluating training programs. The sterile filling department notices a significant loss in production time because of late startups at the beginning of the shift. Upon careful examination of the operation, they determine the cause of the problem to be improper washing of machine parts. As the operators begin to reassemble the machine parts after washing and sterilization, they detect product residue from the previous production run. Consequently, the parts must be rewashed and resterilized before the next product can be filled on the machine. Valuable time is lost because the washing and sterilization process must be repeated. Management decides to implement a training program especially designed for the parts washing personnel.

To evaluate the effect of a training program on the performance of these employees, the multiple baseline design across subjects or groups is used. Three groups of parts washing personnel are selected from different manufacturing facilities. Since the groups are independent of each other, a change in the performance of one group does not affect either of the other two groups. This factor is critical for precise program evaluation. Production downtime in the form of late shift startups is selected as the performance variable to be measured. The baseline for the performance variable is established from the previous production record for each group. In this example, the amount of production time lost because of late startups at the beginning of the shift is plotted on three separate graphs.

A training program is presented to one group of parts washing personnel at a time. The program is divided into two parts, the first of which includes a detailed discussion of the written procedure for cleaning the designated parts. A separate procedure for each product group is established (i.e., one for water-based products and one for oil-based products). The employee receives instruction in the preparation of the appropriate cleaning solutions for each product group. The trainer also discusses the procedure for sterilizing the machine parts. Every aspect of the person's job responsibilities is thoroughly explained. The second part of the program contains a general discussion of the clean room environment. The need for this specialized area is explained in terms of product requirements. Emphasis is placed upon the problems caused by contamination. Each employee must understand the importance of the job and the problems that can arise through carelessness.

The training program is administered to one group of employees at a time. After the initial presentation, the trainer collects data from all three groups. Each of the other two groups is trained at 6-week intervals. After the training, a significant decrease in the amount of production time lost because of late startups is observed with each group. The effect is attributed directly to the training program.

Multiple baseline across settings is used to study one performance variable or one group of individuals in different settings. This design is not useful for the evaluation of the majority of training programs, since the settings selected must be independent of each other, and therefore will not be discussed in the content of this chapter.

Because of the simplicity of design and the ease with which data may be analyzed, the multiple baseline design is considered a good practical method for evaluating the effect of training on employee performance.

C. Advantages of a Training Program

Following is a list of the benefits that can be attributed to a well-developed training program [25, 26]:

1. Improved product quality
2. Increased productivity
3. Greater overall efficiency
4. Improved technical abilities and increased competency of the trainees
5. Reduction in rework time and reject rate
6. Reduction in operating costs
7. Reduction in work stoppage
8. Reduction in waste
9. Improved work schedule
10. Enhanced organizational effectiveness

Training also improves individual human performance and employee morale and motivation. Management can utilize training as a two-way communication net-

work in which the company both gives and receives information relating to the operation. Employees see the training program as a sincere effort by management to
provide them with the knowledge to do their jobs to the best of their ability. Furthermore, employees perceive management's commitment to the clean room in the
recognition and subsequent elimination of contamination problems. If, however,
this formal program of communication is eliminated, personnel performance gradually deteriorates. Workers forget why the clean room is necessary. They revert
to behavior typical of employees who work outside the clean area. Employees assume that if they cannot see it, it does not exist, and no harm can come from something which is nonexistent. The results from this type of thinking can be harmful to
the product, but more importantly, are extremely hazardous to the patient.
". . . although it may take a little extra effort to convey the information, the desire
for knowledge by production people was and is there. After all, it is the hourly
worker, in particular, who must keep the facility in the condition you desire, and he
is the one who must understand why and what it means to him in his daily work now
and in the future" [27].

Managers and first-line supervisors play a very significant role in the development of good operators. How the operators are treated and what management expects of them determines, to a large extent, the level of performance achieved.
Therefore, the influence of management on the operating personnel will determine
the success or failure of the company's compliance with the federal regulations.
Management must keep in mind the legal and moral obligations of the company to
manufacture a product that meets all of the specified requirements. Proper training and motivation are necessary and will prove beneficial to the overall operation.
With people who are highly motivated, and who understand and actively participate
in the operation, these moral and legal obligations can be fulfilled.

Training programs are also designed to change or shape people's behavior.
The difference in the way employees react after the training determines the effectiveness of the program. If the program presented has truly been an educational
experience for the employees, they will approach the responsibilities of their jobs
in a more positive manner. This is evidence that the training program is a success
and that learning has taken place.

VII. MANAGEMENT ROLE IN CLEAN ROOM OPERATIONS

Clean room employees play a significant role in the manufacture of parenteral products. However, management personnel contribute equally to the success of clean
room operations. Their direction and guidance of the operation will determine its
success or failure. There are many ways in which management can influence clean
room operations and clean room employees. The principal factors involved are discussed below.

A. Motivation of Employees

Motivation of employees is a requirement for the efficient operation of any clean
room. Violations of procedures usually occur from poorly trained, unmotivated,
uninvolved operators. In most cases, a single occurrence of contamination is
caused by poor employee behavior—an employee did something incorrectly or failed
to do something he should have done. An employee who is inadequately prepared
for a new job will not possess a favorable attitude toward the job or the supervisor. The employee realizes management's failure to provide the essential knowl-

edge needed to perform the required task. Thus the person develops a feeling of resentment toward the individuals deemed responsible. As a result, performance is likely to be unsatisfactory.

Proper education and training can help to resolve this problem since they contribute significantly to the motivation of manufacturing personnel. Many pharmaceutical companies are presently using a Quality Circles program to achieve this goal. However, this program has more than employee motivation as its purpose. The objectives of a Quality Circles program are to

1. Reduce errors and improve quality
2. Inspire more effective teamwork
3. Promote job involvement
4. Increase employee motivation
5. Create a problem-solving capability
6. Build an attitude of "problem prevention"
7. Improve company communications
8. Develop harmonious manager/worker relationships
9. Promote personal and leadership development
10. Develop greater safety awareness

The Quality Circles approach to on-the-job problem solving is based upon motivational theories of participation and recognition. A Quality Circle is composed of a group of people who voluntarily participate in the identification, analysis, and resolution of specific problems in their work area. The number of members may vary, but the ideal number seems to be seven or eight. Members of the circle should be from the same or similar work areas. Thus the problems they select will be familiar to everyone in the group.

For the most part, the Quality Circles process is composed of the following steps:

1. Identification of a problem by circle members, staff, or management
2. Selection of a particular problem relevant to the work environment
3. Analysis of the problem (with technical assistance from the appropriate technical staff if necessary)
4. Formulation of a solution to the problem
5. Making a formal recommendation directly to management in what is termed "the management presentation"
6. Review of the circle's proposed solution by involved managers and technical specialists to decide whether to implement the solution
7. Implementation of the solution by the organization
8. Evaluation of the success of the solution by the circle and the organization

The members of the circle may be recognized or rewarded for the successful resolution of a problem in a variety of ways: (1) presentations to management; (2) write-ups in the organization's activity report; (3) recognition in the company newspaper; (4) photographs posted on bulletin boards; (5) certificates; (6) trophies or pins; and (7) monetary rewards based upon a percentage of the money saved by the implementation of the circle's suggestion. However, each company must select its own method(s) of recognition for circle members.

The key difference between Quality Circles and quality control programs such as Zero Defects is that management must respond to the recommendations of the circle. If management rejects the recommendation, the reasons for the rejection must be given. This policy of a required management response will enhance communications between management and hourly personnel. However, one critical aspect must be emphasized—a successful Quality Circles program requires total management commitment. Without this, the program will be ineffective and ultimately doomed to failure.

To minimize the problem of motivation, management should incorporate the following as part of the education and training of clean room employees:

1. Keep personnel informed of new government regulations. This should be an ongoing program since personnel must understand what consequences can arise as a result of noncompliance. A training session is the perfect opportunity to present such information.
2. Actively involve personnel in the preparation of batch records. Give them an opportunity to ask questions about any of the procedures associated with these documents.
3. Involve operating personnel in the decision-making and problem-solving process. Sometimes a problem occurs when manufacturing personnel are not informed or inadequately trained. Inviting key persons to participate in discussions dealing with the operation may resolve the problems more quickly.

Providing employees with the information required to perform their jobs is not sufficient unless the proper motivating factors are also present. Neglect and indifference can destroy the most technologically advanced operation. Clean room personnel should be made to realize the responsibility they assume by accepting a job working in the clean room. Management must develop this sense of responsibility by setting a good example for the operating employees, communicating the appropriate information, and reinforcing the practices and procedures discussed during the training sessions.

B. Development of a Positive Attitude

One of the perennial problems that industry has to combat is the attitude of people toward the clean room concept. This problem starts at the top level of management. The clean room operation is undergoing vast technological changes. Some individuals are inflexible to these changes, and have a difficult time justifying in their own minds the need for them and the corresponding cost increase. Management closely scrutinizes the cost factor of any operation, but especially that of the clean room. They argue that production time is lost because personnel must wash their hands and put on a clean garment before entering the controlled area. This is something not encountered in a work area outside the clean room.

Furthermore, personnel attitude is one of the single most important factors influencing the effective utilization of the laminar flow clean room. Laminar airflow cannot compensate for carelessness and improper handling of equipment and components. Proper lighting and color, below-average noise levels, and the appropriate velocity of air have improved the attitude of operating personnel. The employees seem more interested in their jobs and make more suggestions to improve work procedures.

The attitude and competence of first-line supervisors directly influence the operation of the clean room since these individuals are in close contact with the operating personnel. If they are aware of the need for cleanliness in the controlled area, and if they are committed to the clean room concept, that attitude will be passed along to the employees and will be evident in the quality of the work. However, if supervisors are careless about their own practices in the clean room and set a poor example, this attitude will be transferred even faster, thereby destroying the company's investment in the clean room operation. The performance of supervisors, in turn, is influenced by management at higher levels in the organization.

Negative management attitudes filter down through the ranks, creating poor habits among the personnel performing the jobs in the clean area. Poor attitudes may be reflected in improper gowning procedures, incorrect use of personnel cleaning facilities, and the improper handling of parts and equipment. These violations occur because management becomes lax and does not supervise the operation properly.

Management must strive toward the development of positive employee attitudes and discipline in the clean room. They must believe that the clean room is necessary to manufacture the high quality product required by the customer. Employees should see and appreciate the efforts of management to ensure the integrity of the product. They must instill a feeling of pride and confidence in the clean room operators. An appropriately designed training program can provide management with the means to accomplish this goal. During training sessions, the company should stress their dependence on people doing the job correctly, and the important part they play in the manufacture of a reliable product. They must also stress the concept of teamwork—everyone working together to achieve the desired end result. People should be made to feel that being chosen for such a critical job function is truly an honor. After the completion of the training program, employees should understand the clean room operation and procedures required for the satisfactory performance of their specific jobs. Consequently, the success of the clean room operation relies on the transmission of a positive attitude from the uppermost levels of management to the operators performing each job function.

The clean room is constantly being bombarded by contaminants from a variety of sources. However, "when all other factors have been evaluated, and the best possible facilities, equipment, and processes have been set up to do the required job, the most important factor must be considered. This key factor is still people. People can make or break any operation, but nowhere is this responsibility more critical than in the clean room" [28].

REFERENCES

1. Heuring, H., Contam. Control, 9:18-20 (July/Aug. 1970).
2. Austin, P. R., Contam. Control, 4:45, 47, 49, 51 (Oct. 1965).
3. Noble, W. C., J. Environ. Sci., 21(2):25-28 (Mar./Apr. 1978).
4. Cown, Wm. B., and Kethley, T. W., Contam. Control, 6:10-14 (June 1967).
5. Noble, W. C., Br. J. Dermatol., 93:477-485 (1975).
6. Noble, W. C., Habbema, J. D. F., von Furth, R., Smith, I., and deRaay, C., J. Med. Microbiol., 9:53-61 (1976).
7. McDade, J. J., Third Annu. Tech. Conf. Am. Assoc. Contam. Control, 1964.
8. Useller, J. W., Clean Room Technology, NASA SP-5074, Washington, D.C., 1969.
9. Kladko, M., Pharm. Tech., 6(5):72, 75, 77-78, 80, 82 (May 1982).
10. Munkacsy, M., Contam. Control, 5:12-14, 18 (Jan. 1966).
11. Mitchell, N. J., and Gamble, D. R., Lancet, 2:1133-1136 (Nov. 9, 1974).
12. Dyment, J., in Dust Control and Air Cleaning (R. G. Dorman, ed.), Pergamon Press, Oxford, 1974.
13. Austin, P. R., Contam. Control, 5:11, 15, 16, 19 (Jan. 1966).

14. Austin, P. R., Contam. Control, 4:45, 47, 49, 51 (Oct. 1965).
15. Austin, P. R., Contam. Control, 5:26, 27, 32 (June 1966).
16. DeVecchi, F. A., Pharm. Tech., 2:40-44 (Aug. 1978).
17. Austin, P. R., Design and Operation of Clean Rooms, Business News Publishing Co., Birmingham, Mich. 1970.
18. Fed. Regist., 43:45077-45087 (Sept. 29, 1978).
19. McGirr, C. J., 27th Annu. Tech. Meet. IES, Los Angeles, May 4-8, 1981.
20. Kitt, M. J., J. Parenter. Drug Assoc., 33:341-345 (Nov./Dec. 1979).
21. Austin, P. R., Contam. Control, 8:28-31, 34 (Feb. 1969).
22. Austin, P. R., Contam. Control, 5:28, 32 (Nov. 1966).
23. Munkacsy, M., Contam. Control, 5:12-14, 18 (Jan. 1966).
24. Brown, M. G., Train Dev. J., 34:11-16 (Oct. 1980).
25. Scherman, I. A., Train Dev. J., 34:50-55 (Jan. 1980).
26. Donnell, D. E., Sixth Annu. Tech. Meet. Am. Assoc. Contam. Control, 1967.
27. Howarth, Wm., Bull. Parenter. Drug Assoc., 26:147-152 (May/June 1972).
28. Heuring, H., Contam. Control, 9:18-20 (July/Aug. 1970).

Index

A

Absorbance spectra, 98
Absorption rate constant, 77, 80
Acylation, 123
Added substances, 155
Additive programs, in hospitals, 35
Administration of parenteral drugs,
    13–45
  complications of, 35, 37, 42
  cost of, 41
  devices for, 42–44
    cannulas, 43
    catheters, 43
    controllers, 43
    heparin locks, 43
    pumps, 42
  general indications, 2
  hazards of, 35–42
    air emboli, 41
    anaphylaxis, 40
    bleeding, 40
    extravasation, 41
    fever, 41
    hypersensitivity, 40
    incompatibilities, 40
    infiltration, 41
    overdosage, 41
    particulate matter, 40
    phlebitis, 40
    sepsis, 37
    thrombosis, 39
    toxemia, 39

[Administration of parenteral drugs]
  pharmaceutical factors affecting, 14–16
    formulation ingredients, 16
    osmolality, 15
    pH, 15
    solubility, 15
    vehicle characteristics, 15
  precautions, 35
  problems, 35
Administrative areas, 365
Air, 405
  clean, 405
  compressed, 405, 409
    heat control, 409
    moisture control, 409
    system, 406, 407
  compressor, 408
  conditioning, 385–397
  filtration, 390–397, 410
    mechanisms of, 391
Air inlet tubes, 309
Amphotericin B, 97
Antimicrobial agents:
  efficacy, 215, 219
  in formulation, 166, 182
Antioxidants, 160, 161
Area under the curve, 69, 75, 78, 83
Arrestance, 395
Arteriovenous system, 60
Aseptic formulation, 243
Aseptic formulation operation, 233
Aseptic subdivision operation, 237, 244,
    250

Assay, stability-indicating, 193
Atmospheric dust, 391
Autoclave, 242

B

Bacterial aerosols, from personnel,
    428
Bacteria-retaining filters, 39
Ball milling, 240
Ball valves, 383
Batch mixing, 284-287
Batch operations, 359
Batch records, 206
Beer's law, 102
Benzocaine, 107
Binding, to macromolecules, 54
Bioavailability, 69
Bioburden, 287
Biopharmaceutics, 47-86
Blood flow, 48, 61, 63, 65
Buffer capacity, 155
Buffers, 155

C

Caffeine, 107
Calibration, records of, 345
Cap assemblies, aluminum, 310
Capsolut washer, 221
Cefotaxime, 101
Ceramic filters, 289
Cerebrospinal fluid flow, 32
Change rooms, 375-376
Chelating agents, 165
Chlorothiazide, 100
Chromophores, 90
Circulation time, 61
Circulatory system, 59
Clean area, 363
Clean room classes, standards of,
    386, 388
Clean room garments, 436, 440
  criteria for, 437
  stockings, 436
  synthetic filament, 437
Clean room personnel, 433
  characteristics of, 433
    aptitudes, 434
    condition of health, 433
      skin diseases, 433
        upper respiratory diseases, 433

[Clean room personnel]
    personal hygiene, 433
    psychological, 434
    skills, 434
  selection of, 433
Clean room procedures, 441
Clean rooms, 210
  performance of, 400
Closures:
  rubber, 125, 307, 309
Cloth filters, 289
Colloidal systems, 270
Communication instruments, 375
Compatibility, 114-121
  drug-excipient, 114-121
    factorial design, 120
    Plackett-Burman design, 115
Complaint file, 207
Component processing record, 207
Compressed gases, 306, 411
Computers, 323
Concentration gradient, 49
Conduction, 273
Containers, 307-310
  glass, 307
  plastic, 310
Container size, 361
Contaminants, 427
  microbial, 427
  nonviable, 427
  particulate, 427
  viable, 427
Contamination Control Index, Austin's,
    438, 445
Contamination indices, 438
Contamination level, 435, 438, 445
  effect of clothing on, 436
  effect of personnel bathing on, 435
  effect of suntan on, 436
Continuous operations, 359
Convection, 273
Cosolvents, 154
Cozzoli tabletop piston filler, 255
Cozzoli washer, 227
Crystal growth, prevention of, 172
Crystallization, aseptic, 172

D

Decarboxylation, 122
Density, 270
Descaling, 280

Diaphragm valves, 383
Dielectric constants, 142
Differential scanning calorimetry, 95
Differential thermal analysis, 94, 180
Dilution operation, 235
Dioctyl phthalate (DOP) test, 396
Dissociation constant, 148
Distillation, 279, 417
Distribution of parenterally admin-
    istered agents:
  physiological, 33, 34
    degradation, effect on, 34
    formulation ingredients, effect on,
      34
    particle size, effect on, 34
    partition coefficient, effect on, 34
    rate of blood flow, effect on, 34
    solubility, effect on, 34
Distribution rate constant, physio-
    logical, 74
Distribution records, 207
Documentation, in training, 447
Door hardware, 374
Drug absorption, 56
  from aqueous solution, 56
  from aqueous suspensions, 56
  from emulsions, 57
  from oil-in-water emulsions, 57
  from oleaginous solutions, 57
  passive diffusion, 49
  physicochemical factors affecting,
    48
  physiological factors affecting, 59
    anatomical site, 62
    body temperature, 63
    disease state, 64
    effect of vasoactive agents, 65
    mediator enzymes, 64
    muscle movement, 63
    patient age, 64
    tissue condition, 63
  solubility effect on, 49
  from water-in-oil emulsions, 58
Drug degradation, 121-125
  by acylation, 123
  by decarboxylation, 122
  by hydrolysis, 121
  by oxidation, 121
  by polymorphism, 123
  by racemization, 123
  by solvate formation, 124
Drug delivery system, 65

Drug substances, physicochemical
    properties of, 90
Dry solids, preparation of, 174
Dust holding capacity, 396
D values, 242

E

Elastomers, 191
Elimination rate constant, 67, 74,
    77, 80
Employee services, 367
Emulsions, formulation of, 174
Endotoxin, 39
Energy, 357
Engineering and maintenance, 367
Environmental control, 361, 364, 368
  functional groupings, 364
  proximity groupings, 368
  zone groupings, 362-364
Environmental monitoring, records of,
    339
Epinephrine, 111, 123
Equipment cleaning, records of, 211, 345
Equipment maintenance, records of, 345
Ergonovine Maleate, 94
Ethylene oxide sterilization, records of,
    338
Eutectic temperatures, 180
  determination by differential thermal
    analysis, 180
  determination by electric resistivity,
    180
  determination by thermal analysis, 180
Evaluation, 447
  of training, multiple-baseline design,
    448
Expiration date, 192
Extravascular injection:
  one-compartment model, 75
  two-compartment model, 81
Extravascular route, 62

F

Facility area use planning, 358-369
Facility design, 208
Facility design concepts, 369-424
Factorial design, 120
Fick's law, 49
Filling area, 363
Filling equipment, 254

Filling line, 363
Filling, records of, 337
Filling suites, 370–372
Filling ticket, 207
Filter criteria, 294
Filters, 294
  bubble point testing, 299
  cartridges, 302
  cellulose ester, 295
  choice of, 294
  efficiency of, 395
  membrane, 295, 300
  polycarbonate, 296
  support system (holders), 301
  testing of, 296, 395
  utilization of, 294
Filtration, 287–303
  with cake filters, 289
  with depth filters, 289, 292–294
  rate of, 290
  with screen filters, 288, 292–294
  sterilization by, records of, 172, 338
  theory of, 289
Filtration operation, 233
First order:
  degradation plot, 197
  kinetics, 67
  process, 66
Flocculation, 172
Floor plan, 208
Floors, construction of, 373
Fluid dynamics, 266–273
Fluid flow, in autoclaves, 272
Formulation, 185–192
  container effects on, 185
  process effects on, 198
Formulation manufacturing record, 207
Formulation operation—nonsterile,
    230, 233, 235
Fourier's law, 274
Freeze-dried powder formula, 244
Freeze-drying, 178, 244
  eutectic temperatures in, 180
  formulation for, 179
  freezing and thawing curves, 181
F_0 values, 242, 269

G

Gases, compressed, 411
Gentamicin sulfate, 96

Glass containers, 127, 224
  effect on formulation, 186
  fluoride treatment of, 225
  handling of, 308
  siliconization of, 228
  sterilization of, 227
  sulfur treatment of, 225
  washing of, 224, 308
Glass types, 188
Good manufacturing practice require-
    ments, 321

H

Half-life, $t_{1/2}$, 68, 82
Heat exchangers, 404
Heating, 385–397
Heat of solution, 146, 151
Heat transfer, 273
Henderson-Hasselbach equation, 51, 53,
    158
Henry's Law, 272
HEPA filters, 392, 396
High-performance liquid chromatography,
    114
Homogenization, aseptic, 244, 245
Hotpack hot air sterilizer, 228
Housekeeping, 209
Huber stopper washer, 221
Humidity, 388
Hydrogen bonding, 140, 145
Hydrolysis, 121
Hypak prefilled syringe system, 260
Hypodermoclysis, 20, 21

I

Incompatibilities, 40
Inert gas treatment, 254
Inspection, 127, 261
Integrated operations, 360
Intracutaneous route, 26
Intradermal route, 26
Intrahepatic injection, 22
Intramuscular route, 17
Intrapleural route, 28
Intrathecal route, 29
Intravenous catheters, 20
Intravenous fat emulsion, 285
Intravenous injection:
  one-compartment model, 66, 83

[Intravenous injection:]
  two-compartment model, 72
Intravenous route, 18, 61
Intravitreal injection, 27
Inventory practices, 282
Ionic strength, 160
Ionization, 51
Ionization constant, 110
Isoosmotic, 55, 170
Isotonic, 55
Isotonicity, 140, 168
  in formulation, 140

K

Ketamine, 95
King rotary chemical pump, 256

L

Label control report, 207
Labeling, 261
Lactated Ringer's 5% dextrose
    injection, 284
Laminar air flow, 397-400
Large volume parenteral (LVP),
    265-313
  containers, 311
    filling of, 311
    sealing of, 311
  drug administration vehicles, 312
  manufacturing of, 265
Leak testing, records of, 338
Lighting fixtures, 374
Lymphatic system, 61
Lyophilization, 244
Lyophilization operation, 250
Lyophilized product, formulation, 247

M

Maintenance procedures:
  annual, 215
  biannually, 214
  daily, 211
  monthly, 213
  routine, 216
    clean room area, 216
    sterile areas, 218
  weekly, 212
Management role, 451

[Management role]
  in training, 451
    attitude, 453
    motivation, 451
    quality circles, 452
Master file, 206
Material logs, 207
Materials management, 205
Mechanical services, 377
Melting point, 92
Membrane filters, 289
Metromatic washer, 226
Metronidazole, 109
Micelles, in solubilization, 141
Microbial load, 212
Microorganisms, 429
  on human skin, 429
    aerobic bacteria, 430
    anaerobic bacteria, 430
    carriers, 432
    gram negative bacteria, 429
    gram positive bacteria, 429
    shed rate, 431
      sex, effect of, 431
    total counts, 432
Microscopes, optical, 92
Microscopes, polarizing, 92
Microscopes, scanning electron, 92
Minimum inhibitory concentrations,
    168
Molality, 141
Molarity, 141
Molecular structure, 90
Molecular weight, 90
Multiple baseline design, 448

N

Needles, 20
Needle selection, 19
Newton's law, 267
Nitrogen gas:
  storage system, 412
Non-Newtonian liquids, 267

O

Optical rotation, 110, 111
Osmolality, 55
Oxidation, 121
Oxidation potential, 163

Oxidation-reduction reaction, 161
Oxygen gas, 413

P

Packaging and sealing, 254-261
Packaging components, 125, 220
  closure selection, 125
  glass selection, 127
  screening of, 125
Packaging, records of, 341
p-Aminosalicylic acid, 122
Parenteral dosage forms, 1-12
  distinctive characteristics, 2
  history of, 4
    events tabulated, 10
    filtration, 6
    pyrogenic reactions, 7
    radiopharmaceuticals, 7
    routes of administration, 4-6
    standards and regulations, 8
    sterilization, 7
    ultraclean facilities, 8
    vaccines, 5
  perspectives, 3
  selection of, 1
Particles, airborne, 429
Particulate matter, 40
Partition coefficient, 50, 108
Passivating, 280
Passive diffusion, 49
Pass-throughs, 375
Peritoneal dialysis, 22
Perry liquid filling machine, 257
Perry powder filler, 253, 257, 258
Personnel, 369
  clean room, 433
Personnel management, 206
Personnel practices and procedures,
    439
  gowning, 440
Personnel training program:
  objectives of, 442
pH, 51
Pharmacokinetic models, 65-85
  one-compartment, 65, 66, 75, 83
  two-compartment, 65, 72, 81
Phase solubility, 142
Phenol, 122
pH-solubility profile, 103
pH-stability profile, 114
Physicochemical properties, 90-112
  absorbance spectra, 98

[Physicochemical properties]
  color, 90
  hygroscopicity, 96
  ionization constant, 110
  melting point, 92
  molecular structure, 90
  molecular weight, 90
  odor, 91
  optical activity, 110
  particle characteristics, 91
  partition coefficient, 108
  solubility, 100
  thermal analytical profile, 100
Piping system, 380, 382
  joining techniques, 382
  materials of, 380
  valving, 382
pK_a, 51
Plackett-Burman design, 115
Plant exterior, 364
Plant layout, 356, 360, 362
Plastic containers, 229
Plastic ophthalmic dispensers, 229
Plastic syringes, 229
Plug valves, 383
Polymorphic changes, 172
Polymorphic forms, 124
Polymorphism, 123, 151
Polysorbate 80 solution operation, 242
Potentiometric titration, 110
Powder filler, auger type, 259
Powder filling, 176
Prefilters, 289, 293, 393
Preformulation research, 89-135
  physicochemical properties, 90-
    112
Preformulation worksheet,
    128-135
Preservative solution operation,
    242
Procaine Hydrochloride, 121
Process equipment, 303-306
  cleaning of, 303
  sanitization of, 305
Process logs, 207
Prodrugs, 109
Production, 364
Production area, 364
Product release sheets, 207
Propane gas, 413
Pseudomonas diminuta, 298
Purified water, 277
Pyrogens, 212

Q

Quality control, 366
Quarantine areas, 282

R

Racemization, 123
Radiation, 274
Raoult's law, 271
Raw materials, 281-284
  distribution of, 284
  inventory control of, 284
  receiving of, 282, 334
  records of, 334-336
Reconciliation, 343
Record content, 317
  conditions of performance, 320
  location, 319
  person(s) responsible for, 317
  point in time for, 318
  work performed, 319
Record maintenance, 321
  good manufacturing practice require-
      ments, 321
  retention, 322
  subject to inspection, 321, 322
Record retrieval, 321
  automated systems, 323
  manual systems, 323
Records, 315-349
  business purpose of, 316
  of inspection results, 353
  regulatory purpose of, 316
  scientific purpose of, 315
Record systems, 324
  administrative records, 348
    of consultants, 348
    of health, 348
    job descriptions, 348
    of training, 348
  batch production records, 324
  calibration records, 345
  control records, 325
    batch-related information, 325
    instrument calibration, 326
    reference standards, 326
    stability testing, 326
  distribution records, 347
  environmental monitoring, 339
  equipment cleaning, 345
  in-process control records, 336
    filling, 337
    leak testing, 338

[Record systems]
  [in-process control records]
    of lyophilization, 339
    material and equipment verifica-
        tion, 336
    of sterilization, 338
      ethylene oxide, 338
      steam, 338
      sterilizing filtration, 338
  maintenance records, 345
  master production records, 324
  packaging and labeling, 341
    material examination and usage, 342
    record review, 344
  personnel records, 348
  raw materials, 334
    approved vendors, 336
    inventory of, 335
    receiving, 334
    sampling, 334
    testing of, 335
    usage of, 335
  reprocessing records, 346
  returned goods records, 347
  salvaging records, 347
  sanitation records, 346
  standard operating procedures, 330
    operations requiring, 331
    preparation of, 332
    procedure conformance, 333
    procedure distribution, 333
    for procedure review, 332
  validation records, 327
    of analytical, 330
    of processes, 328
    protocol, 327
    of suppliers, 330
    system for change, 328
Reports, 349-353
  of adverse reactions, 352
  of complaints, 352
  of internal audits, 351
  of investigation of deviations, 349
  of quality analysis, 350, 352
  of recalls, 351
  trend analysis, 350
Residual detergent, 214
Retrobulbar injection, 27
Retrograde administration, 43
Returned goods record, 207
Revalidation, 328
Reverse osmosis, 278
Reynold's number, 273

Routes of administration, 16-33
    influence of formulation on, 140
    intra-abdominal injection, 21
    intra-arterial route, 22
    intra-articular route, 24
    intracardiac route, 24
    intracisternal route, 25
    intracutaneous route, 26
    intradermal route, 26
    intralesional route, 26
    intramuscular route, 17
    intraocular route, 27
    intraperitoneal injection, 21
    intrapleural route, 28
    intrathecal route, 29
    intrauterine route, 30
    intravenous route, 18
    intraventricular route, 31
    subcutaneous route, 20
Rubber closures, 166
    compatibility of, 192
        effect on formulation, 166, 190
    physical properties of, 191
    siliconization of, 224
    sterilization of, 223
    washing of, 220

S

Safety procedures, 442
Safety tests, 194
Sampling, of raw materials, 334
Sanitary design, of water systems,
        280
Sanitation, 346
    records of, 423
Sanitizing, 280
Saturated salt solutions, humidity
        control, 97
Sealing ampuls, 260
Sealing bottles, 260
Sealing cartridges, 260
Sealing syringes, 260
Sealing vials, 260
Security, 368
Sheppard-Andrade equation, 269
Silicone oil, 224
Site selection criteria, 355-358
Skin, 429
    bacterial load on, 429
    resident organisms on, 428
    transient organisms on, 428

Skin cells, 428
    shed rate, 429
        aseptic technique, effect on,
        429
Small volume parenterals, 139,
        203-263
    classes of, 139
    manufacturing overview, 204
    processing of, 203-262
        documentation control, 206
        equipment and facilities manage-
        ment, 207
        materials management, 205
        personnel management, 206
Sodium Carboxymethylcellulose
        solution operation, 240
Sodium chloride equivalent method,
        169
Sodium chloride solution operation,
        240
Solubility, 34, 100, 141
    expression of, 141
    measurement of, 100
    methods of improving, 104-108
        complexation, 106
        cosolvents, 105
        prodrug approach, 107
        salt formation, 104
    pH-solubility profile, 103
Solubilization, 141
    bonding forces in, 142
    molecular structure, effect of,
        149
    pH effect on, 146
    temperature, effect on, 151
Solution filtration operation, 249
Solution formulation, 231
    nonsterile, 249
    stability of, 193
Solvate formation, 124
Solvents
    aqueous, 153
    nonaqueous, 154
    water-miscible, 154
Specific gravity, 270
Sporicidal action, 219
Spray drying, 176
Sprinkler systems, 374
Stability, 192-198
    evaluation of, 192, 196
Stability evaluation—accelerated,
        112-121

[Stability evaluation—accelerated]
  to autoclaving, 114
  to heat, 112
  to light, 112
  to oxygen, 113
  to pH, 114
Stability factors, 281
Stability testing records, 326
Stainless steel, 381
  passivating of, 280
  surface finish, 381
Steady-state concentration, 84
Steam, clean, 401, 404
Steam sterilization, 408
  records of, 402
Sterile crystallization, 239
Sterile dry fill powder, preparation
    of, 251
Sterile filtration operation, 237
Sterile lyophilized product, process
    flow diagram, 248
Sterile processing room, 210
Sterile solids, stability of, 194
Sterile solution production,
    schematic, 232, 234, 236
Sterile subdivision operation, 232,
    235
Sterile suspension, process flow
    chart, 241
Sterile Water for Injection opera-
    tion, 242
Sterilization:
  ethylene oxide, records of, 338
Sterilization operation, 231, 235
  thermal, 233, 235
  with steam, 266
    factors of control, 266-276
Storage, 282
Storage and handling, 35
Subconjuntival injection, 27
Subcutaneous route, 20
Subdivision operation, 252
Subdivision sampling operation, 252
Surface active agents, 141, 152
Surface tension, 270
Suspension formulation, 237, 239
Suspensions, 238, 256
  formulation of, 171
  stability of, 195
  sterilization of, 238
  syringeability of, 173
Syringeability, 173

T

Terms, general, glossary of, 9
Thermal analytical profile, 94
Thermal conductivity, 274-276
Thermal resistance, 274
Thermogravimetric analysis, 95
Thin-layer chromatography, 114
Tonicity, 168
Total parenteral nutrition, 174
Training:
  on-the-job, 447
  supervisory, 443
  technical, 446
Training methods, 444
Training program:
  advantages of, 450
  three-step, 445
    classroom/orientation, 445
Training specialist, 444
Training syllabus:
  media, 443

U

Utilities, 366, 377-385
  distribution system, 379
  location of, 377
  requirements of, 378
  service connections, 384

V

van der Waals forces, 142, 144, 146
Vapor pressure, 271
Ventilation, 385-397
Venting, 421
Viscosity, 267, 290, 291
Volume of distribution, 70, 78, 83
Volume of injection, 56

W

Wall junctions, construction of, 374
Walls, construction of, 372
Warehouse, 376-377
Warehousing, 364, 365
Waste disposal, 358, 422
Water, 277
  pretreatment of, 357
Water for Injection, 153, 277, 303,
    416

[Water for Injection]
  distribution, 419
    control, 421
    loop system, 420
  storage, 417
  testing of, 303
Water systems:
  cleaning of, 303
  microbial limits for, 303
  sanitization of, 304

Water treatment, 413–416
  deionization, 414
  distillation, 414–416
    multiple effect still, 415
    vapor compression still, 415
  filtration, 414
  softening, 414
Weighing, mixing, and transfer area,
    363
Weighing room, 285